Biomaterials and medical tribology

Published by Woodhead Publishing Limited, 2013

Woodhead Publishing Series in Biomaterials: Number 65

Biomaterials and medical tribology

Research and development

EDITED BY
J. PAULO DAVIM

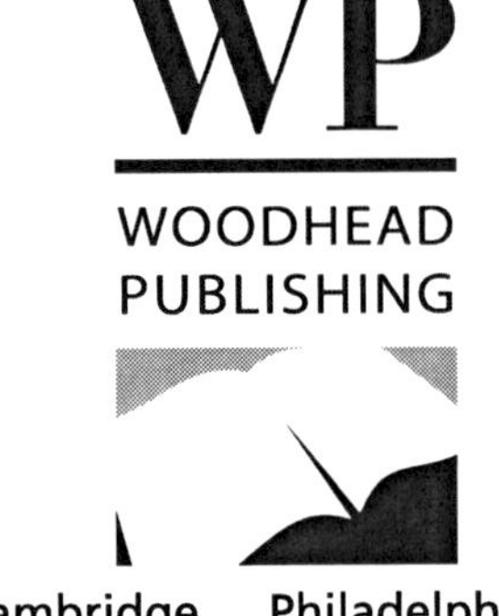

Oxford Cambridge Philadelphia New Delhi

Published by Woodhead Publishing Limited, 2013

Published by Woodhead Publishing Limited,
80 High Street, Sawston, Cambridge CB22 3HJ, UK
www.woodheadpublishing.com
www.woodheadpublishingonline.com

Woodhead Publishing, 1518 Walnut Street, Suite 1100, Philadelphia,
PA 19102-3406, USA

Woodhead Publishing India Private Limited, G-2, Vardaan House, 7/28 Ansari Road,
Daryaganj, New Delhi – 110002, India
www.woodheadpublishingindia.com

First published 2013, Woodhead Publishing Limited

British Library Cataloguing in Publication Data
A catalogue record for this book is available from the British Library.

Library of Congress Control Number: 2013932738

ISBN 978-0-85709-017-1 (print)
ISBN 978-0-85709-220-5 (online)
ISSN 2049-9485 Woodhead Publishing Series in Biomaterials (print)
ISSN 2049-9493 Woodhead Publishing Series in Biomaterials (online)

Typeset by RefineCatch Limited, Bungay, Suffolk

Contents

Published by Woodhead Publishing Limited, 2013

Published by Woodhead Publishing Limited, 2013

Published by Woodhead Publishing Limited, 2013

Published by Woodhead Publishing Limited, 2013

Published by Woodhead Publishing Limited, 2013

About the contributors

(* corresponding author)

Editor

***J. Paulo Davim** received his PhD in mechanical engineering from the University of Porto in 1997 and the Aggregation from the University of Coimbra in 2005. He is at present aggregate professor in the Department of Mechanical Engineering of the University of Aveiro and Head of MACTRIB – Machining and Tribology Research Group. He has more than 25 years of teaching and research experience in manufacturing, materials and mechanical engineering with special emphasis in machining and tribology. He has also, recently, taken an interest in sustainable manufacturing and industrial engineering. He is the editor of six international journals, and guest editor, editorial board member, reviewer and scientific advisor for many international journals and conferences. Presently, he is an editorial board member of 20 international journals and acts as reviewer for than 70 prestigious ISI Web of Science journals. He has also published more than 40 book chapters and 350 articles as author and co-author in refereed international journals (more than 180 cited in ISI Web of Science, h-index = 25+) and conferences.

Published by Woodhead Publishing Limited, 2013

Department of Mechanical Engineering
University of Aveiro
Campus Santiago
3810–193 Aveiro
Portugal

E-mail: pdavim@ua.pt

Authors

Chapter 1

Suad Rashdan is an assistant professor of Chemistry in the College of Science at the University of Bahrain, Kingdom of Bahrain. She received her PhD in Organic Chemistry from the University of Southampton, UK, in October 2007. Her research interests are in the fields of supramolecular, host–guest chemistry and synthesis of nanomaterials for biomedical applications.

L. Selva Roselin is presently working at Yuan Ze University, Taiwan. She received her PhD degree in Chemistry from Anna University, India, in 2002. She carried out her postdoctoral research in the area of nanocatalysis with Professor Feg-Wen Chang at National Central University (2004–2007) and thermodynamic approaches in biorecognition processes with Professor Wen-Yih Chen in the same university (2007–2009). She joined Don Bosco Institute of Technology as assistant professor in 2009. She worked as visiting professor at Lunghwa University of Science and Technology, Taiwan for 3 months. Her present research interest is centered on nanomaterials for catalytic applications and energy storage materials.

Published by Woodhead Publishing Limited, 2013

Rosilda Selvin is an associate professor at Lunghwa University of Science and Technology, Taiwan with research interests in the design, synthesis and study of nanomaterials, including their application in catalysis. She obtained her BSc in Chemistry from Holy Cross College, Nagercoil, India, and her Master's degree from Alagappa University, India. She received her MPhil in 1994 and PhD in 2000 from Anna University, Chennai, India, under the supervision of Professor K. Rengaraj. Her research was focused on various zeolite catalysts for fine chemical synthesis. From 2003 to 2005, she was a postdoctoral scholar in the laboratory of AST Chiang at the National Central University, Taiwan, where she developed a rapid synthesis procedure for non-agglomerated nanozeolites.

O. M. Lemine is an associate professor of Physics in the College of Science at Al-imam University, Saudi Arabia. He received his MSc (1995) and PhD (1999) in Materials Science from Henri Poincaré University, Nancy, France. His research interests are in magnetic nanoparticles and their biomedical application, and thin film preparation and characterization.

*__Mohamed Bououdina__ is the director of the Nanotechnology Centre at the University of Bahrain. He obtained his PhD in Condensed Matter Physics from University Joseph Fourier, France in 1995. He has over 15 years of experience and has worked at various places in France, UK, Japan, etc. He is the author and co-author of more than 90 papers published in international journals and has contributed to a number of book chapters. He is an associated editor for numerous international journals such as *International Journal of Hydrogen Energy, International Journal of Nanoscience, International Journal of Nanoparticles, International Journal of Materials Engineering Innovation, International*

Published by Woodhead Publishing Limited, 2013

Journal of Biomedical Nanoscience & Nanotechnology, etc. He has broad areas of expertise including renewable energy (hydrogen), advanced materials, nanoscience and nanotechnology, etc.

Nanotechnology Centre
University of Bahrain
PO Box 32038
Kingdom of Bahrain

Department of Physics
College of Science
University of Bahrain
PO Box 32038
Kingdom of Bahrain

E-mail: mboudina@gmail.com, mboudina@sci.uob.bh

Chapter 2

*Jean Geringer** obtained a Master's degree with honors from Ecole Nationale Supérieure de Chimie de Toulouse-France in 1997. After working in secondary schools as a professor, he earned the 'Agrégation' of physics and chemistry, the highest-rated competitive academic examination in the French system in 2001. He studied as a PhD student till 2005. He held the position of assistant professor at the Ecole Nationale Supérieure des Mines de Saint-Etienne-France in 2006. He is now visiting scholar at Penn State University, USA. He is working on biomaterials for orthopedic implants with specific emphasis on fretting corrosion of 316L involved in the lifetime of hip implants. Understanding of synergistic effects occurring during fretting corrosion is the major focus of his research activity.

Published by Woodhead Publishing Limited, 2013

Ecole Nationale Supérieure des Mines de Saint-Etienne
158 Cours Fauriel
42023 Saint-Etienne Cedex 02
France

E-mail: geringer@emse.fr

M. Mathew is working as an instructor in the Department of Orthopedic Surgery, Rush University Medical Center, Chicago. He has other appointments in the Dental School and Bioengineering, University of Illinois, Chicago. He has a BSc in Mechanical Engineering and holds a doctoral degree from the University of Strathclyde (2005). His postdoctoral experience was at the University of Minho, Portugal during 2005–2008, before joining Rush University. His main areas of research are electrochemistry, tribocorrosion and wear/corrosion synergism aspects of implants in orthopedics and dentistry. As the behavior of a metal implant in a body environment is a complex issue, the objective of this research is to find an optimum solution related to longevity, biocompatibility and stability by adopting an interdisciplinary approach.

M. Wimmer received his Diploma in Engineering from the Technical University of Munich, after completing 5 years of studies in Mechanics and Materials Science. He then earned a doctorate (PhD) in Biomechanics at Hamburg University of Technology. He is currently working as the director of the Section of Tribology at Rush University Medical Center, one of the United States' premier medical centers. Before that, he was a researcher at the AO Foundation in Switzerland, where he studied functional tissue engineering for articular cartilage. His research focuses on the phenomena between interacting surfaces in natural and artificial joints. Lately, he has paid

Published by Woodhead Publishing Limited, 2013

particular attention to tribocorrosion issues of metal-on-metal hip implants, which have been published in *Science* among other highly ranked journals.

D. D. Macdonald gained his BSc and MSc degrees in Chemistry at the University of Auckland, New Zealand, and his PhD degree in Chemistry from the University of Calgary in Canada (1969). He has served as assistant research officer at Atomic Energy of Canada Ltd, lecturer in Chemistry at Victoria University of Wellington, New Zealand, director and professor of the Fontana Corrosion Center, Ohio State University, SRI International, Menlo Park, California, and has been professor and later distinguished professor of Materials Science and Engineering at Pennsylvania State University since 1991. He has received numerous awards and honors. From 1993 to 1997 he was a member of the US Air Force. He has published nearly 800 papers in scientific journals, books and conference proceedings, plus one book (*Transient Techniques in Electrochemistry*), and has 10 patents and numerous patent disclosures credited to his name.

Chapter 3

***Yong Luo** received his PhD in Mechanical Engineering from the China University of Mining and Technology in 2008. Currently, he is an associated professor in the School of Material Science and Engineering of China University of Mining and Technology. He has more than 10 years of teaching and research experience in surface modification, biomaterials, tribology and artificial joints. He is editorial board member, reviewer and scientific advisor for international journals and conferences. He has also published more than 30 articles and three books.

Published by Woodhead Publishing Limited, 2013

School of Material Science and Engineering
China University of Mining and Technology
Xuzhou 221116
China

E-mail: sulyflying@yahoo.com

Li Yang received her Bachelor's degree in Material Engineering from the China University of Mining and Technology in 2011. Currently, she is a graduate student in the School of Material Science and Engineering of China University of Mining and Technology. Now she is working in the fields of biomaterials and artificial joints.

Maocai Tian received his Bachelor's degree in Material Engineering from the China University of Mining and Technology in 2011. Currently, he is a graduate student in the School of Material Science and Engineering of China University of Mining and Technology. Now he is working in the fields of biomaterials and surface modification.

Chapter 4

***Robert Sonntag** is a scientist and lecturer at the Laboratory of Biomechanics and Implant Research of Heidelberg University Hospital, Germany. He graduated in mechanical engineering at the University of Karlsruhe and the Ecole Nationale Supérieure d'Arts et Métiers (ENSAM) at Paris in 2007 and is a member of the German Society of Biomechanics (DGfB). Within the field of arthroplasty, he focuses on issues of biotribology, radiostereometric migration analysis (RSA) and implant failure, and is author and co-author of different essays on arthroplasty mechanics and tribology.

Published by Woodhead Publishing Limited, 2013

Laboratory of Biomechanics and Implant Research
Heidelberg University Hospital
Schlierbacher Landstrasse 200a
96118 Heidelberg
Germany

E-mail: robert.sonntag@med.uni-heidelberg.de

Joern Reinders is a scientist at the Laboratory of Biomechanics and Implant Research of Heidelberg University Hospital in Germany. He graduated in Biomechanical Engineering in 2009. His research focuses on tribological *in vitro* investigations of the large joints. Recently, he has specialized in soft tissue modeling and wear simulation of the ankle joint.

Jens Gibmeier is a senior scientist/lecturer and since 2008 head of the section 'Structure and Stress Analysis' at the Institute of Applied Materials (IAM-WK) at the Karlsruhe Institute of Technology (KIT), Germany. He graduated in Mechanical Engineering in 1999 and received his PhD from the Department of Mechanical Engineering of the University of Kassel in 2004. From 2006 to 2008 he worked as a research associate at Hahn-Meitner-Institute Berlin (now Helmholtz-Centre-Berlin) and was the responsible beamline scientist at the materials research synchrotron beamline EDDI@BESSY II. He specializes in the development, establishment and application of measuring and evaluation strategies for phase and residual stress analysis by diffraction and mechanical methods.

J. Philippe Kretzer is the technical director of the Laboratory of Biomechanics and Implant Research of Heidelberg University Hospital, Germany. He graduated in Biomedical

Published by Woodhead Publishing Limited, 2013

Engineering in 2004 and received his PhD in 2008 from the University of Heidelberg. He specializes in biomechanics and tribology of arthroplasty, and he has written extensively in professional journals and book chapters. Currently, he is a co-chairman of the German Research Network on Musculoskeletal Biomechanics (MSB-Net) and the coordinator of the Research Cluster on Tribology (associated to the MSB-Net). He received the Young Investigator Award of the German Society of Biomechanics in 2009, another award by the International Society for Technology in Arthroplasty (ISTA) in 2010 and the Science Award of the German Working Group Arthroplasty (Arbeitsgemeinschaft Endoprothetik) in 2011.

Chapter 5

***Sebastian Jaeger** is a scientist at the Laboratory of Biomechanics and Implant Research of Heidelberg University Hospital in Germany. He graduated in Physical Science and Technology, Specialization Medical Technology, in 2009. His research focuses on implant stability analysis and cementing technique. Recently, he has specialized in failure analysis of implants.

Laboratory of Biomechanics and Implant Research
Heidelberg University Hospital
Schlierbacher Landstrasse 200a
96118 Heidelberg
Germany

E-mail: sebastian.jaeger@med.uni-heidelberg.de

Joern Reinders (see Chapter 4).

Published by Woodhead Publishing Limited, 2013

Johannes S. Rieger is a scientist at the Laboratory of Biomechanics and Implant Research of Heidelberg University Hospital in Germany. He graduated in Medical Engineering in 2009. His field of activity is the evaluation of implant stability of endoprosthesis. The focus of his research lies on the diagnosis of loosened implants using the methods of Roentgen stereophotogrammetry (RSA) and vibration analysis.

J. Philippe Kretzer (see Chapter 4).

Chapter 6

***Zenon Pawlak** is a professor at the University of Economy, Bydgoszcz, Poland. His research expertise is in the lubrication of engine oils, lubrication of human joints, environmental engineering and radiochemistry. He is a fellow of the American Chemical Society, Polish Chemical Society and Polish Tribological Society. He has published over 190 papers in refereed scientific papers in international journals and conferences. He is author of the book *Tribochemistry of Lubricating Oils* (Elsevier, 2003).

Tribochemistry Consulting
Salt Lake City
UT 84117
USA

Biotribology Laboratory
University of Economy
Garbary 2
85-229 Bydgoszcz
Poland

E-mail: zpawlak@xmission.com

Published by Woodhead Publishing Limited, 2013

Wieslaw Urbaniak is a doctor of engineering in the Faculty of Kazimierz Wielki University, Bydgoszcz, Poland. He is a fellow of the Polish Tribological Society. His research expertise is in biotribology, dynamic methods, compaction of porous materials and impregnation of porous materials. He has published about 30 scientific and technical papers in international journals and conference proceedings.

Adekunle Oloyede is a professor at Queensland University of Technology, Brisbane, Australia. He is an applied mechanist with established and renowned expertise in the area of connective tissue research; in particular, articular cartilage biomechanics. He has published notable concepts contributing to fundamental opinions in the field. His research has led to seven patents and over 140 refereed scientific papers in international journals and conferences. He is the developer of an arthroscopy device, SMARTHROSCOPE, which is currently undergoing prototyping.

Chapter 7

***Zenon Pawlak** (see Chapter 6).

Wieslaw Urbaniak (see Chapter 6).

Tadeusz Kałdoński is a professor at the Military University of Technology, Warsaw, Poland. He specializes in tribology, fuels and lubricants. He has published about 400 scientific and technical papers in international journals and conferences proceedings. He is also the author of seven monographs and five patents.

Adekunle Oloyede (see Chapter 6).

Published by Woodhead Publishing Limited, 2013

Chapter 8

*Eugeniusz Sajewicz is associate professor in the Mechanical Engineering Faculty at Bialystok University of Technology, Poland. The main research interests are biotribology focused on dental tribology, design of medical devices, prosthetics and orthotics.

Division of Materials and Biomedical Engineering
Faculty of Mechanical Engineering
Bialystok University of Technology
Wiejska 45C
15-351 Bialystok
Poland

E-mail: e.sajewicz@pb.edu.pl

Chapter 9

Iftikhar Khan is a PhD student in the Institute of Nanotechnology and Bioengineering, University of Central Lancashire, Preston, UK. He graduated from the University of Peshawar in Pakistan in Pharmacy and obtained his Master's from Sheffield Hallam University. His research project is based on 'Nanotechnology Formulations for Pulmonary Drug Delivery' at the University of Central Lancashire.

*Waqar Ahmed is professor of Advanced Manufacturing and Nanotechnology at the University of Central Lancashire, and is currently the head of the Institute of Nanotechnology and Bioengineering. He was previously professor of Nanotechnology at the University of Ulster and

Published by Woodhead Publishing Limited, 2013

at Manchester Metropolitan University. He gained his degrees from the University of Salford, and his research interests are focused on nanotechnology, chemistry, bioengineering and surface engineering.

Institute of Nanotechnology and Bioengineering
School of Computing, Engineering and Physical Sciences
University of Central Lancashire
Preston PR1 2HE
UK

E-mail: wahmed4@uclan.ac.uk

Abdelbary Elhissi is a senior lecturer in Pharmaceutics and the head of the Drug, Gene and Protein Delivery Research Group at the Institute of Nanotechnology and Bioengineering, School of Pharmacy and Biomedical Sciences, University of Central Lancashire. He graduated from the Faculty of Pharmacy, October 6th University, Egypt in 1999 with Hons distinction and had the highest grade in his year. He joined the School of Pharmacy, University of London as a PhD student and completed his PhD in Pharmaceutics in 2005 under the supervision of Professor Kevin Taylor and also worked as a postdoctoral research fellow in Clinical Pharmaceutics. In November 2006 he joined Lipoxen as a senior scientist. Currently, he is leading research into drug delivery and has established one of the largest groups in this field within the Institute of Nanotechnology and Bioengineering, University of Central Lancashire. His group is currently working on the development of lipid and polymer-based formulations for respiratory drug delivery and cancer treatment in collaboration with UCL-School of Pharmacy, University of London and West China School of Pharmacy, Sichuan University.

Published by Woodhead Publishing Limited, 2013

Mahmood Shah is a senior lecturer at the Lancashire Business School, and is a leading expert in information security and e-banking. He is a key member of the Institute of Nanotechnology and Bioengineering, University of Central Lancashire, UK.

Published by Woodhead Publishing Limited, 2013

Woodhead Publishing Series in Biomaterials

1 Sterilisation of tissues using ionising radiations
Edited by J. F. Kennedy, G. O. Phillips and P. A. Williams
2 Surfaces and interfaces for biomaterials
Edited by P. Vadgama
3 Molecular interfacial phenomena of polymers and biopolymers
Edited by C. Chen
4 Biomaterials, artificial organs and tissue engineering
Edited by L. Hench and J. Jones
5 Medical modelling
R. Bibb
6 Artificial cells, cell engineering and therapy
Edited by S. Prakash
7 Biomedical polymers
Edited by M. Jenkins
8 Tissue engineering using ceramics and polymers
Edited by A. R. Boccaccini and J. Gough
9 Bioceramics and their clinical applications
Edited by T. Kokubo
10 Dental biomaterials
Edited by R. V. Curtis and T. F. Watson
11 Joint replacement technology
Edited by P. A. Revell
12 Natural-based polymers for biomedical applications
Edited by R. L. Reiss et al.
13 Degradation rate of bioresorbable materials
Edited by F. J. Buchanan
14 Orthopaedic bone cements
Edited by S. Deb
15 Shape memory alloys for biomedical applications
Edited by T. Yoneyama and S. Miyazaki

16 **Cellular response to biomaterials**
Edited by L. Di Silvio
17 **Biomaterials for treating skin loss**
Edited by D. P. Orgill and C. Blanco
18 **Biomaterials and tissue engineering in urology**
Edited by J. Denstedt and A. Atala
19 **Materials science for dentistry**
B. W. Darvell
20 **Bone repair biomaterials**
Edited by J. A. Planell, S. M. Best, D. Lacroix and A. Merolli
21 **Biomedical composites**
Edited by L. Ambrosio
22 **Drug-device combination products**
Edited by A. Lewis
23 **Biomaterials and regenerative medicine in ophthalmology**
Edited by T. V. Chirila
24 **Regenerative medicine and biomaterials for the repair of connective tissues**
Edited by C. Archer and J. Ralphs
25 **Metals for biomedical devices**
Edited by M. Ninomi
26 **Biointegration of medical implant materials: science and design**
Edited by C. P. Sharma
27 **Biomaterials and devices for the circulatory system**
Edited by T. Gourlay and R. Black
28 **Surface modification of biomaterials: methods analysis and applications**
Edited by R. Williams
29 **Biomaterials for artificial organs**
Edited by M. Lysaght and T. Webster
30 **Injectable biomaterials: science and applications**
Edited by B. Vernon
31 **Biomedical hydrogels: biochemistry, manufacture and medical applications**
Edited by S. Rimmer
32 **Preprosthetic and maxillofacial surgery: biomaterials, bone grafting and tissue engineering**
Edited by J. Ferri and E. Hunziker
33 **Bioactive materials in medicine: design and applications**
Edited by X. Zhao, J. M. Courtney and H. Qian

Published by Woodhead Publishing Limited, 2013

34 Advanced wound repair therapies
Edited by D. Farrar
35 Electrospinning for tissue regeneration
Edited by L. Bosworth and S. Downes
36 Bioactive glasses: materials, properties and applications
Edited by H. O. Ylänen
37 Coatings for biomedical applications
Edited by M. Driver
38 Progenitor and stem cell technologies and therapies
Edited by A. Atala
39 Biomaterials for spinal surgery
Edited by L. Ambrosio and E. Tanner
40 Minimized cardiopulmonary bypass techniques and technologies
Edited by T. Gourlay and S. Gunaydin
41 Wear of orthopaedic implants and artificial joints
Edited by S. Affatato
42 Biomaterials in plastic surgery: breast implants
Edited by W. Peters, H. Brandon, K. L. Jerina, C. Wolf and V. L. Young
43 MEMS for biomedical applications
Edited by S. Bhansali and A. Vasudev
44 Durability and reliability of medical polymers
Edited by M. Jenkins and A. Stamboulis
45 Biosensors for medical applications
Edited by S. Higson
46 Sterilisation of biomaterials and medical devices
Edited by S. Lerouge and A. Simmons
47 The hip resurfacing handbook: a practical guide to the use and management of modern hip resurfacings
Edited by K. De Smet, P. Campbell and C. Van Der Straeten
48 Developments in tissue engineered and regenerative medicine products
J. Basu and J. W. Ludlow
49 Nanomedicine: technologies and applications
Edited by T. J. Webster
50 Biocompatibility and performance of medical devices
Edited by J-P. Boutrand
51 Medical robotics: minimally invasive surgery
Edited by P. Gomes
52 Implantable sensor systems for medical applications
Edited by A. Inmann and D. Hodgins

Published by Woodhead Publishing Limited, 2013

53 **Non-metallic biomaterials for tooth repair and replacement**
Edited by P. Vallittu

54 **Joining and assembly of medical materials and devices**
Edited by Y. Norman Zhou and M. D. Breyen

55 **Diamond-based materials for biomedical applications**
Edited by R. Narayan

56 **Nanomaterials in tissue engineering: characterization, fabrication and applications**
Edited by A. K. Gaharwar, S. Sant, M. J. Hancock and S. A. Hacking

57 **Biomimetic biomaterials: structure and applications**
Edited by A. Ruys

58 **Standardisation in cell and tissue engineering: methods and protocols**
Edited by V. Salih

59 **Inhaler devices: fundamentals, design and drug delivery**
Edited by P. Prokopovich

60 **Bio-tribocorrosion in biomaterials and medical implants**
Edited by Yu Yan

61 **Microfluidics for biomedical applications**
Edited by X.-J. James Li and Y. Zhou

62 **Decontamination in hospitals and healthcare**
Edited by J. T. Walker

63 **Biomedical imaging: applications and advances**
Edited by P. Morris

64 **Characterization of biomaterials**
Edited by M. Jaffe, W. Hammond, P. Tolias and T. Arinzeh

65 **Biomaterials and medical tribology: Research and development**
Edited by J. Paulo Davim

Published by Woodhead Publishing Limited, 2013

Preface

Nowadays, it is difficult to obtain an exact definition of biomaterials. However, it is currently possible to use, for example, the following sentence: '. . . a synthetic material used to replace part of a living system or to function in intimate contact with living tissue', or a formal definition by the Clemson University Advisory Board for Biomaterials: '. . . a systemically and pharmacologically inert substance designed for implantation within or incorporation with living systems'. All types of biomaterials are addressed, including metals and alloys, polymers, ceramics, and composites.

Tribology is a branch of mechanical engineering that deals with the design, friction, wear and lubrication of interacting surfaces in relative motion. By extension it is usual to define medical tribology as the tribological phenomena occurring in the human body. Humans possess a wide variety of sliding and frictional interfaces.

This research book aims to provide information on biomaterials and medical tribology. Chapter 1 provides information on nanoparticles for biomedical applications (current status, trends and future challenges). Chapter 2 is dedicated to synergism effects during friction and fretting corrosion experiments (focusing on biomaterials used in orthopedic implants).

Chapter 3 presents the application of biomedical-grade titanium alloys in trabecular bone and artificial joints. Chapter 4 covers fatigue strengthening of an orthopedic

Ti6Al4V alloy. Chapter 5 is dedicated to wear determination on retrieved metal-on-metal hip arthroplasty (an example of extreme wear).

Chapter 6 contains information on natural articular joints (that is, the model of 'lamellar-roller-bearing lubrication' and the nature of the cartilage surface). Chapter 7 describes the importance of bearing porosity in engineering and natural lubrication. Chapter 8 covers tribological characterization of human tooth enamel. Finally, Chapter 9 is dedicated to liposome-based carrier systems and devices for pulmonary drug delivery.

This book can be used as a research volume for final-year undergraduate engineering students or as a topic on biomaterials and medical tribology at postgraduate level. It can also serve as a useful reference for academics, biomechanical researchers, medical doctors, mechanical, materials and biomedical engineers, and professionals related to engineering, medicine and the biomedical industry. The interest of the scientific community in the subject area of this book is evident from the many important centers of research, laboratories and universities existing throughout the world.

The Editor acknowledges Woodhead Publishing for this opportunity, and for their enthusiastic and professional support. Finally, I would like to thank all the chapter authors for making themselves available to contribute to this work.

J. Paulo Davim
University of Aveiro, Portugal

1

Nanoparticles for biomedical applications: current status, trends and future challenges

S. Rashdan, University of Bahrain, Kingdom of Bahrain, L. Selva Roselin and Rosilda Selvin, Lunghwa University of Science and Technology, Taiwan, O. M. Lemine, Imam University, Saudi Arabia and Mohamed Bououdina, University of Bahrain, Kingdom of Bahrain

DOI: 10.1533/9780857092205.1

Abstract: This chapter highlights the application of nanoparticles for biomedical applications including cancer therapy and diagnosis, antibacterial treatment, etc. It provides an overview on synthesis routes and characterization followed by some specific applications of various types of nanoparticles, more particularly (i) gold nanoparticles, including labeling and visualizing, drug delivery, biosensors, and as a heat source; (ii) silver nanoparticles for antibacterial activity; (iii) iron oxides (Fe_3O_4); and (iv) some natural nanoparticles and other

Published by Woodhead Publishing Limited, 2013

types of nanoparticles. The chapter also covers some toxicity aspects and includes concluding remarks.

Key words: nanoparticles, synthesis, characterization, biomedical applications.

1.1 Introduction

In recent decades, the synthesis of materials at the nano-scale has attracted great interest due to their novel and unique properties, offering new potential and wide technological applications: the physical, chemical, mechanical and biological properties are strongly dependent on their size and the shape. It is found that the properties at the nano-scale are tremendously enhanced compared with the bulk. Hence, nanoscience (discovery and study of materials at the nano-scale) and nanotechnology (manipulation and engineering of nanomaterials) have become widespread and are of great importance worldwide. Therefore, new sciences and disciplines have emerged, in particular nanomedicine, which is the use of nanotechnology for the diagnosis and treatment of human diseases. The National Science Foundation (NSF) estimated the market value of nanotechnology by 2015 will be around US$1 trillion.

There are a variety of nanoparticle systems currently being investigated and explored for biomedical applications, with particular emphasis for cancer therapeutics; hence some precious metals (mainly gold (Au) and silver (Ag) systems) and some magnetic oxides (in particular magnetite Fe_3O_4) have received much interest, together with quantum dots and what are also termed 'natural nanoparticles'.

Khlebtsov and Dykman (2010) published a very interesting overview on the various chemical routes for synthesis and

Published by Woodhead Publishing Limited, 2013

surface functionalization by the attachment of specific biomolecules, optical properties and biomedical applications of noble metal nanoparticles with various sizes, desirable shapes (nanospheres, nanorods, nanoshells, etc.), different structures and hence tunable plasmonic properties.

Bhattacharya and Mukherjee (2008) discussed some novel and unique biological properties of Au, Ag and platinum (Pt) nanoparticles: these metals interact with selective proteins and inhibit their activities, hence offering localized therapy of some diseases such as cancer, multiple myeloma, B-chronic lymphatic leukemia, arthritis, etc. Moreover, Kateb et al. (2011) presented nanoplatforms under development in nanomedicine for imaging (such as lymph node magnetic resonance imaging (MRI), nanocontrast agents for differential tissue imaging, etc.), cancer treatment and drug delivery using micelles, metal complex nanoparticles (Au and Ag), liposomes, quantum dots, superparamagnetic iron oxide nanoparticles (Fe_3O_4), peptides and proteins, etc. Fukumori and Ichikawa (2006) reviewed the design and use of nanoparticles for cancer therapy and diagnosis. The authors focused on the most investigated inorganic nanoparticles, magnetite Fe_3O_4 (which is used directly or dispersed in a polymeric matrix as cores), quantum dots (Cd, ZnS), core–shell CdSe/ZnS, etc. More particularly, Kim et al. (2011) outlined some nanotechnology approaches for the diagnosis and therapy of ovarian cancer, which is often fatal because of its late initial diagnosis. Similarly, Byrne et al. (2008) showed how more effective delivery of nanoparticles will result in the development of novel methods for tumor cell targeting for the most common types of cancer (breast, colorectal, lung and prostate) via two methods:

(i) *Passive targeting*, where the nanoparticles exploit the characteristics of tumor growth. The tumor becomes diffusion-limited at a volume above 2 mm^3, which impacts nutrition intake, waste excretion and oxygen delivery. However, this can be overcome by increasing the surrounding vasculature in a process called angiogenesis.

(ii) *Active targeting*, which involves the use of peripherally conjugated targeting moieties for enhanced delivery of nanoparticle systems.

Nowadays, chemotherapy is widely used in cancer treatment. Paclitaxel, cisplatin, carboplatin, doxorubicin (DOX), decitabine or their combinations are considered as first-line chemotherapeutic agents for various cancers. The lack of specificity and poor pharmaco-bioavailability exhibited by the chemotherapeutic agents provoke toxicity, major side-effects and cancer recurrence due to tumor resistance to the chemotherapeutic agents. Therefore, to minimize or completely eliminate side-effects, new therapeutic modalities need to be developed, such as the use of natural dietary phytochemicals (Yallapu et al., 2010).

Early-stage diagnosis is one the major and critical approaches to cancer therapy, which prevents tumor cell metastasis (Bharali and Mousa, 2010). It is known that most types of cancer can be treated effectively with full recovery of the patient if they are detected at an early stage. Unfortunately, early-stage diagnosis remains a significant challenge, as clinical symptoms rarely manifest before cancer progresses to a fatal stage. Moreover, the majority of anticancer therapeutics need to be dissolved in an organic solvent, usually toxic and having side-effects, in order to be administered as an injectable solution (Bharali and Mousa, 2010).

Moreover, the low molecular weight of anticancer drugs results in rapid excretion and a poor therapeutic index, requiring the administration of escalating doses to the cancer

Published by Woodhead Publishing Limited, 2013

patient, and therefore increasing the incidence of cytotoxicity and other adverse events. In addition, chemotherapeutic drugs, when administrated alone, lack specificity and cause significant damage to non-cancerous tissues, resulting in undesirable side-effects, including bone marrow suppression, hair loss (alopecia) and sloughing of gut epithelial cells (Bharali and Mousa, 2010).

It is important to know that the incorporation of anticancer drugs into nanoparticles not only has the potential to decrease their adverse cytotoxic effects, but also in many cases may increase the accumulation of the drug in the tumor vasculature – a phenomenon known as enhanced permeability and retention (Bharali and Mousa, 2010). Doxil® and Abraxane® are two nanotechnology-based anticancer drug formulations that are approved by the US Food and Drug Administration for ovarian and metastatic breast cancer, respectively (Bharali and Mousa, 2010).

The feasibility of thermotherapy of prostate cancer using biocompatible superparamagnetic magnetite nanoparticles has been investigated (Johannsen et al., 2007). Tests were carried out on 10 patients. The magnetic fluid was injected transperineally into the prostate and six thermal therapies of 60 min at weekly intervals using an external alternating (AC) magnetic field were applied. Hyperthermic (40–45 °C, which causes apoptosis, known as a form of cell death in which a programmed sequence of events leads to the elimination of cells without releasing harmful substances into the surrounding area) and thermoablative temperatures (higher than 45 °C, which causes killing of cells) were achieved.

Responsiveness of systems can be defined as their autonomous reaction to environmental features (stimuli) by tuning their properties (Tirelli, 2006). Nanoparticle responsiveness can be influenced by several parameters, including size (can modulate rapidity, sensitivity and in some cases intensity of the response, but does not generally change its nature: the size of an object is inversely related to its diffusion coefficient and its surface-to-volume ratio), surface (response is fast and homogeneous if the active groups are attached on the surface of the nanoparticles; however, when the active groups are encapsulated in the core, the surface may act as a barrier, thus modulating the stimulus and determining kinetics and extent of the response) and core composition (such as response of metal or metal oxides to electromagnetic fields). Nanoparticles show various types of passive and active responsiveness to physicochemical and biological stimuli, such as electromagnetic fields, temperature, pH, etc. (Tirelli, 2006). An external (magnetic) field can drive metal and metal oxide nanoparticles to specific macro- or microtargets (infection sites or tumoral masses) or even submicron targets (ion channels on cell membranes). Moreover, nanoparticles subjected to an external AC magnetic field cause heat-induced necrosis of the tissues called 'hyperthermia'. Also, metal nanoparticles can be localized through magnetic resonance and then activated through near-infrared (NIR) light irradiation (Tirelli, 2006).

1.2 Nanoparticles of interest

1.2.1 Biomedical applications of gold nanoparticles

Au nanoparticles have been used technologically since ancient times. Recently, much emphasis has been placed on their synthesis, modification and potential biomedical applications. Au nanoparticles have a much larger surface area-to-volume ratio than their bulk counterparts, which is

Published by Woodhead Publishing Limited, 2013

the basis of the novel physicochemical properties exhibited by these nanomaterials. These new properties include optical, magnetic, electronic and structural properties, making nanosized Au particles (generally 1–100 nm) very promising for a wide range of biomedical applications, such as labeling, delivering, heating and sensing (Sperling et al., 2008).

Several varieties of nanoparticles with biomedical relevance are available, including polymeric nanoparticles, metal nanoparticles, liposomes, micelles, quantum dots, dendrimers and nanoassemblies. Au nanoparticles are used for biomedical applications because of their facile synthesis and surface modification, strongly enhanced and tunable optical properties as well as excellent biocompatibility in the clinic setting. For biomedical applications, surface functionalization of Au nanoparticles is essential in order to target them to specific disease areas and allow them to selectively interact with cells or biomolecules (Fu et al., 2005). In this section, we will summarize the current state-of-the-art of Au nanoparticle synthesis methods and their biomedical applications.

Synthesis of gold nanoparticles

The synthesis of small, monodisperse nanoparticles is a major challenge in nanotechnology research. Significant efforts have been devoted over the past 40 years to the fabrication of Au nanoparticles with monodispersity and controlled size. The homogeneity of the obtained particles depends on the homogeneity of nucleation and particle growth. Both of these processes are determined by the temperature, solvent and local concentration of the reactants. The synthesis of Au nanoparticles is well established in aqueous solution as well as in organic solvents. Many different protocols exist for the synthesis of pure Au

Published by Woodhead Publishing Limited, 2013

nanoparticles by chemical reduction of metal ions or complexes. Au nanoparticles with varying core sizes are prepared by the reduction of Au salts in the presence of appropriate stabilizing agents that prevent particle agglomeration. In the preparation of Au nanoparticles by citrate reduction, citrate acts as both reducing and stabilizing agent. The adsorption of citrate on the particles as a stabilizer significantly affects the particle size and the multirole of citrate increases the complexity of the particle. It is generally accepted that a high citrate concentration allows the fast and complete stabilization of small Au nanoparticles, while, for lower citrate concentrations, the coverage of citrate is incomplete and the aggregation process leads to the formation of larger particles. Ji et al. (2007) found that the nucleation rate at a citrate/$HAuCl_4$ ratio of 2:1 is faster than that at a ratio of 7:1. They relied on the behavior of citrate as a pH mediator to explain the tendency of particle size. Citrate is known as a weak base that can change the solution pH to a certain extent through its concentration. The pH of the solution increases as the citrate concentration increases. Subsequently, the less reactive complexes $[AuCl_2(OH)_2]^-$ and $[AuCl(OH)_3]^-$ are formed by the hydrolysis of $AuCl_4^-$; consequently, the nucleation rate becomes slower and the amount of Au precursor remaining in the solution will become larger. The final particle size is determined by the diffusional growth of Au precursor on the surface of Au nuclei. As a result of using an excessive amount of citrate, in the second stage the final particle size increases a little or becomes relatively constant. Figure 1.1 shows transmission electron microscopy (TEM) images and the tendency of the average sizes of Au nanoparticles synthesized using different citrate/$HAuCl_4$ ratios. Herein, we present various other methods for the synthesis of Au nanoparticles.

Published by Woodhead Publishing Limited, 2013

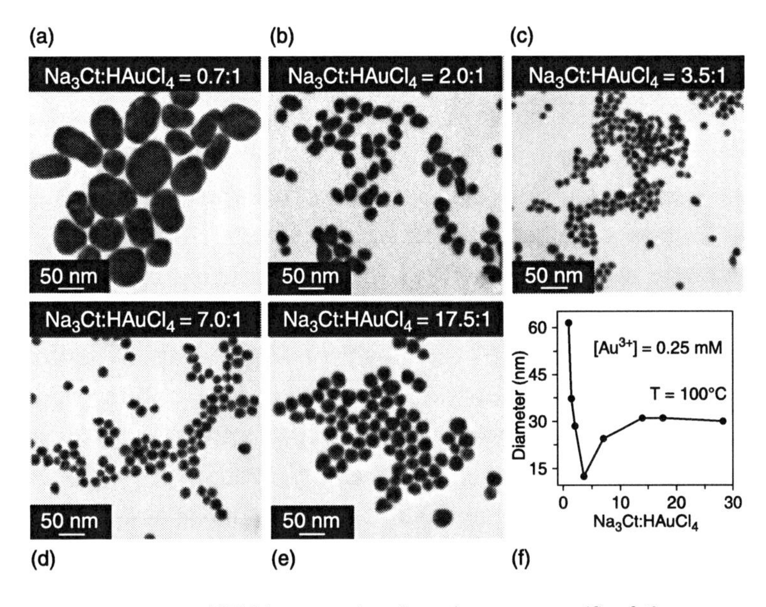

Figure 1.1 TEM images (a–e) and summary (f) of the average sizes of Au nanocrystals synthesized using different $Na_3Ct/HAuCl_4$ precursor ratios as labeled in each image.

Source: Adapted with permission from Ji et al. (2007).

In most of the reported procedures, the reaction is usually initiated by mixing the reactant solutions and this strongly affects the nucleation process. The actual mechanisms of Au nanoparticle formation often remain unclear due to limited accessibility to *in situ*-derived time-resolved information about precursor conversion and particle size distribution. To overcome such limitations, a method is presented that analyzes the formation of nanoparticles via *in situ* small-angle X-ray scattering (SAXS) and X-ray absorption near-edge spectroscopy (XANES) using synchrotron radiation. The method is applied to study the classical Au nanoparticle synthesis route via the reduction of tetrachloroauric acid by trisodium citrate at different temperatures and reactant

Published by Woodhead Publishing Limited, 2013

concentrations. A mechanism of nanoparticle formation is proposed comprising different steps of particle growth via both coalescence of nuclei and further monomer attachment. The coalescence behavior of small nuclei was identified as one essential factor in obtaining a narrow size distribution of the formed particles (Polte et al., 2010).

Simple reduction of metal salts by reducing agents in a controlled fashion generally produces spherical nanoparticles, because spheres are the lowest-energy shape. Several methods including reduction of Au chloride by citrate, phase transfer agent, followed by reduction with borohydride, microemulsion methods, and seeding methods are reported in the literature (Rosi and Mirkin, 2005; Burda et al., 2005; Murphy et al., 2005, 2006). Sanpui et al. (2008) used purified recombinant Green Fluorescent Protein (GFP), expressed in *Escherichia coli* bacteria, for single-step synthesis of Au nanoparticles with extraordinary size specificity in aqueous medium. They observed that in the presence of $AuCl_4^-$ alone the proteins produced spherical Au nanoparticles of 5–70 nm, whereas uniform spherical particles smaller than 5 nm were formed in the additional presence of $AgNO_3$ (Sanpui et al., 2008). In another method, Knauera et al. (2011) presented a two-step micro-continuous flow-through method for synthesizing colloidal dispersions of Au core–shell and multishell nanoparticles in aqueous solutions in the presence of cetyltrimethylammonium bromide (CTAB). The synthesis is based on the reduction of the metal salts $HAuCl_4$ and $AgNO_3$ at the surface of seed particles by ascorbic acid. In the micro fluidic system, constant residence times and an effective mixing were achieved by applying the segmented flow principle. The colloidal solutions were analyzed by differential centrifugal sedimentation, UV/Vis spectrophotometry and scanning electron microscopy (SEM). The size distribution of the Au/Ag core–shell and

Published by Woodhead Publishing Limited, 2013

multishell nanoparticles synthesized by the micro flow-through technique was very narrow. In the case of Au/Ag core–shell nanoparticles, an average diameter of 20 nm with a distribution half-width of 3.8 nm and for Au/Ag/Au multishell nanoparticles, an average diameter of 46 nm with a distribution half-width of 7.4 nm were obtained. The optical spectra of the particle solutions exhibited drastic changes with the deposition of each additional metal shell (Knauera et al., 2011).

NIR-sensitive Au–Au_2S nanocolloids were prepared by mixing $HAuCl_4$ and Na_2S in aqueous solutions (Rena and Chow, 2003). Monosized core–shell Fe_3O_4/Au magneto-optic multifunctional nanoparticles were synthesized by Liu et al. (2010) using a modified nanoemulsion process. The formation of the core–shell nanostructure was accomplished in the presence of poly(vinylpyrrolidone) (PVP) as the surfactant in two consecutive steps. The comparison Fourier transform IR (FTIR) study proves the PVP coating on the surface of the resultant nanoparticles, whereas the morphological analysis illustrates the nanoparticle shape, nanostructuring, size and size distribution, and shows the excellent monodispersity (below 10%). The crystal structure of the core–shell nanoparticles is revealed by the X-ray diffraction (XRD) patterns, with the single-crystallinity of such individual nanoparticles illustrated by the lattice imaging. Moreover, the nanoparticles manifest soft ferromagnetic behavior with a small coercivity of around 40 Oe at room temperature and ensuing excellent susceptibility. The magnetic hysteresis curves of the nanoparticles were elucidated by a modified Langevin equation, giving an estimate of the effective magnetic dimension of the nanoparticles and reflecting the enhanced susceptibility response as a result of the surface covering. The UV/Vis spectroscopic examination reveals the well-behaved surface plasmon at around 590 nm. Thus, the use of PVP evidently led to the improved structure and properties, anticipating potential applications of the nanoparticles.

A novel dendritic nanostructure of Fe_3O_4/Au nanorods (SPIONs-AuNRs) was fabricated by a facile route. The dendritic SPIONs-AuNRs showed a mean particle size of 35 nm, intense NIR absorbance at 754 nm and strong superparamagnetism, implying potential applications in the fields of optical/magnetic resonance bimodal imaging (Zhu et al., 2010). Chandran et al. (2007) demonstrated a seed-mediated procedure for the synthesis of hydrophobic Au_{core}–Ag_{shell} nanoparticles in toluene. The reaction proceeds by way of the interfacial reduction of Ag ions by 3-pentadecylphenol followed by their deposition on hydrophobized Au nanoparticles. Such a hitherto unreported interfacial seeded growth reaction leads to the formation of phase-pure Au_{core}–Ag_{shell} nanoparticles that retain the hydrophobicity of the seed particles and remain stable in toluene. Such core–shell structures are, however, not formed in the aqueous phase. The core–shell architecture was verified using TEM analysis and the formation process was studied by recording the UV/Vis spectra of the organic phase nanoparticles as a function of time. TEM kinetics also showed a gradual increase in the Ag layer thickness. Conclusive evidence was, however, obtained on examination of the high-resolution images of the products formed. Elemental analysis using X-ray photoelectron spectroscopy of the Au_{core}–Ag_{shell} nanostructure revealed the presence of metallic Ag. Moreover, changing the surface capping of the Au seed did not affect the formation of the Au_{core}–Ag_{shell} nanostructure. Tang et al. (2008) combined the reversible addition-fragmentation chain transfer (RAFT) polymerization method with Au nanoparticle fabrication to synthesize Au nanoparticles grafted with functionalized copolymers.

Published by Woodhead Publishing Limited, 2013

Dynamic light scattering (DLS) and TEM were used to probe the structure and thermo-responsiveness of these particles, and SAXS provided a wealth of information on the particle structure, especially polymer chain packing. The large change in size and good reversibility of the polymer coating layer dimensions is a significant finding of this report, which suggests a series of applications of these smart nanoparticles in biosensors, drug delivery, and photothermal therapy.

The layer-by-layer (LBL) assembly method, combined with the seeded growth technique, has been used to deposit Au shells on the surface of hematite (a-Fe_2O_3) spindles (Spuch-Calvar et al., 2007). This method of preparing Au nanorods assembled on hematite spindles provided a flexible way to tune the optical properties of the resulting composite colloids. Spherical Au nanoparticles of approximately 16 nm were synthesized using a sonochemical reduction method and were shown to have more affinity towards sonochemically synthesized Au nanoparticles compared with Au nanoparticles synthesized using other methods (Naveenraj et al., 2010).

Sardar et al. (2007) synthesized Au nanoparticle dimers by a solid-phase approach using a simple coupling reaction of asymmetrically functionalized particles. The method may be used to generate dimers with a wide size range and containing two nanoparticles of different sizes. The dimers demonstrated remarkable stability in ethanol. In addition, the distance between nanoparticles could be controlled, generating a molecular ruler, by simply varying the chain length of the linker molecules.

Sub-100-nm hollow Au nanoparticle superstructures were prepared in a direct one-pot reaction. An Au-binding peptide conjugate, C6-AA-PEPAu (PEPAu = AYSSGAPPMPPF), was constructed and used to direct the simultaneous synthesis and assembly of Au nanoparticles. TEM and electron tomography revealed that the superstructures were uniform and consisted of monodisperse Au nanoparticles arranged into a spherical monolayer shell (Song et al., 2010). In another study (Lee and Park, 2011), the hydroxyphenol compounds and their derivatives could be used as versatile reducing agents for facile one-pot synthesis of Au nanoparticles with diverse morphological characters by reducing precursor Au(III) ions into an Au crystal structure via a biphasic kinetically controlled reduction process. It was found that the biphasic reduction of hydroxyphenols generated single-crystalline branched Au nanoparticles having high-index facets on their surface. The kinetically controlled self-conversion of hydroxyphenols to quinones was mainly responsible for the generation of morphologically different branches on the Au nanoparticles. Different hydroxyphenol derivatives with additional functional groups on the aromatic ring could produce totally different nanostructures, such as nanoprisms, polygonal nanoparticles and nanofractals, possibly by inhibiting self-conversion or by inducing self-polymerization. In addition, polymeric hydroxyphenol derivatives generated stably polymer-coated spherical Au nanoparticles with controlled size, usefully applicable for biomedical applications.

A facile synthesis of stable Au nanoparticle clusters densely functionalized with DNA (DNA–AuNP clusters) using dithiothreitol and monothiol DNA and their thermally reversible assembly properties has been reported (Kim and Lee, 2009). The size of the clusters exhibits a very narrow distribution and can be easily controlled by adjusting the stoichiometry of dithiothreitol and DNA, leading to a variety of colors due to the surface plasmon resonance (SPR) of the Au nanoparticle clusters. Importantly, the DNA–AuNP clusters exhibit highly cooperative melting properties with distinctive and diverse color changes depending on their size. The selective and sensitive colorimetric detection of target sequences was demonstrated based upon the unique properties of the DNA–AuNP clusters. The synthesis of Au nanoparticles supported on silica with average Au particle sizes ranging from 3.7 to 6.6 nm using supercritical carbon dioxide ($scCO_2$) was reported (Wong et al., 2007). The flexibility of this supercritical fluid processing technique was also demonstrated by successfully incorporating Au nanoparticles into polyamide, polypropylene and poly(tetrafluoroethylene) (PTFE). Under the conditions employed, it was found that dimethylacetylacetonato Au(III) ($Au(acac)Me_2$) produced samples with sufficiently high metal loadings that allowed in-depth sample analysis. To date, $scCO_2$ processing is the only method known to us to be capable of both depositing and impregnating a wide range of substrates with Au nanoparticles. Yao et al. (2011) developed a practical and mild sol–gel self-assembly method that was successfully developed for the synthesis of plain and Au-nanoparticle-modified silica nanowires. In this new method, 3-mercaptopropyltrimethoxysilane (MPTMOS) was used as the key linker through disulfide bonds and mediated the reorganization of the particles into elongated clusters.

Biomedical applications of gold nanoparticles

Au nanoparticles are one of the materials that are frequently mentioned in respect of biomedical research. The unusual optical and electronic properties of small Au particles and their high chemical stability have made them the choice for different areas of biologically related research (Jennings and Strouse, 2007). A field that has shown fast growth over the past decades is the use of Au nanoparticles in the life sciences. These bioapplications can be classified into four areas: labeling, delivery, heating and sensing.

Published by Woodhead Publishing Limited, 2013

Gold nanoparticles for labeling and visualizing

Although Au nanoparticles have several applications in the biomedical field, they are conventionally used for labeling applications. In this regard, the particles are directed and enriched at the region of interest, and they provide contrast for the observation and visualization of this region. Au nanoparticles are a very attractive contrast agent as they can be visualized with a large variety of different techniques. The most prominent detection techniques are based on the interaction between Au nanoparticles and light (Huang et al., 2007b). When a metal particle is exposed to light, the oscillating electromagnetic field of the light induces a collective coherent oscillation of the free electrons (conduction band electrons) of the metal. This electron oscillation around the particle surface causes a charge separation with respect to the ionic lattice, forming a dipole oscillation along the direction of the electric field of the light (Figure 1.2a). The amplitude of the oscillation reaches a maximum at a specific frequency, called the SPR (Mie, 1908; Kerker, 1969; Papavassiliou, 1979; Bohren and Huffman, 1983; Kreibig and Vollmer, 1995). The SPR band is much stronger for plasmonic nanoparticles (noble metals, especially Au and Ag) than other metals. Au particles strongly absorb and scatter visible light. Upon light absorption the light energy excites the free electrons in the Au particles to a collective oscillation. The SPR band is affected by the particle size (Link and El-Sayed, 1999) (Figure 1.2b). As the color of the light scattered by Au particles depends on their sizes and shapes, Au particles can be used for labeling with different colors (Jin et al., 2001; Sonnichsen et al., 2002). When Au nanoparticles absorb light, heating of the particles and particle environment occurs. This can be detected by differential interference contrast microscopy and a microphone in photothermal and

Published by Woodhead Publishing Limited, 2013

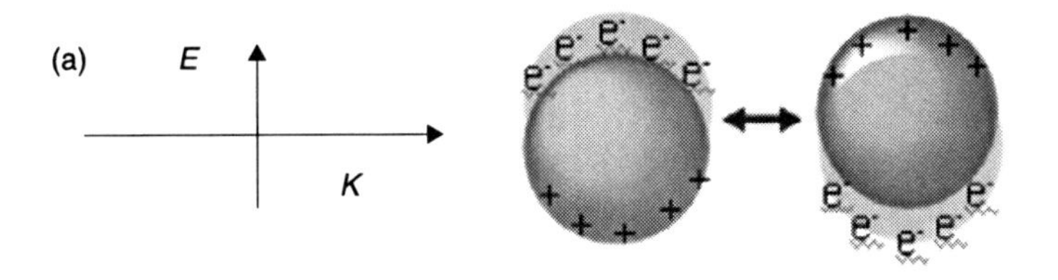

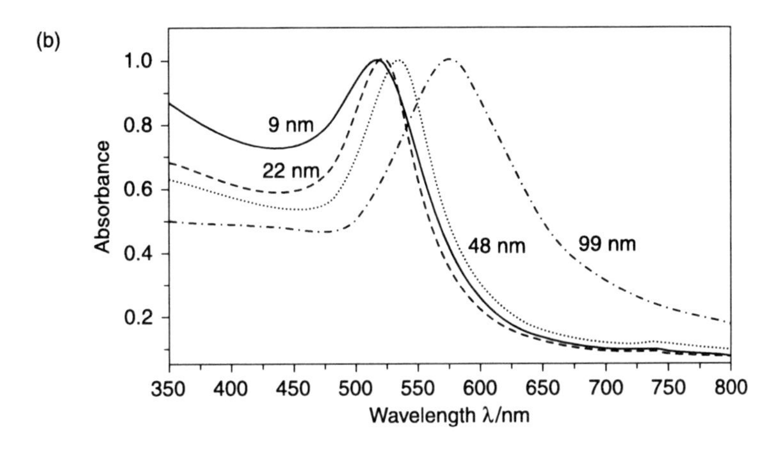

Figure 1.2 (a) Schematic illustration of SPR in plasmonic nanoparticles. (b) Extinction spectra of Au nanoparticles of different sizes. The electric field of incident light induces coherent collective oscillation of conduction band electrons with respect to the positively charged metallic core. This dipolar oscillation is resonant with the incoming light at a specific frequency that depends on the particle size and shape. For Au nanoparticles, the SPR wavelength is around 520 nm depending on the size of the nanoparticles.

Source: Adapted with permission from Huang et al. (2010) and Link and El-Sayed (1999).

photoacoustic imaging studies (Boyer et al., 2002; Berciaud et al., 2004; Kim et al., 2007; Mallidi et al., 2007). The feasibility of Au nanoparticles for cancer imaging has been demonstrated in recent years (Sokolov et al., 2003a,b; Loo

Published by Woodhead Publishing Limited, 2013

et al., 2004, 2005; El-Sayed et al., 2005; Huang et al., 2006a,b).

An improvement of cancer imaging based on the scattering properties of Au nanoparticles was made by El-Sayed et al. using dark field microscopy in 2005 (El-Sayed et al., 2005). In this case, the nanoparticles are excited by white light from a halogen lamp, which is also the same lamp used for bright field imaging. In the dark field (Figure 1.3a and b), a dark field condenser delivers and focuses a very narrow beam of white light on the top of the sample with the center illumination light blocked by the aperture. The objective with an iris for adjusting the light collection zone is used to collect only the scattered light from the samples and thus presents an image of a bright object in a dark background. As the nanoparticles scatter light most strongly at the wavelength of the SPR maximum, the nanoparticles appear in brilliant color, which depends on the size and shape of the particles, and nanoparticles bind specifically to the cancer cells. As a result, the well-organized scattering pattern of the nanoparticles bound to the cancer cells could be clearly distinguished from the random distribution of the nanoparticles around healthy cells (Figure 1.3b). As the SPR of the nanoparticles is located around 540 nm on the cell monolayer, the nanoparticles scatter strongly in the green-to-yellow color range. In the following year, Huang et al. (2006a) conjugated anti-epidermal growth factor receptor (EGFR) antibodies to Au nanorods via a poly(styrenesulfonate) linker and demonstrated that Au nanorods could also be used as imaging contrast agents for cancer cell diagnosis with a conventional optical microscope (Figure 1.3c). In addition to the interaction with visible light, the interaction with both electron waves and X-rays can also be used for visualization of Au nanoparticles (Roth, 1996; Hainfeld et al., 2006). Au nanoparticles can also be radioactively

Published by Woodhead Publishing Limited, 2013

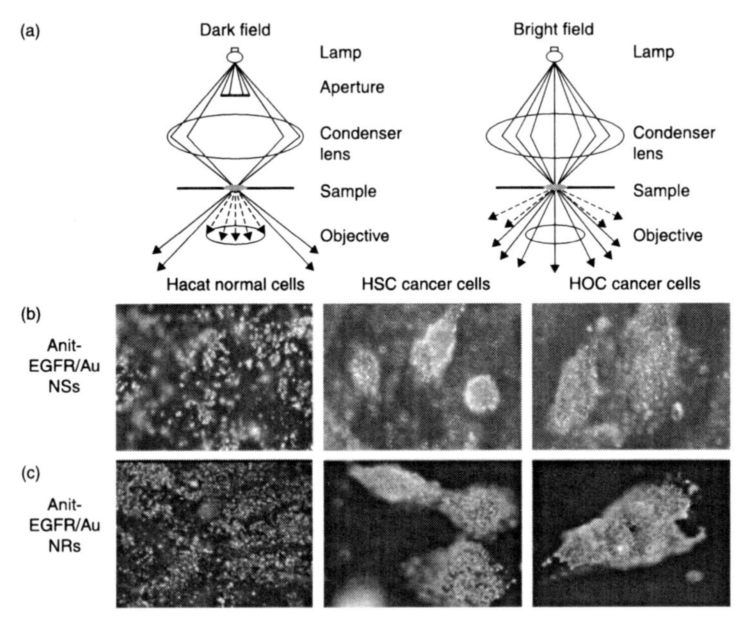

Figure 1.3 **(a) Schematic illustration of dark field (left) and bright field (right) imaging. (b) Cancer cell diagnostics using dark field light scattering imaging of spherical Au nanoparticles. (c) Cancer cell diagnostics using dark field light scattering imaging of Au nanorods.**

Source: Adapted with permission from Huang et al. (2006a, 2010).

labeled by neutron activation and can be detected in this way by γ-radiation (Gosselin, 1956).

Gold nanoparticles in delivery applications

In recent years, significant effort has been devoted to develop Au nanoparticles for drug and gene delivery applications. Due to their inherent properties such as tunable size and low polydispersity, long-term stability and weak toxicity, easy functionalization and large surface-to-volume ratio, Au

Published by Woodhead Publishing Limited, 2013

nanoparticles could find promising applications in drug delivery technologies (Jain et al., 2007; Ghosh et al., 2008). The concept of drug targeting stems from the idea of minimizing the risk-to-benefit ratio. Au nanoparticles can be used to deliver the drug to the central nervous system due to their smaller size and higher barrier permeability. Efficient release of these therapeutic agents could be triggered by internal or external stimuli.

Use of Au nanoparticles involves using thiolated compounds to stabilize Au nanoparticles through thiol linkages (Zhang et al., 2009). The monolayer ranges from small organic compounds to macromolecules and can be further functionalized in various ways to improve drug delivery functionalities. Inside cells the molecules will eventually detach themselves from the Au particles.

Currently, the type of Au nanoparticle most suitable for drug delivery applications is still debatable. It was found that the intracellular uptake of different sized and shaped Au nanoparticles is highly dependent upon their physical dimensions (Chithrani et al., 2006). The absorption/scattering efficiency and optical resonance wavelengths have been calculated for three commonly used classes of Au nanoparticles: nanospheres, nanoshells and nanorods (Jain et al., 2006b). It was found that the nanorod with a higher aspect ratio and a smaller effective radius is a better photo-absorbing nanoparticle, suitable for therapeutic applications.

Au nanoparticles can also be used for drug delivery applications. In general, the amount of antibiotics used in therapy is much higher than the actual dose required for pathogenic destruction. The excess amount of antibiotics can cause adverse effects (Geller et al., 1986). Therefore, the conjugation of Au nanoparticles with antibiotics in combination with some type of targeting would be a possible way to improve antibiotic efficacy. Au nanoparticles can be

Published by Woodhead Publishing Limited, 2013

directly conjugated with antibiotics or other drug molecules via ionic or covalent bonding, or by physical absorption. It has been shown that conjugates of Au nanoparticles with antibiotics provide promising results in the treatment of intracellular infections (Thirumurugan and Dhanaraju, 2001; Gu et al., 2003; Chen et al., 2007; Saha et al., 2007). For example, methotrexate (MTX) has been conjugated to 13-nm colloidal Au (Chen et al., 2007) (Figure 1.4a). MTX is an analog of folic acid that has the ability to destroy folate metabolism of cells and has been commonly used as a cytotoxic anticancer drug. The carboxylic groups on the MTX molecule can bind to the surface of Au nanoparticles after overnight incubation. At the same volume, it has been reported that the concentration of the MTX conjugated to Au nanoparticles is higher than that of the free MTX. The cytotoxic effect of free MTX is about seven times lower than that of MTX conjugated to Au nanoparticles in the case of Lewis lung carcinoma cells. The conjugated forms of the antibiotics were claimed to provide a greater degree of inhibition of the growth of bacteria than the free forms of the antibiotics. However, the bluish color of the conjugates suggested that there was some aggregation after conjugation (Burygin et al., 2009). Therefore, it is likely that modification of the surface of the Au nanoparticles to prevent aggregation would improve the efficacy of such drug delivery systems further.

Several studies have highlighted the attractive properties of polymer-modified Au nanoparticles (Liao and Hafner 2005). The amphiphilic characteristics of poly(ethylene glycol) (PEG) in particular ensure that particles coated with it have a high degree of biocompatibility and an affinity for cell membranes. The use of PEG to modify the surface of Au nanoparticles strongly increases the efficiency of cellular uptake compared with unmodified Au nanoparticles (Choi et al., 2003; Niidome T et al., 2006; Paciotti et al., 2006).

Published by Woodhead Publishing Limited, 2013

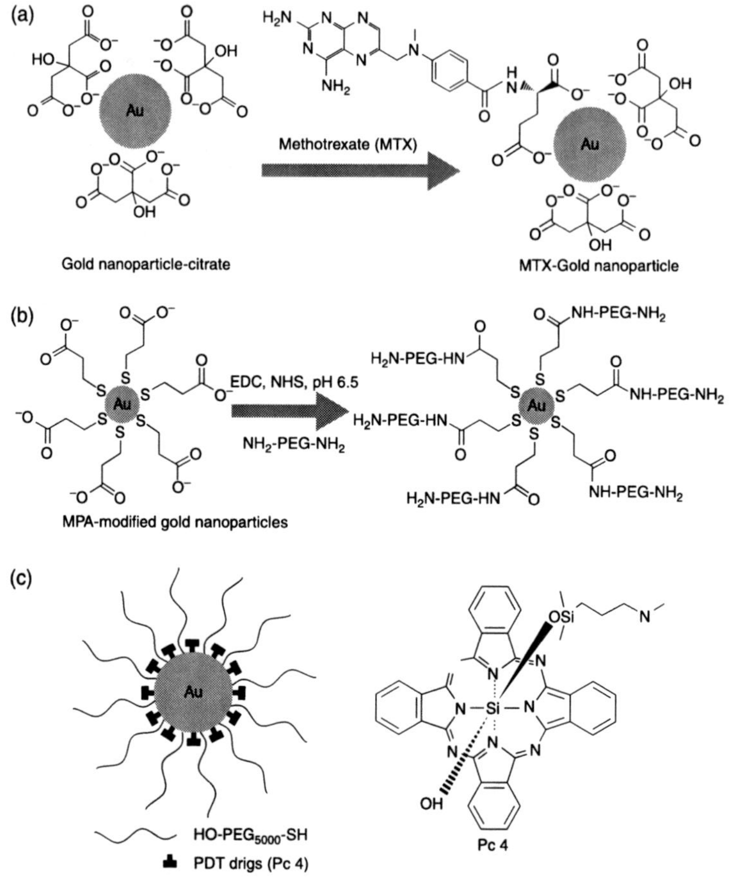

Figure 1.4 **Schematic representation of MTX conjugated to the surface of spherical Au nanoparticles (a), the surface modification of Au nanoparticles using MPA and PEG-amines (b), and photodynamic therapy drugs (c) conjugated to PEGylated spherical Au nanoparticles.**

Source: Adapted with permission from Pissuwan et al. (2011).

Gu et al. (2009) demonstrated a new form of surface functionalized Au nanoparticle that has the capability to target a payload to the cell nucleus. The surfaces of spherical Au nanoparticles of 3.7 nm diameter were modified with

Published by Woodhead Publishing Limited, 2013

3-mercaptopropionic acid (MPA) to form a self-assembled monolayer. NH_2-PEGNH_2 was then conjugated to the MPA layer via amidation between the amine end-groups on the PEG and the carboxylic group on the Au nanoparticles (Figure 1.4b). This conjugation results in good stability in an electrolyte environment and a high efficiency of intracellular transport – both factors being useful for delivery targeted to the nucleus. In another example, Au nanoparticle conjugates could be bound to silicon phthalocyanine-4 (pc-4) (Figure 1.4c). The attachment is through N–Au bonding of the amine group on the pc-4 axial ligand to the PEGylated Au surface. After the PEGylated Au nanoparticle–pc-4 conjugates attained the tumor site, irradiation with light of about 670 nm was used to liberate the pc-4 molecules from the surface of the nanoparticle and initiate phototherapy (Cheng et al., 2008).

Au nanoparticles are also attractive to carry nucleic acids (Felnerova et al., 2004). Generally, the use of nucleic acids to treat and control diseases is termed 'gene therapy'. This type of therapy can be carried out by using viral and non-viral vectors to transport foreign genes into somatic cells to remedy defective genes there or provide additional biological functions (Roy et al., 1999). Many reports are found in the literature for gene therapy (McIntosh et al., 2001; Niidome et al., 2004; Han et al., 2005, 2006; Bonoiu et al., 2009). DNA can be released from the modified Au nanoparticle after treatment with glutathione (GSH) (Han et al., 2005). Recently, studies have shown that the combination of phototherapy with conventional gene therapy offers a high possibility to improve the efficiency of gene delivery into cells (Mariko et al., 2005; Niidome Y et al., 2006).

Au nanorods have demonstrated strong and tunable surface plasmon absorption in the NIR range. Therefore, a controlled release system for genes using Au nanorods offers significant possibilities in gene therapy (Takahashi et al., 2005; Chen et al., 2006; Pissuwan et al., 2008; Wijaya et al., 2008). Wijaya et al. (2008) used Au nanorods to selectively release multiple DNA oligonucleotides. They separately conjugated two different DNA oligonucleotides to short and long Au nanorods. The aspect ratio of the short and long Au nanorods was 4.0 and 5.4, corresponding to longitudinal plasmon resonances with light at 800 and 1100 nm, respectively. When the mixture of the two different sizes of Au nanorods was irradiated with a laser at a wavelength of 800 nm, only the short Au nanorods were melted, but not the long ones. Alternatively, when a laser at a wavelength of 1100 nm was used to irradiate the mixture, the long rods transformed to spherical shapes, but not the short ones. TEM images showed that the shapes remaining after irradiation at 1100 nm were short rods, spheres and a 'candy-wrap' shape. They further studied the selective release of two DNAs, FAM-DNA and TMR-DNA, in the mixture of short and long Au nanorods, respectively. After laser irradiation at a wavelength of 800 nm, about 70% of the FAM-DNA attached to the short rods was released while only about 10% of the TMR-DNA conjugated to long rods was released. This showed that the selective release from Au nanorods could be a new and powerful technique to improve gene delivery (Figure 1.5).

Gold nanoparticles as a heat source

Au nanoparticles absorb light millions of times more strongly than organic dye molecules. The SPR of Au nanoparticles can be exploited to promote light-to-heat conversion. Au nanoparticles are regarded as an effective medium in the conversion of light to heat owing to their strong SPR absorption in the NIR region (Chen et al., 2009). When Au

Published by Woodhead Publishing Limited, 2013

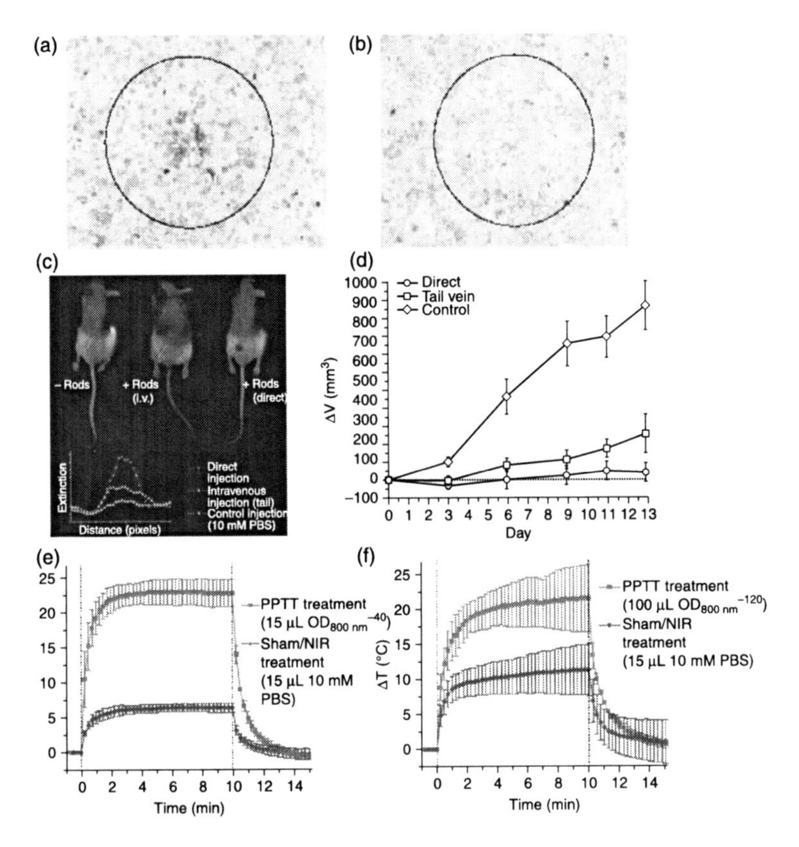

Figure 1.5 (a and b) Selective *in vitro* photothermal cancer therapy using Au nanorods. HSC-3 cancer cells undergo irreversible photodestruction indicated by Trypan blue staining (a); the HaCat normal cells are not affected (b). (c) *In vivo* NIR tumor imaging and (d) *in vivo* photothermal tumor therapy using Au nanorods. Temperature measurements during photothermal treatment with Au nanorods administered by intratumoral injection (e) and intravenous injection (f).

Source: Adapted with permission from Huang et al. (2006a) and Dickerson et al. (2008).

particles are irradiated with light in the 'water window' (800–1200 nm) the free electrons in the Au particles are excited. The excited electrons and the crystal lattice of the Au particles interact, which makes the electron relax, and the thermal energy is transferred to the lattice. Subsequently the heat from the Au particles is dissipated into the surrounding environment (Govorov et al., 2006). Nearly 100% absorbed light is converted to heat, as described above (Hirsch et al., 2003; Pitsillides et al., 2003; Loo et al., 2005; El-Sayed et al., 2006; Huang et al., 2006a,b). The ability of Au nanoparticles to convert strongly absorbed light efficiently into localized heat can be exploited for the selective photothermal therapy of cancer.

Human cells are very sensitive to small increases in temperature and a rise of a few degrees can lead to cell death. Au nanoparticles can be heated by absorption of light, whereby the absorbed light energy is converted into thermal energy. Thus, the idea is to enrich cancerous tissues with Au nanoparticles and to illuminate the tissue. Due to the heat mediated by the Au particles to the surrounding tissue, cancerous tissues can be destroyed locally without exposing the entire organism to elevated temperatures (Huang et al., 2006b; Lowery et al., 2006; Huff et al., 2007).

Photothermal therapy using spherical Au nanoparticles (Pitsillides, 2003; Zharov et al., 2003, 2004, 2005a,b; El-Sayed et al., 2006; Khlebtsov et al., 2006; Huang et al., 2006a,b, 2007a,b; Pissuwan et al., 2007; Hleb et al., 2008; Liu X et al., 2008; Pustovalov et al., 2008) can be achieved with pulsed or cw (continuous wave) visible lasers due to the SPR absorption in the visible region and thus such treatments are suitable for shallow cancers (e.g. skin cancer). Tissue absorbs light in the visible region and infrared (IR) light can only penetrate relatively thin tissue. For this reason Au nanoparticles are needed that absorb light in the IR rather

Published by Woodhead Publishing Limited, 2013

than in the visible range, such as Au rods or hollow structures (Huang et al., 2008; Chen et al., 2007). The light penetration depth can be up to a few centimeters in the spectral region 650–900 nm, also known as the biological NIR window, depending on the tissue type (Weissleder, 2001). A study using pulsed laser and Au nanospheres was performed in 2003 by Lin's group for selective and highly localized photothermolysis of targeted lymphocyte cells (Pitsillides et al., 2003). Their numerical calculations showed that the peak temperature lasting for nanoseconds under a single pulse exceeds 2000 K at a fluence of 0.5 J/cm^2 with a heat fluid layer of 15 nm. Cell death is attributed mainly to the cavitation damage induced by the generated micro-scale bubbles around the nanoparticles. Zharov et al. (2003) performed similar studies on the photothermal destruction of K562 cancer cells. Photothermal properties of Au nanoparticles of different shapes and structures were reviewed in a recent review (Huang and Al-Sayed, 2010). Compared with nanoshells, the use of Au nanorods enables effective treatment at three times lower laser intensity. This is because nanorods exhibit higher absorption efficiency than nanoshells with the SPR at the same wavelength (Jain et al., 2006a). In recent studies, it has been shown that, when the linearly polarized light is converted into circularly polarized light, the light absorption by the Au nanorods is enhanced, which leads to an ultra-low-energy threshold for cancer killing (five times lower) (Li J A et al., 2008).

In photothermal therapy, a cw Ti:Sapphire laser at 800 nm, overlapping maximally with the SPR absorption band of the nanorods, was used for electromagnetic irradiation of labeled cells. Under laser exposure for 4 min, it was found that the cancer cells required half the laser energy (10 W/cm^2) to be photothermally damaged as compared with normal cells (20 W/cm^2), attributed to the selective targeting of the overexpressed EGFR on the cancer cell surface by the anti-EGFR-conjugated Au nanorods (Figure 1.5a), while the normal cells were not affected (Figure 1.5b). In the recent studies by El-Sayed's group in an ENT cancer xenograft model (Dickerson et al., 2008), the nanorods were conjugated to mPEG-SH 5000, and injected into mice both intravenously and subcutaneously. Using transmission imaging of the NIR laser with a customized camera, the tumor could be well identified due to the NIR light absorption by the nanorods in the tumor (Figure 1.5c). The spectral profiling of the images clearly shows the difference of the delivery efficiency of Au nanorods by the two methods. After exposure to a cw NIR diode laser at 808 nm with an intensity of 1–2 W/cm^2 for 10 min, tumor growth is significantly inhibited for both treated groups (Figure 1.5d). The intravenously treated tumors show lower photothermal efficiency due to the fewer nanoparticles accumulated inside the tumor, as shown in the NIR spectral imaging. Thermal transient measurements show that temperature increase by over 20 °C is sufficient to induce tumor destruction (Figure 1.5e and f). Au nanorods have two significant advantages making them more feasible for future clinic settings – their synthetic procedure is relatively facile and they possess superior long blood circulation time due to the anisotropic geometry. For tissues deep inside the body heating with magnetic particles with radiofrequency (RF) fields is favorable (Hiergeist et al., 1999; Pankhurst et al., 2003). The excitation of magnetic nanoparticles works at lower frequencies (RF).

Gold nanoparticles as sensors

Sensors are a class of device that produce measurable responses to changes in physical or chemical properties. Biosensors are generally defined as sensors that consist of biological recognition elements, often called bioreceptors or

Published by Woodhead Publishing Limited, 2013

transducers (Clark and Lyons, 1962; Vo-Dinh and Cullum, 2000). With the recent advances in nanotechnology, nanomaterials have received great interest in the field of biosensors due to their exquisite sensitivity in chemical and biological sensing (Jain, 2003). Among the nanomaterials used as components in biosensors, Au nanoparticles have received most interest because they have several kinds of interesting properties (Wang et al., 2001, 2002).

Au nanoparticle-based biosensors can be classified into optical biosensors, electrochemical biosensors and piezoelectric biosensors. The optical properties of Au nanoparticles provide a wide range of opportunities for the construction of optical biosensors. Optical biosensors generally measure changes in light or photon output. There are several optical sensing modalities for Au nanoparticles and SPR is the one that has attracted most intensive research. The plasmon resonance frequency is a very reliable intrinsic feature present in Au nanoparticles that can be used for sensing (Klar, 2007). The plasmon resonance frequency is dramatically changed when the average distance between Au particles is reduced so that they form small aggregates (Jain et al., 2006a). SPR, which is an optical phenomenon arising from the interaction between an electromagnetic wave and the conduction electrons in a metal, is used for probing and characterizing physicochemical changes of thin films on metal surfaces (Daniel and Astruc, 2004; Hu et al., 2006). The binding of specific molecules onto the surface of metallic films can induce a variation in the dielectric constant, which can cause a change in the reflection of laser light from a metal–liquid surface (Figure 1.6). This effect of plasmon coupling can be used for colorimetric detection of analytes. The method is the well-known example of an Au-based sensor (Mirkin et al., 1996; Elghanian et al., 1997; Moller and Fritzsche, 2007). A sensing method for the detection of

Published by Woodhead Publishing Limited, 2013

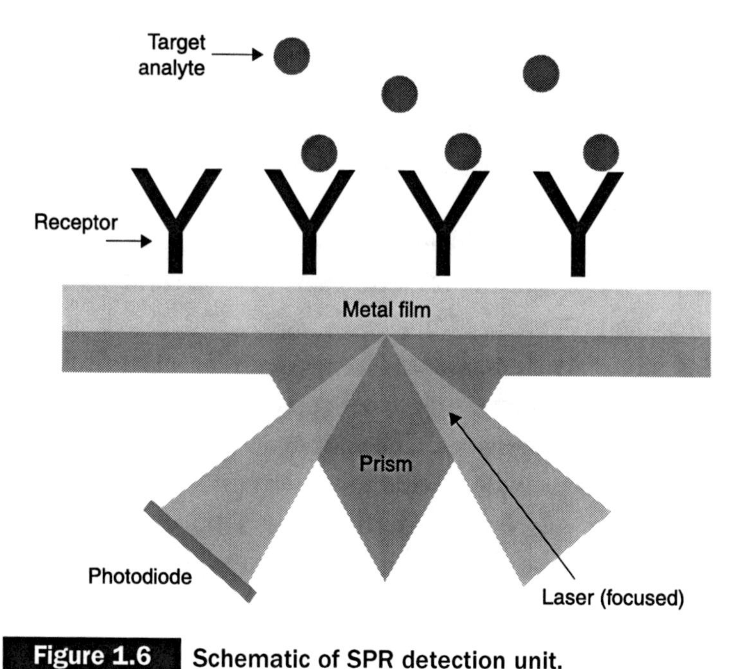

Figure 1.6 **Schematic of SPR detection unit.**

Source: Adapted with permission from Li et al. (2010).

DNA hybridization by Au nanoparticle-enhanced SPR was demonstrated by He et al. (2000). As each Au nanoparticle bears several oligonucleotides, hybridization results in the formation of small aggregates of Au particles, which will lead to a change in the plasmon resonance and the colloidal solution appears a violet/blue color. Several DNA assays have been derived from this concept and nowadays the method is established in a way that quantitative detection of DNA sequences of very low concentrations is possible (Nam et al., 2004). Based upon the signal amplification effect, Yang et al. (2007a,b) developed a sensitive bioanalytical method for DNA detection utilizing catalytic growth of Au nanoparticle-enhanced SPR.

Electrochemical biosensors, which convert the biological binding events into useful electrical signals, have received

Published by Woodhead Publishing Limited, 2013

considerable attention in the past few years because they may provide fast, simple and low-cost detection capabilities (Katz et al., 2004). The excellent biocompatibility, conductivity and catalytic properties make Au nanoparticles candidates to amplify the electrode surfaces, enhance the electron transfer between redox centers in proteins and act as catalysts to increase electrochemical reactions. In many bioelectrochemical reactions, the electron transfer between the redox protein and the electrode surface is the key subject to be detected. Au nanoparticles can also be used for the transfer of electrons in redox reactions (Willner et al., 2006). The idea of such assays is to detect analytes that are substrates to redox enzymes. However, the introduction of Au nanoparticles has several advantages. (i) An electrode covered with a layer of nanoparticles has a much higher surface roughness and thus larger surface area, which leads to higher currents. (ii) Due to the small curvature of small Au particles the contact of the Au particle with the enzyme can be more 'intimate', i.e. located in close proximity to the reactive center, which can facilitate electron transport (Zhao et al., 1992; Yu et al., 2003). Natan's group have proved the direct electron transfer between the electrode and the protein by Au nanoparticles (Brown et al., 1996). Since then, a series of papers has reported the electron communication between the biocatalysts and electrodes using Au nanoparticles as promoter (Jia et al., 2002; Shumyantseva et al., 2005; Zhang et al., 2005; Carralero et al., 2006; Xu et al., 2006; Xue et al., 2006; Lin et al., 2007; Tangkuaram et al., 2007; Zhang et al., 2007; Liu et al., 2008). Willner's group studied the electron transfer turnover rate of a reconstituted bioelectrocatalyst using Au nanoparticles (Xiao et al., 2003).

As shown in Figure 1.7, they constructed a reconstituted Au nanoparticle–glucose oxidase (GOX)-monolayer

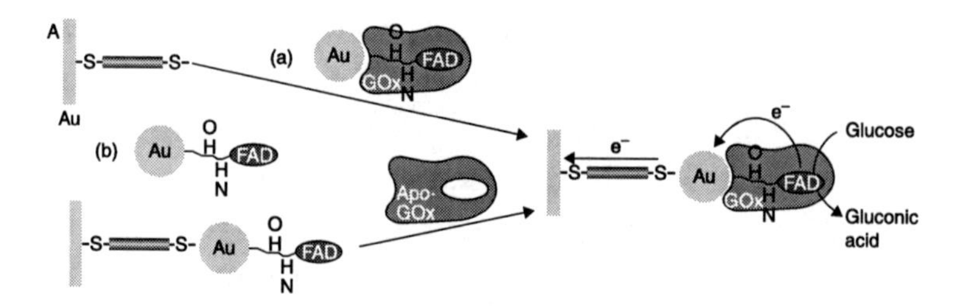

Figure 1.7 **Two construction methods of Au nanoparticle-reconstituted GOX electrode: (a) adsorption of Au nanoparticle-reconstituted GOX to a dithiol monolayer associated with an Au electrode and (b) adsorption of GPNs functionalized with FAD on the dithiol-modified Au electrode followed by the reconstitution of apo-GOX on the functional Au nanoparticles.**

Source: Adapted with permission from Xiao et al. (2003).

electrode by two different ways: (i) functionalizing 1.4-nm Au nanoparticles with N^6-(2-aminoethyl)-flavin adenine dinucleotide (FAD), reconstituting apo-GOX with the FAD-functionalized Au nanoparticle and then assembling the Au nanoparticle-GOX on an Au electrode or (ii) assembling the FAD-functionalized Au nanoparticle on the electrode and reconstituting apo-GOX subsequently. Both enzyme electrodes exhibited very fast electron transfer between the enzyme redox center and the electrode in the presence of the Au nanoparticles. The electron transfer rate was found to be about 5000 s^{-1}, while the rate between GOX and its natural substrate, oxygen, was around 700^{-1}. Au nanoparticles dispersed in polymeric matrices are also used to construct electrochemical biosensors with increased stability, and improved processability, reusability and solubility in a variety of solvents (Shenhar et al., 2005). The nanocomposite of Au nanoparticles and biopolymer, such as chitosan and poly(*p*-aminobenzene sulfonic acid), has been employed as

Published by Woodhead Publishing Limited, 2013

an excellent matrix for fabricating novel biosensors (Xu et al., 2006; Gao et al., 2007; Njagi and Andreescu, 2007; Li W et al., 2008; Yang et al., 2008).

Piezoelectric biosensors measure the mass change arising from the biological recognition process. The piezoelectric effect, which described the relation between mechanical stress and electrical change in solid, was first discovered in 1880 by Jacques and Pierre Curie. They observed that, when a mechanical stress was applied on crystals, electrical changes appeared and this voltage was proportional to the stress. They also verified the converse piezoelectric effect, i.e. that a voltage across these crystals caused a corresponding mechanical stress. The quartz crystal microbalance (QCM) is one of the most important techniques based on the piezoelectric effect. As the high density and high surface-to-volume ratio of Au nanoparticles can amplify the mass change on the crystals during the analysis, numerous research groups have focused on improving the analytical sensitivity by coupling Au nanoparticles with the QCM sensing process. In 2000, Jiang's group (Lin et al., 2000) and Li's group (Zhou et al., 2000) reported an amplified DNA microgravimetric sensor by Au nanoparticles (Figure 1.8). Jiang's group immobilized Au nanoparticles onto the Au surface of the QCM, followed by immobilization of 17mer oligonucleotide probes onto the Au nanoparticles (Figure 1.8a). The target DNA was detected by hybridization reaction with the probes. The relatively large surface area of the Au nanoparticles was considered to immobilize more probes onto the Au surface of the QCM and thereby enhance the sensitivity (Lin et al., 2000). Li's group developed a sandwich-type ternary complex consisting of an oligodeoxynucleotide immobilized on a QCM electrode, a target DNA and an Au nanoparticle-modified DNA, in which the latter two oligonucleotides were both complementary to the oligodeoxynucleotide (Zhou et al., 2000) (Figure 1.8b).

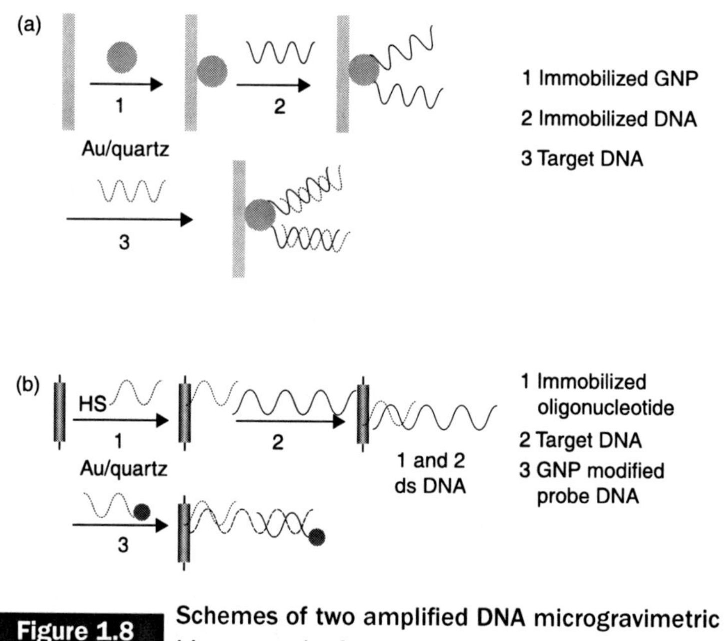

Figure 1.8 **Schemes of two amplified DNA microgravimetric biosensors by Au nanoparticles. (a) Immobilization of Au nanoparticles on the Au surface of the QCM and (b) modification of DNA with Au nanoparticles.**

Source: Adapted with permission from Li et al. (2010).

A piezoelectric sensor is a mass-sensitive device, which means any strategies that amplify the mass change will improve the analytical sensitivity. The quantity and activity of biological recognition elements immobilized on the sensing surface of piezoelectric biosensors determine sensitivity as well as the regeneration ability. The high surface area-to-volume ratio and biocompatibility of Au nanoparticles, which provide a very large number of interaction sites, make Au nanoparticles potential candidates to amplify the sensing surface area and maintain the sensing bioactivity, thereby enhancing the quantity and activity of biological recognition elements (Lin et al., 2000; Hongqiu

Published by Woodhead Publishing Limited, 2013

et al., 2001; Weizmann et al., 2001). Moreover, the excellent biocompatibility can improve the stability of the biological recognition and the relatively high density of Au nanoparticles allows application as a mass enhancer (Zhou et al., 2000; Zhao et al., 2001; Willner et al., 2002; Pang et al., 2006; Chen et al., 2008; Liu et al., 2009).

1.2.2 Antibacterial activity of silver nanoparticles

The high specific surface area and high fraction of surface atoms of the metal nanoparticles will lead in general to high antimicrobial activity compared with bulk metal. Nanoparticles with bactericidal activity can have many applications in several fields, i.e. medical instruments, devices, water treatment and food processing. Several groups have studied the antibacterial activities of metal nanoparticles (Lin et al., 1998; Kumar et al., 2004; Sondi and Salopek-Sondi, 2004; Cho et al., 2005; Jain and Pradeep, 2005; Lok et al., 2006; Porter et al., 2006; Williams et al., 2006; Ruparelia et al., 2008; Sathishkumar et al., 2009; Akhavan and Ghaderi, 2010; Sadeghi et al., 2010; Tran et al., 2010a,b; Chamakura et al., 2011). It was found that Ag nanoparticles have important antimicrobial properties, but for other metal nanoparticles such as Pt, Au, iron oxide, silica and its oxides, and nickel there are no bactericidal effects in studies with *E. coli* (Lok et al., 2006; Williams et al., 2006). We will focus our attention on the recent results of antibacterial activities of Ag nanoparticles.

In the investigations of the antibacterial activities of any kind of nanoparticles, there are two parameters: the minimum inhibitory concentration (MIC) and the minimum bactericidal concentration (MBC) are the lowest concentrations (mg/ml) at which a tested compound can, respectively, inhibit

Published by Woodhead Publishing Limited, 2013

bacterium growth or kill more than 99% of the added bacteria (Lok et al., 2006; Sadeghi et al., 2010). If the tested material does not kill but inhibits the growth of bacteria (bacteriostatic), bacteria will grow when taken out from the solution and colonies will be observed. If the tested material is bactericidal, no bacterial colonies will be observed. It will be interesting also to notice that different research groups used several methods to prepare the Ag nanocrystallines, but most of them studied the bactericidal activity against *E. coli*.

Sathishkumar et al. (2009) were interested by the green synthesis of nanocrystalline Ag particles and their bactericidal activity. They reported the biosynthesis of Ag nanoparticles from Ag precursors using the bark extract and powder of novel *Cinnamon zeylanicum*. They used aqueous 1 mM $AgNO_3$ solutions and different dosages of *C. zeylanicum* bark powder (CBP) for the bioreduction of nano-scale Ag particles. This reduction of Ag ion to nanosize Ag particles is explained by the presence of water-soluble organics. Sathishkumar et al. (2009) performed UV/Vis, TEM and XRD measurements for different CBP dosages. They showed that the particle size increased with increasing dosage due to the amount of reductive biomolecules. The important role of pH in controlling the shape and size of the Ag nanocrystalline was also shown. Finally, Sathishkumar et al. (2009) tested the bactericidal activity of the Ag nanoparticles against Gram-negative *E. coli* strain BL-21. They used different Ag nanoparticle concentrations of 2, 5, 10, 25 and 50 mg/l producing inhibition of 10.9, 32.4, 55.8, 82 and 98.8%, respectively.

Using wet chemical synthesis involving the reaction between sodium borohydrides and Ag ions, Ruparelia et al. (2008) synthesized Ag nanoparticles with an average particle size of 3 nm. In a second step of their study, the antimicrobial properties of Ag nanoparticles were investigated using

Published by Woodhead Publishing Limited, 2013

E. coli (four strains). It was reported that MIC ranged from 40 to 180 μg/ml and MBC ranged from 60 to 220 μg/mL for various strains of *E. coli*. They reported a growth inhibition of around 50% in 18 h for the *E. coli* when grown with 100 mg/l Ag nanoparticles. This is in agreement with the 55.8% inhibition at the same concentration of Ag nanoparticles obtained by Sathishkumar et al. (2009).

Lok et al. (2006) investigated the mode of antibacterial action of nano-Ag against *E. coli*. They synthesized Ag nanoparticles by the borohydride reduction of $AgNO_3$ in the presence of citrate as a stabilizing agent. $NaBH_4$ (50 mg) was added to a vigorously stirred $AgNO_3$ solution (16 mg in 1 l) and sodium citrate (0.7 mM) at room temperature. Then the solution was concentrated further to 100 ml under vacuum. TEM revealed that Ag nanoparticles are spherical with a diameter of 9.3 ± 2.8 nm. Lok et al. (2006) identified a possible mode of action underlying the antibacterial action of Ag nanoparticles through proteomic analyses. The proteomic signatures of nano-Ag-treated *E. coli* cells are characterized by an accumulation of envelope protein precursors. This indicated that the Ag nanoparticles may target the bacterial membrane, leading to a dissipation of the proton motive force (Lok et al., 2006).

Tran et al. (2010a) synthesized monodisperse chitosan-based Ag nanoparticles and then investigated their antibacterial activities. The authors used a 'green' synthesis method to prepare Ag nanoparticles using non-toxic chitosan agent. They added 25 ml of fresh solution of 0.1 M $AgNO_3$ to 100 ml of chitosan and then dissolved it in a solution of 1 wt% acetic acid to reach an appropriate concentration. TEM measurement revealed that the nanoparticle size was in the range of 5–7 nm. Tran et al. (2010a) also studied the bactericidal effect against Gram-negative (*E. coli* and *Pseudomonas aeruginosa*) and Gram-positive (*Lactobacillus*

Published by Woodhead Publishing Limited, 2013

fermentum, Staphylococcus aureus and *Bacillus subtilis*) bacterial strains, and yeast (*Candida albicans*). They showed that the bactericidal activity of Ag nanoparticles was affected by the cell membrane structure: Gram-negative bacteria were inhibited more strongly than Gram-positive bacteria (Tran et al., 2010a).

Sadeghi et al. (2010) reported the antibacterial activity of Ag nanoparticles against *S. aureus* and *E. coli.* They synthesized Ag nanoparticles by a chemical method using reduction of $AgNO_3$ in the presence of $NaBH_4$. To investigate the antimicrobial activity of Ag nanoparticles on the bacterial growth, the authors determined the MIC of Ag nanoparticles for *S. aureus* and *E. coli* by optical density of the bacterial culture solution containing different concentrations of Ag nanoparticles after 24 h (Figure 1.9).

In addition, the effect of Ag nanoparticles on the morphological changes of *S. aureus* and *E. coli* was observed by SEM. They showed that the Ag nanoparticles had high antibacterial efficacies, and this activity was quite strong and durable. It was also shown by Sadeghi et al. (2010) that Ag nanoparticles require a lower concentration to inhibit development of the *Streptococcus mutans* and *E. coli* strains,

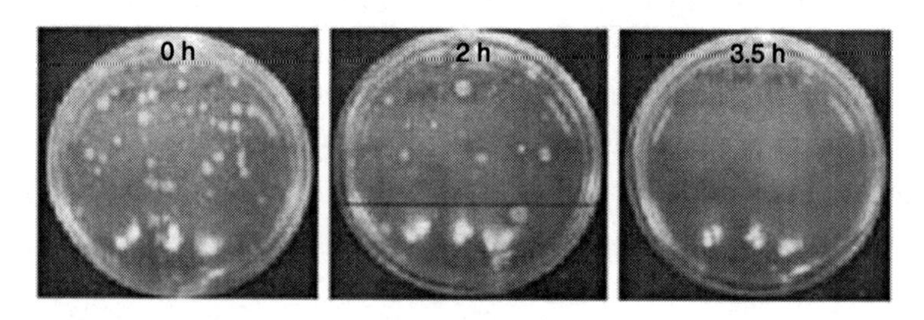

Figure 1.9 **Growth inhibition of *E. coli* colonies after Ag nanoparticle (10 p.p.m.) treatment v. the incubation time (0, 2 and 3.5 h).**

Source: Adapted with permission from Sadeghi et al. (2010).

Published by Woodhead Publishing Limited, 2013

and this result can be explained by the increasing surface area in nanoparticles.

Most of the studies on the antibacterial activity of Ag nanoparticles reported that the concentration of nano-Ag played the main role; however, recently, Chamakura et al. (2011) showed that efficacy is dependent upon the ratio of *E. coli* to nanoparticles rather than the concentration of Ag nanoparticles. Chamakura et al. (2011) synthesized Ag nanoparticles by a chemical reduction method. They used Ag nitrate and various reducing agents (ascorbic acid ($C_6H_8O_6$), sodium citrate ($C_6H_5ONa_3$), sodium borohydride ($NaBH_4$), and dimethylamine borane (DMAB, $C_2H_{10}NB$)) in order to complete the reduction of Ag cations. The authors treated the *E. coli* with different Ag nanoparticle concentrations and proposed a summary of known modes of inactivation of the bacteria by Ag nanoparticles (Figure 1.10).

They also compared the effect of Ag nanoparticles with other chemical disinfectants. It was found that higher ratios of Ag nanoparticles to bacteria resulted in a faster bactericidal effect, and that Ag nanoparticles exhibit persistent and efficient bactericidal activity even at the lowest concentration compared with the chemical disinfectant.

Other research groups were interested by the synthesis of Ag nanoparticles accumulated on the surface and studied their bactericidal activities. For example, Kumar et al. (2004) studied the generation of Ag nanoparticles on active carbon by an electrochemical deposition method and they were also interested in the utilization of Ag nanoparticles in controlling the microorganisms in water. The Ag nanoparticles were generated electrochemically by passing a DC current through Ag electrodes dipped in distilled water. A 2 wt% of Ag deposited on activated carbon (AgC-EC) was prepared by suspending around 5 g of carbon in distilled water with vigorous stirring and maintaining 40 V DC current through

Published by Woodhead Publishing Limited, 2013

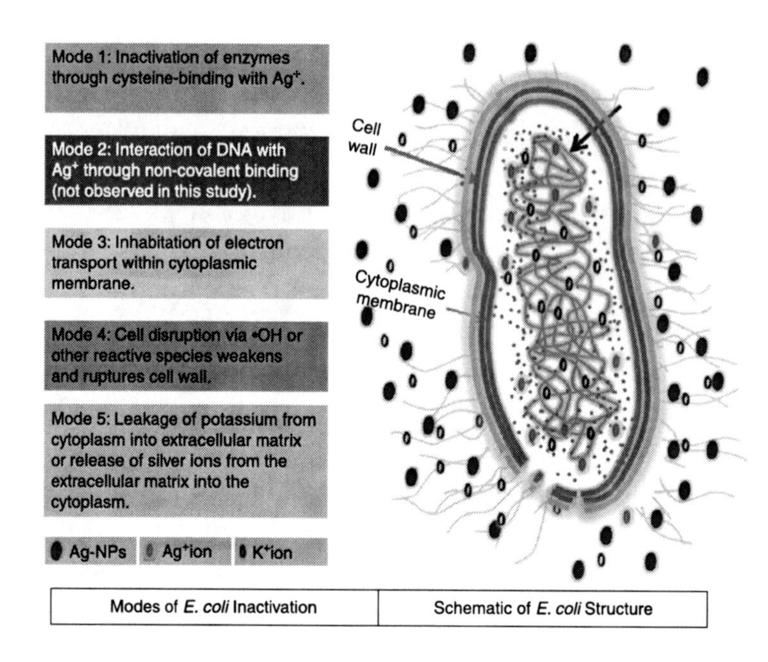

Figure 1.10 **Summary of known modes of *E. coli* inactivation by Ag cations.**

Source: Adapted with permission from Chamakura et al. (2011).

the Ag electrodes for a sufficient amount of time. SEM results showed the formation of Ag nanoparticles (50–200 nm) after a run time of 5 min. Kumar et al. (2004) also qualitatively studied the antibacterial activity of the Ag nanoparticles by testing the presence of coliforms in water after contact with the catalyst, using a Readycult reagent. They showed that the Ag nanoparticles increased the intrinsic activity (activity per site) and hence had superior activity. The high intrinsic activity of this catalyst is evidenced from its effectiveness in controlling the microorganism in water with lower weight. Akhavan and Ghaderi (2010) reported the antibacterial activity of a sol–gel synthesized Ag–TiO_2 nanocomposite layer against *E. coli* bacteria. Their TEM images showed that the size of Ag nanoparticles is in the range of 5–10 nm.

Published by Woodhead Publishing Limited, 2013

They showed that Ag–TiO_2/(a)TiO_2 nanocomposite thin films have excellent antibacterial activity against *E. coli* bacteria. By comparing the antibacterial activity of Ag–TiO_2/TiO_2 nanocomposite and TiO_2 thin films, they showed that the relative rate of reduction of the viable bacteria by Ag–TiO_2/(a)TiO_2 nanocomposite thin film was greater than the corresponding value for the parent TiO_2 thin film.

Finally, it is interesting to note that the exact mechanism for the growth inhibition by Ag nanoparticles is not yet clear. For example, Kumar et al. (2004) proposed a mechanism that involves the association of Ag with oxygen and its reaction with sulfhydryl (S–H) groups on the cell wall to form R–S–S–R bonds, thereby blocking respiration and causing cell death. Lin et al. (1998) claimed that the Ag ions from nanoparticles are attached to the negatively charged bacterial cell wall and rupture it, which leads to denaturation of protein and finally cell death. Chamakura et al. (2011) supposed that the mechanism of *E. coli* inactivation using Ag nanoparticles could involve multiple processes, including: (i) indirect generation of reactive oxygen species (ROS), and (ii) direct interaction of Ag with proteins and lipids in the cell wall and proteins in the cytoplasmic membrane involved in transport and respiration metabolism, compromising their function.

1.2.3 Iron oxide nanoparticles

Iron oxide nanoparticle properties

The most common forms of iron oxides in nature are magnetite (Fe_3O_4), maghemite (γ-Fe_2O_3) and hematite (α-Fe_2O_3). The three types of iron oxides all have specific close-packed planes of oxygen anions and iron cations, e.g. in hematite the oxygen ions are in hexagonal sites and the Fe(III) cations are in octahedral sites. In magnetite the oxygen

Published by Woodhead Publishing Limited, 2013

ions are in the cubic close-packed arrangement and iron cations are distributed randomly between octahedral and tetrahedral sites and Fe(II) ions are in octahedral sites. Maghemite has a similar structure to magnetite but with some vacancies in some sites. The iron atom has a strong magnetic moment because it contains four unpaired electrons in its 3d orbitals. The saturation magnetization *M* is the vector sum of all the magnetic moments of the atoms in the material per unit volume of the material. The magnetization curve is a hysteresis loop because when an external field *H* with a magnetic strength *M* is applied to a ferromagnet crystal the magnetization increases until a saturation magnetization M_s is reached (Figure 1.11). When *H* is

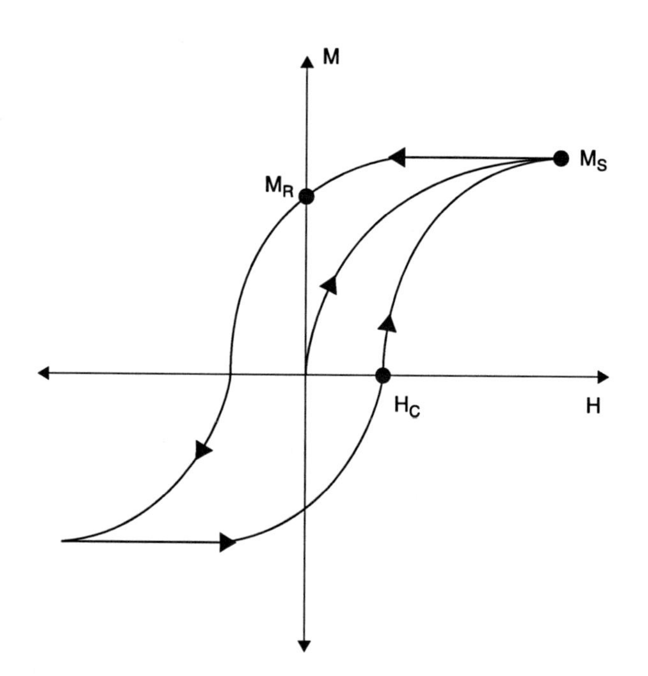

Figure 1.11 **Magnetization *M* as a function of an applied magnetic field *H*.**

Source: Adapted with permission from Teja and Koh (2009).

decreased not all domains return to their original orientation – some remnant magnetization remains and can only be removed by applying a coercive field H_c in the opposite direction to the external field (Teja and Koh, 2009).

Fe_3O_4 has unique electric and magnetic properties due to the transfer of electrons between Fe^{2+} and Fe^{3+} ions in the octahedral sites. A crystal of Fe_3O_4 has a spinel structure, space group Fd3m and a lattice constant of about 8.39 Å (Teja and Koh, 2009).

There are three types of interaction among the nanoparticles: London–Van der Waals forces, magnetic forces and reacting forces of the double electronic layer. To make the particles disperse well in the solvent, the surface of the nanoparticles should be modified by a layer of surfactant; thus the repulsion force from the surfactant can inhibit the affinities between the particles (Yan et al., 2009). Different magnetic materials display dissimilar performances; diamagnetic atoms (Figure 1.12a) in solids have negligible magnetic moments, in paramagnetic solids magnetic atoms are not ordered because of thermal energy that shakes each atom randomly (Figure 1.12b), in a ferromagnetic material displacement of the domain walls results in open hysteresis cycles (Figure 1.12c) and for a superparamagnetic state the whole magnetic moment of each particle is shaken in the same way as in paramagnetic material (Goya et al., 2008).

Synthesis of iron oxides

The preparation method of nanomaterials is one of the important challenges that determine the particle size, morphology and shape, the size distribution, the surface chemistry of the particles, the degree of impurities in the particles and their magnetic properties, and consequently their applications. Many attempts have been made to develop

Published by Woodhead Publishing Limited, 2013

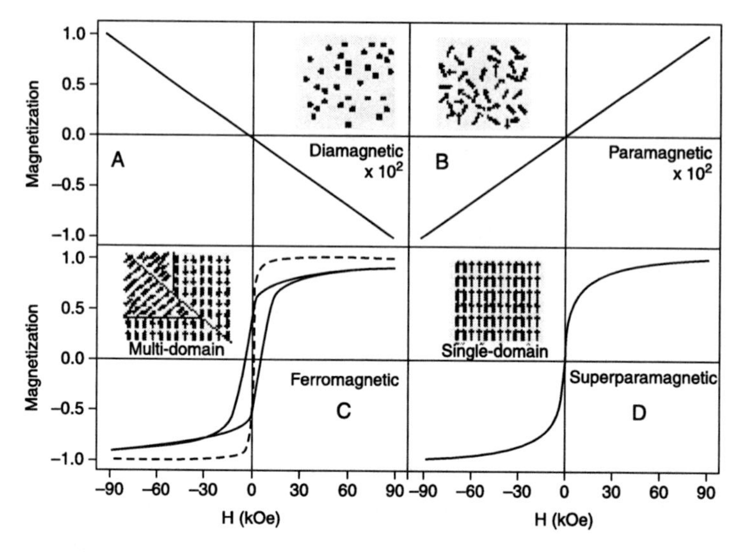

Figure 1.12 **Performances of different magnetic materials: (a) diamagnetic, (b) paramagnetic solid, (c) ferromagnetic and (d) superparamagnetic materials.**

Source: Adapted with permission from Goya et al. (2008).

techniques to produce highly uniform and monodispersed nanoparticles. Two main approaches are often used for the preparation of magnetic nanoparticles: top-down and bottom-up. In the *top-down* strategy, the starting bulk material is reduced to nanometric scale in one (thin films), two (nanowires) or three (nanoparticles or quantum dots) dimensions. This route is often based on physical processes like mechanical alloying, laser machining, laser chemical etching, reactive ion etching, etc. On the contrary, the *bottom-up* approach uses atomic or molecular units as starting materials to grow larger, nanometric structures. Bottom-up techniques include chemical vapor deposition (CVD), pulsed laser deposition (PLD), and also wet routes like sol–gel and microemulsion techniques. In the following section, some synthesis methods will be discussed.

Published by Woodhead Publishing Limited, 2013

Precipitation from solution

This process involves the formation of a homogeneous precipitate when the concentration of the reactants reaches critical supersaturation. Some important examples of this process are: coprecipitation, microemulsions and thermal decomposition of iron or organic iron precursors.

Coprecipitation method

In this method the nanoparticles are precipitated from a solution by mixing stoichiometric mixtures of Fe^{3+} and Fe^{2+} salts in aqueous basic solution. The reaction is usually carried out under inert atmospheric conditions to avoid oxidation of Fe_3O_4 into Fe_2O_3. However, several methods have been developed for the formation of Fe_3O_4 in air without protection. The size of the particles and their morphology can be adjusted by changing the pH, concentration of the ionic precursors, type of raw materials and reaction conditions (temperature and time). The general mechanism for the coprecipitation is (Zhao et al., 2009):

$$Fe^{2+} + 2Fe^{3+} + 8OH^{-} \rightarrow Fe_3O_4 + 4\ H_2O \qquad [1.1]$$

Several studies have been reported in the literature concerning the synthesis of Fe_3O_4 nanoparticles using the coprecipitation method with some modifications in order to improve the properties of the prepared nanoparticles.

Hong et al. (2007) studied the effect of solvent and type of base on the properties of the prepared Fe_3O_4 nanoparticles and accordingly they prepared Fe_3O_4 nanoparticles using NH_3 in alcohol or NaOH in water. The saturation magnetizations of the prepared samples were in the range of 34.5–50.6 e.m.u./g and the magnetic properties of Fe_3O_4 prepared using NaOH were lower than those using

Published by Woodhead Publishing Limited, 2013

NH_3 because Na^+ ions enhance the electropositivity of the solution and the collision between Fe^{3+} and Fe^{2+} ions, thus affecting the formation of Fe_3O_4. The average crystallite size of the Fe_3O_4 prepared in NH_3 and alcohol was smaller than that prepared in NaOH solution (Hong et al., 2007).

Fe_3O_4 nanorods have been synthesized by mixing Fe^{3+} and Fe^{2+} solutions containing urea at 90–95 °C for 12 h. It has been suggested that in this synthesis the optimum molar ratio of Fe^{2+}/Fe^{3+} was 0.5 and if the molar ratio is less than 0.5, Fe_2O_3 is produced instead of Fe_3O_4. The obtained magnetic nanorods are composed of uniform rod-like structures with a diameter in the range of 40–50 nm and length of 1 μm (Figure 1.13) with a saturation magnetization (M_s) of 67.6 e.m.u./g. The mechanism of the formation of Fe_3O_4 nanorods can be inferred as (Lian et al., 2004):

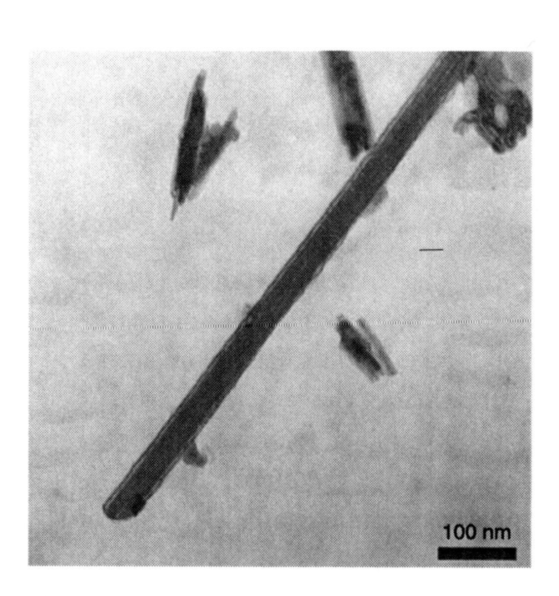

Figure 1.13 Fe_3O_4 nanorods.

Source: Adapted with permission from Lian et al. (2004).

$$(NH_2)_2CO + H_2O \rightarrow 2NH_3 + CO_2 \quad [1.2]$$

$$NH_3 + H_2O \rightarrow NH_4^+ + OH^- \quad [1.3]$$

$$Fe^{3+} + OH^- \rightarrow Fe(OH)_3 \quad [1.4]$$

$$Fe(OH)_3 \rightarrow FeOOH + H_2O \quad [1.5]$$

$$Fe^{2+} + OH^- \rightarrow Fe(OH)_2 \quad [1.6]$$

$$FeOOH + Fe(OH)_2 \rightarrow Fe_3O_4 + H_2O \quad [1.7]$$

A series of Fe_3O_4 nanoparticles was prepared by coprecipitation of different molar ratios of Fe^{3+}/Fe^{2+} ranging from 2.2 to 1.8 in NaOH solution and dodecylbenzene sulfonic acid sodium salt (NaDS) at 80 °C for 10 min. The particles were almost spherical with a diameter ranging from 10 to 20 nm. The saturation magnetization of the prepared samples decreased with the increase of the Fe^{3+}/Fe^{2+} molar ratio. An increase in the temperature of these particles between 42 and 98 °C was observed when the particles were suspended in physiological saline and then exposed to an external AC magnetic field (80 kHz and 30 kA/m) for 29 min (Figure 1.14) (Zhao et al., 2009).

Fe_3O_4 nanoparticles were synthesized by hydrolysis of an aqueous solution containing iron salts and 1,6-hexanediamine at room temperature under atmospheric conditions (Iida et al., 2007). In this study the type of iron salt and the molar ratio of Fe^{2+} to Fe^{3+} were varied while holding the total molar concentration constant at about 0.05 mol/dm^3. The average diameter for the samples prepared with Fe^{2+} alone was larger than that for the samples prepared with both Fe^{2+} and Fe^{3+} (Figure 1.15). The saturation magnetizations of the samples synthesized with Fe^{2+} ions (80–87 e.m.u./g) were lower than that prepared by both ions (47–55 e.m.u./g), which is due to the increase in the thermal fluctuation near the surface of Fe_3O_4 nanoparticles (Iida et al., 2007).

Published by Woodhead Publishing Limited, 2013

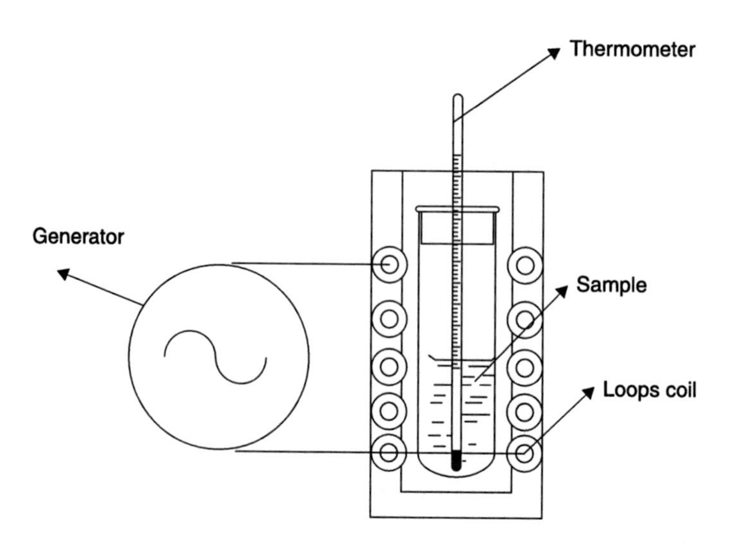

Figure 1.14 **Set-up for measuring heat properties using an AC magnetic field generator.**

Source: Adapted with permission from Zhao et al. (2009).

Yangde et al. (2008) prepared Fe_3O_4 by reacting Fe^{2+} and Fe^{3+} ions in hydrochloric acid and PEG 2000 under atmospheric conditions. The PEG was used to prevent agglomeration by replacing water molecules on the surface of particles and thus reducing the surface free energy. The average crystallite size of prepared Fe_3O_4 nanoparticles was about 42.5 nm with saturation magnetization of about 7–8 e.m.u./g.

Rashdan et al. (2010b) obtained a mixture of different ratios of Fe_3O_4 and Fe_2O_3 nanoparticles when mixing $FeCl_3$ and $FeSO_4$ salts in urea and PEG 200 or 3000 at 40–50 °C for 3 h with the addition of NaOH solution. The samples obtained showed a similar crystallite size of around 23.5 nm, but the saturation magnetization of the sample prepared by PEG 3000 (31 e.m.u./g) was about three times higher than that prepared by PEG 200. The group suggested that the mixture of product obtained in this experiment can be

Published by Woodhead Publishing Limited, 2013

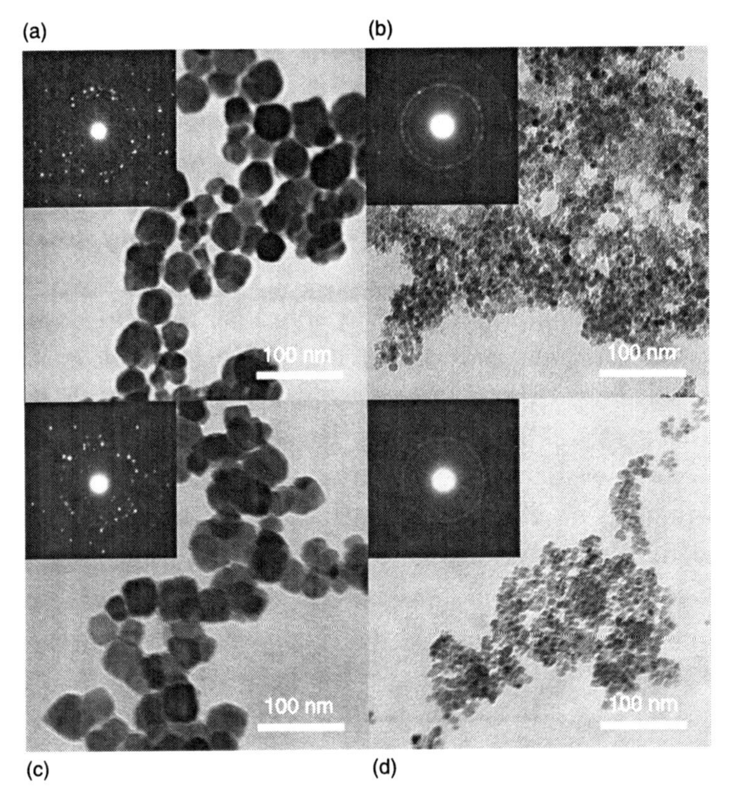

Figure 1.15 TEM images and electron diffraction patterns of samples synthesized with $Fe(SO_4)_2$ (a), $Fe(SO_4)_2$ and $Fe(SO_4)_3$ (b), $FeCl_2$ (c), and $FeCl_2$ and $FeCl_3$ (d).

Source: Adapted with permission from Iida et al. (2007).

attributed to the short reaction time or/and to the lower reaction temperature (Rashdan et al., 2010b). Urea was used because it causes a uniform rise in pH of the solution and thus allows homogeneous nucleation to occur, as suggested by Lian et al. (2004). On the other hand, Grabis et al. (2008) have obtained pure Fe_3O_4 nanoparticles by using the same raw salts and conditions as those used by Rashdan et al. (2010b), and the prepared Fe_3O_4 nanoparticles had an average crystallite size in the range of 16.7–25.1 nm.

Published by Woodhead Publishing Limited, 2013

Faiyas et al. (2010) studied the effect of pH on the phase, morphology and magnetic properties of Fe_3O_4 nanoparticles prepared by mixing ferric and ferrous chlorides in ammonia and mercaptoethanol. Fe_3O_4 nanoparticles were obtained at pH 11, whereas Fe_2O_3 nanoparticles were obtained at a pH lower than 11. The crystallite size of the prepared sample was in the range of 8–22 nm and as the amount of mercaptoethanol increased, the crystallite size decreased. The saturation magnetization of the Fe_3O_4 nanoparticles was generally low at about 34.15×10^3 A/m (Faiyas et al., 2010).

Zheng et al. (2010) found that Fe concentration and molecular weight of PEG play an important role in the morphology of Fe_3O_4 nanoparticles. They show that at high Fe concentrations cubic nanostructures are formed, and at low Fe concentrations rod-like and dendric structures are dominant (Figure 1.16). In addition, when the molecular

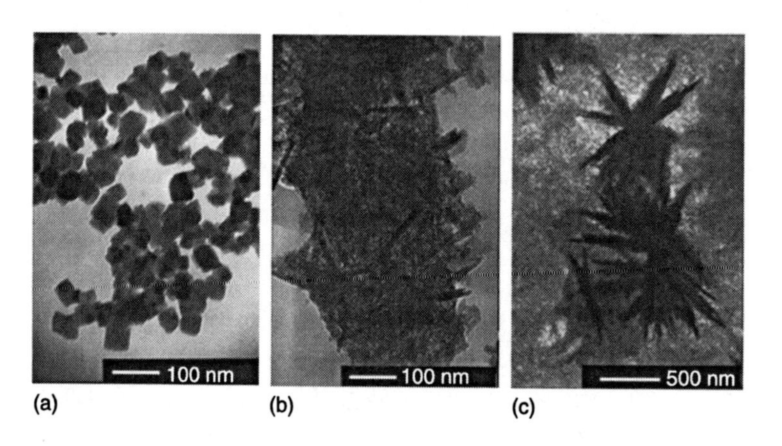

Figure 1.16 TEM images of Fe_3O_4 nanostructures at different concentrations of Fe^{3+} and Fe^{2+} solutions: (a) Fe^{3+}: 0.2, Fe^{2+}: 0.1 mol/l; (b) Fe^{3+}: 2.0×10^{-2}, Fe^{+2}: 1.0×10^{-2} mol/l; and (c) Fe^{3+}: 2.0×10^{-3}, Fe^{2+}: 1.0×10^{-3} mol/l.

Source: Adapted with permission from Zheng et al. (2010).

Published by Woodhead Publishing Limited, 2013

weight of the PEG increases, the size of the nanoparticles increases, e.g. when PEG 400 used the diameter of the obtained Fe_3O_4 was 15 nm, but it was 100 nm when PEG 100 000 was used (Figure 1.17).

Yuanbi et al. (2008) reported the synthesis of Fe_3O_4 nanoparticles by coprecipitation of ferric and ferrous chloride ions in basic, inert conditions and PEG 4000 at 50 °C. The particle size of the prepared sample in NH_4OH was smaller than that obtained in NaOH, which can be attributed to the fact that NaOH has a higher concentration of OH^- ions that will accelerate the reaction and lead to large particle size, whereas NH_4OH releases OH^- gradually to form smaller particles. The size of the prepared sample increased as the concentration of Fe^{2+} and Fe^{3+} increased, and the average particle size was about 11.4 nm (Yuanbi et al., 2008).

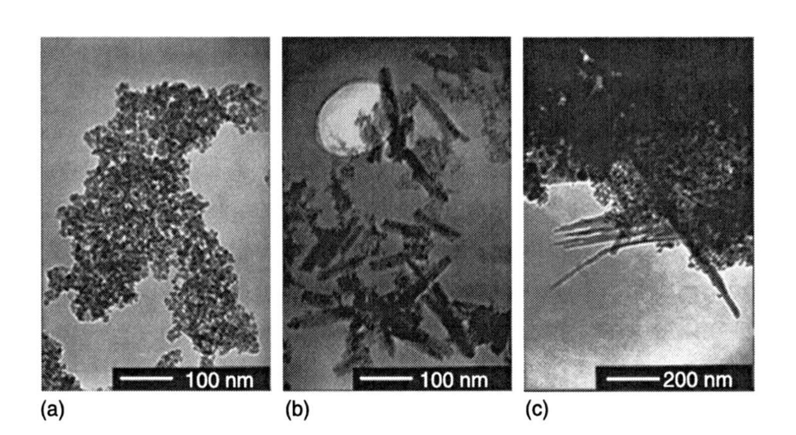

Figure 1.17 TEM images of Fe_3O_4 nanostructures for different molecular weights of PEG: (a) 400, (b) 10 000 and (c) 100 000.

Source: Adapted with permission from Zheng et al. (2010).

Thermal oxidation of iron ions

This process is based on the reduction of dissolved metallic salts, usually ferrous salts, in basic conditions. The general mechanism for the synthesis of Fe_3O_4 nanoparticles by this method is (Iida et al., 2007):

$$Fe^{2+} + 2OH^- \rightarrow Fe(OH)_2 \quad [1.8]$$

$$3Fe(OH)_2 + 1/2O_2 \rightarrow Fe(OH)_2 + 2FeOOH + H_2O \quad [1.9]$$

$$Fe(OH)_2 + 2FeOOH \rightarrow Fe_3O_4 + 2H_2O \quad [1.10]$$

Fe_3O_4 nanoparticles have been synthesized by thermal decomposition of Fe-acetylacetonate (Sun and Zeng, 2002; Sun et al., 2004) with a crystallite size of 4 nm. The particle size can be controlled by a seed-mediated growth method, in which smaller Fe_3O_4 nanoparticles are mixed with more precursor materials; with slow nucleation, larger nanoparticles are formed. For example, mixing 62 mg of 4 nm Fe_3O_4 with 2 mmol of $Fe(acac)_3$ led to 12-nm Fe_3O_4 nanoparticles (Sun and Zeng, 2002; Sun et al., 2004).

Aslam et al. (2007) have reported a one-step synthesis of Fe_3O_4 nanoparticles with a crystallite size in the range of 9–30 nm and saturation magnetization of about 70 e.m.u./g in aqueous solution under ambient conditions using $FeCl_2$ as a precursor and dodecylamine (DDA) as a reducing agent and surface functionalizing agent. The group suggested that the average crystallite size and morphology of the Fe_3O_4 nanoparticles can be controlled by changing the concentration of amine with respect to Fe^{2+} ion concentration. It was found that the higher the molar ratio, the smaller the nanoparticles; as the concentration of amine increases, the particle size becomes more uniform. In addition to the concentration, the particle size was also affected by the time of reaction as the shorter reaction time (3 h) afforded irregularly shaped nanoparticles, whereas at a longer time (12 h) the crystallite

Published by Woodhead Publishing Limited, 2013

size became larger with a broad distribution (Aslam et al., 2007).

Haddad et al. (2008) have prepared superparamagnetic Fe_3O_4 nanoparticles via thermal decomposition of $Fe(acac)_3$ in 1,2-hexadecanodio (reducing agent) and oleyamine (capping ligands) in organic solvent. 2,3-Dimercaptosuccinic acid (DMSA) was added to transfer the magnetic nanoparticles from the organic to aqueous phase. The experiment showed that the smaller particle size is obtained at lower temperature and shorter heating times with a saturation magnetization in the range of 30–60 e.m.u./g. The prepared nanoparticles were incorporated in HeLa cells and tested by the Prussian blue technique, where Fe^{3+} reacts with a mixture of HCl (2%) and $K[Fe(CN)_6]$ (2%) producing $Fe_4[Fe(CN)_6]_3$, which is an insoluble blue product deposited inside the cell at the location of Fe^{3+} ions (Figure 1.18). The intensity of the

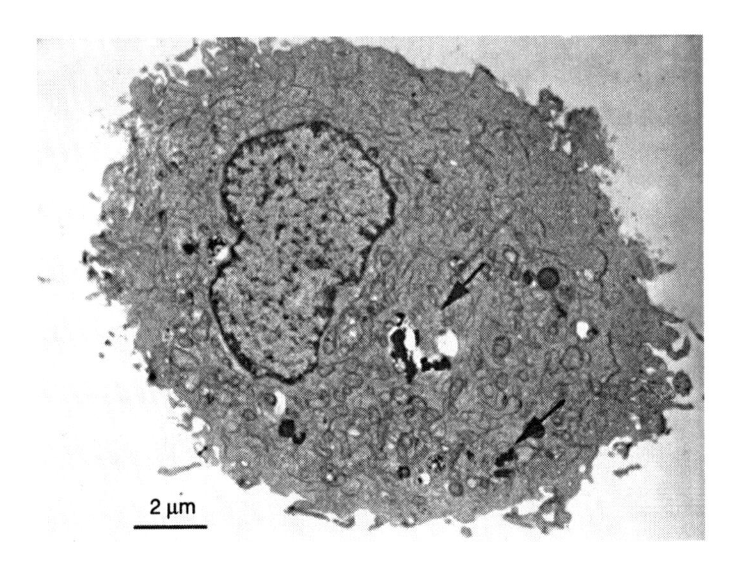

Figure 1.18 Incorporation of Fe_3O_4 nanoparticles (8.1 nm) in the HeLa cells.

Source: Adapted with permission from Haddad et al. (2008).

Published by Woodhead Publishing Limited, 2013

stained area/cell determines the concentration of the Fe^{3+}-containing nanoparticles (Haddad et al., 2008).

Fe_3O_4 nanoparticles have been synthesized by hydrothermal reaction using sodium bis(2-ethylhexyl)sulfosuccinate (AOT) as a surfactant and hydrazine hydrate as a reducing agent. The best Fe_3O_4 sample was prepared at 150 °C for 10 h when the concentrations of AOT and hydrazine were 0.10 M and 20%, respectively. The average particle size of the sample was about 11–12 nm with M_s of 55.8 e.m.u./g (Yan et al., 2009).

Rashdan et al. (2010a) have prepared Fe_3O_4 as a major product when heating an aqueous solution of $FeSO_4$ in urea and PEG 200 at 40–50 °C for 3 h. The sample had a high saturation magnetization of 74.7 e.m.u./g with a crystallite size of 70 nm (Rashdan et al., 2010a).

Yan et al. (2008) have prepared Fe_3O_4 via a solvothermal method of $FeCl_3$ with mixed surfactants of sodium dodecyl sulfate (SDS) and PEG as protective agents. The size of the prepared nanoparticles could be controlled in the range of about 15–190 nm by changing the reaction parameters, such as the protective agents (Figure 1.19) and reaction time (Figure 1.20) (Yan et al., 2008).

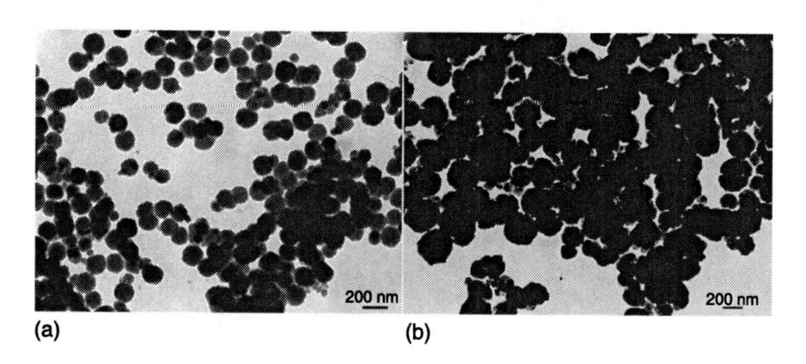

Figure 1.19 **TEM images of Fe_3O_4 nanoparticles prepared with different protective agents (a) SDS and (b) PEG.**

Source: Adapted with permission from Yan et al. (2008).

Published by Woodhead Publishing Limited, 2013

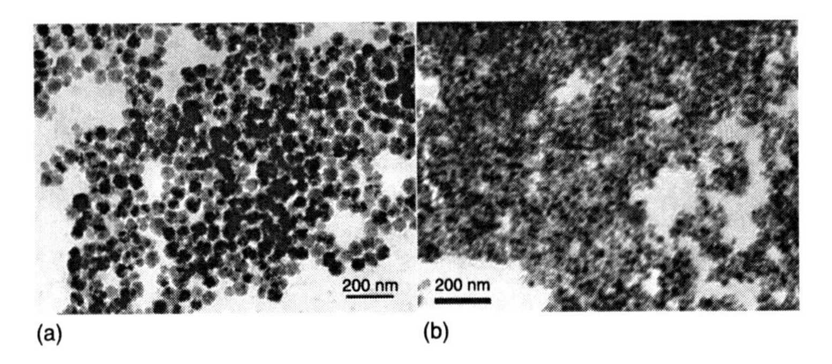

Figure 1.20 TEM images of Fe_3O_4 nanoparticles prepared at different conditions (a) 24 and (b) 6 h.

Source: Adapted with permission from Yan et al. (2008).

A single-crystalline Fe_3O_4 nanobelt was synthesized by mixing PEG 6000 and $FeCl_2$ with NaOH at 180 °C for 17 h (Li et al., 2009). The morphology of the Fe_3O_4 formed was changed by increasing the time, e.g. when the reaction time was 4 h, irregular nanospheres and nanorods were formed of 50–60 nm in diameter (Figure 1.21a), for 8 h some nanobelts were formed (Figure 1.21b) and when the reaction time was

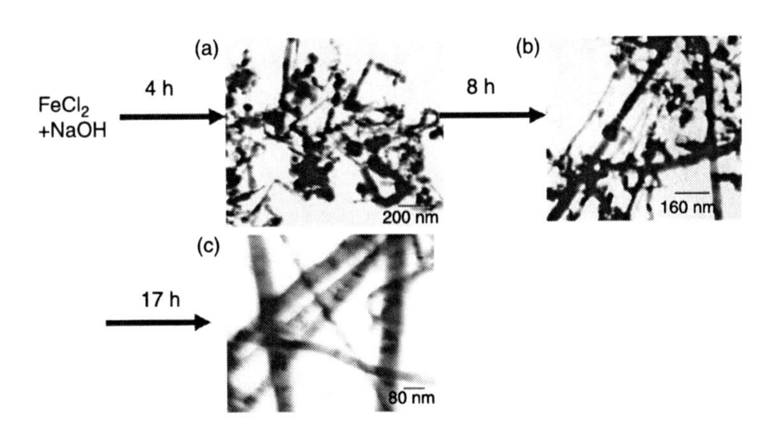

Figure 1.21 TEM images of belt-like Fe_3O_4 synthesized at 180 °C for (a) 4, (b) 8 and (c) 17 h.

Source: Adapted with permission from Li et al. (2009).

Published by Woodhead Publishing Limited, 2013

17h, nanobelts were formed (Figure 1.21c). The M_s of the prepared nanobelt was about 54 e.m.u./g at room temperature (Li et al., 2009).

Microemulsion and reverse microemulsion methods

The microemulsion method is a two-phase method that involves a water-in-oil (w/o) microemulsion consisting of nanosized water droplets trapped within assemblies of surfactant molecules dispersed in an oil phase. The size of the microemulsion droplets can be controlled by changing the water-to-surfactant ratio and the flexibility of the surfactant film (Tavakoli et al., 2007).

Surfactants are molecules that contain a hydrophilic head and long hydrophobic tail. The formation of a micelle occurs when a critical concentration of surfactant molecules is reached. Normal micelles are formed in aqueous medium whereas reverse micelles form in oily medium. When magnetic nanoparticles are synthesized by this method, the iron precursor is dissolved in aqueous solution and then added to the oily reaction mixture that contains surfactant molecules, followed by addition of base and/or inorganic coated molecules. The main drawback of this method is that organic coating is impossible because the monomer will remain in the organic phase outside the micelles.

Water-in-oil microemulsion solutions are transparent, isotropic liquid media containing nanosized water droplets dispersed in an oil phase and stabilized by surfactant molecules at the water/oil interface. These water droplets offer a unique microenvironment for the formation of nanoparticles and prevent agglomeration of the particles. Hollow sphere-like Fe_3O_4 were synthesized in a reverse microemulsion using sodium dodecylbenzene sulfonate as surfactant with diameters between 200 and 400 nm. Formation of the hollow spheres was suggested by this group

Published by Woodhead Publishing Limited, 2013

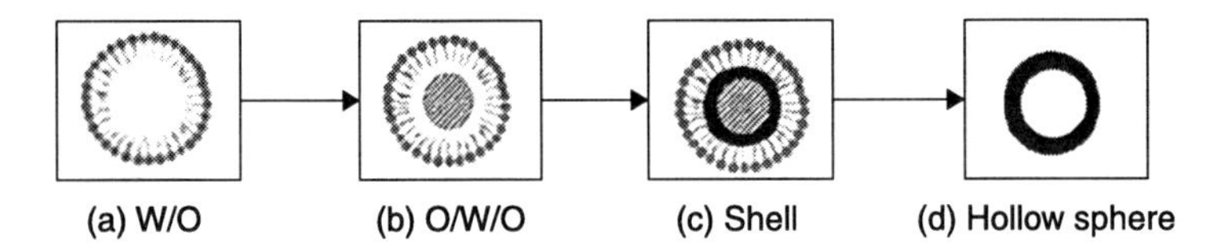

Figure 1.22 Formation mechanism of hollow Fe_3O_4 spheres.

Source: Adapted with permission from Zhang D et al. (2008).

by the mechanism shown in Figure 1.22: first an aqueous droplet is formed in the presence of the surfactant and then an oil droplet is formed inside each aqueous droplet to obtain a stable oil/water/oil structure (o/w/o). Some Fe_3O_4 nanoparticles are formed in the aqueous phase and condensed into solid gel, which consequently forms shells between the outside and the inside of the oil phase through aggregation and assembly of Fe_3O_4 nuclei. Finally, the hollow spheres were obtained after removal of organic oil and surfactant by washing with acetone and water. The obtained hollow particles showed ferromagnetic properties with M_s of 20 e.m.u./g (Zhang D et al., 2008).

Other methods

Gas-phase method

The gas-phase method is a method for preparing nanomaterials that is based on thermal reactions such as decomposition, reduction, oxidation, hydrolysis, etc., to precipitate solid products from the gas phase. An example of this method is CVD, in which a carrier gas stream with precursors is delivered by a gas delivery system to a reaction chamber under vacuum at high temperature (above 1900 °C). The reaction precursors react in the chamber to form nanoparticles that grow and agglomerate via rapid expansion of the two-phase gas stream at the outlet of the reaction

Published by Woodhead Publishing Limited, 2013

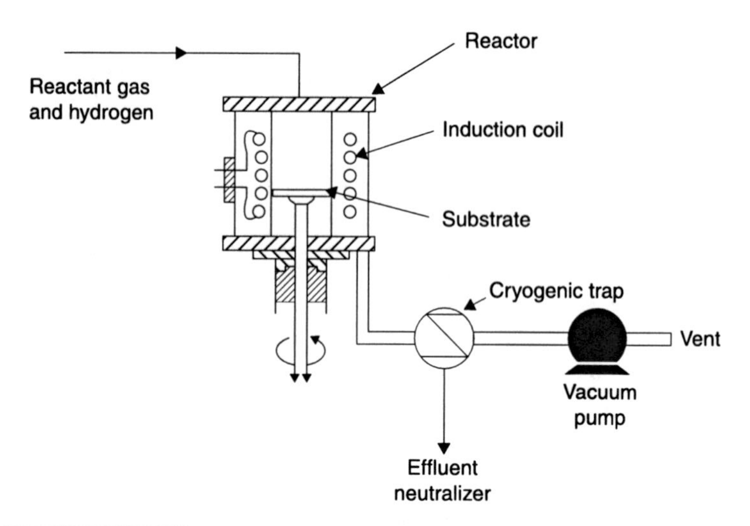

Figure 1.23 Schematic diagram of a CVD apparatus.

Source: Adapted with permission from Tavakoli et al. (2007).

chamber (Figure 1.23). Subsequent heat treatment of the prepared nanoparticles in various high purity gas streams leads to structural modifications, including crystallite size, composition and morphology (Tavakoli et al., 2007).

Chemical vapor condensation

This method is based on heating volatile metal compounds in an inert gas atmosphere that decomposes and eventually forms nanoparticles. Choi et al. (2001) have synthesized magnetic nanoparticles using iron pentacarbonyl with crystallite sizes in the range of 5–13 nm. The disadvantages of this method are that it requires specific equipment, the starting $Fe(CO)_5$ is toxic, and it produces byproducts that are difficult to handle.

Aerosol/vapor methods

This method involves two techniques: spray and laser pyrolysis. These methods are direct and high-yield processes,

Published by Woodhead Publishing Limited, 2013

but the size of the particles produced by spray pyrolysis is larger than those produced by laser pyrolysis. Spray pyrolysis involves spraying a solution into a series of reactors where the aerosol droplets undergo several reactions (evaporation, condensation, drying and thermohydrolysis) to precipitate the nanoparticles at high temperature (Tartaj et al., 2003).

Laser pyrolysis

Laser pyrolysis is based on the interaction between laser photons, a gaseous reactant species and a sensitizer. The sensitizer acts as an energy transfer agent that is excited by absorption of CO_2 laser radiation and transfers the energy to the reactants through collision. Iron pentacarbonyl decomposes into iron and CO_2, which initiate a chemical reaction until a critical concentration of nuclei and homogenous nucleation of particles occurs. The nucleated particles formed are then retrained by the gas stream and are collected at the exit. The particle size can be controlled by changing the oxygen content (Tartaj et al., 2003).

Chen L et al. (2011) have synthesized pure mesoporous Fe_3O_4NPs by direct pyrolysis of ferric nitrate–ethylene glycol gel under atmospheric conditions without any template, additives and carrier gas at 400 °C for 12 h, and a mixture of phases was obtained when the temperature was higher than 500 °C (Figure 1.24). The obtained magnetic nanoparticles showed ferromagnetic properties at room temperature with M_s of 26 e.m.u./g and an average diameter of 6 nm (Chen et al., 2011).

Fe_3O_4 nanoparticles in the range of 4–18 nm in diameter have been synthesized by heating iron oleate in oleic acid. The iron oleate is prepared by ion exchange between Na oleate and Fe tetrachloride hexahydrate (Chiu et al., 2007).

Published by Woodhead Publishing Limited, 2013

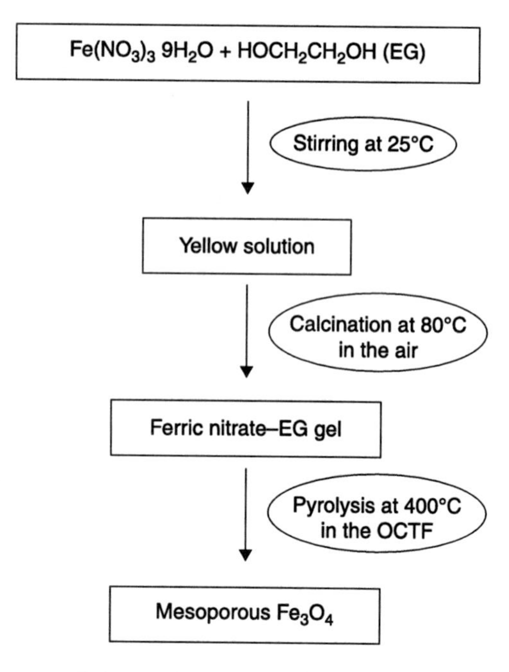

Figure 1.24 **Schematic illustration of the synthesis of mesoporous Fe_3O_4.**

Note: EG is ethylene glycol; OCTF is a one-end closed horizontal tube furnace
Source: Adapted with permission from Chen L et al. (2011).

Sol–gel method

The sol–gel method involves hydrolysis and condensation of metal alkoxides, leading to dispersion of oxide particles in a sol, which is then dried by solvent removal or chemical reaction to form a gel. The most common solvent used in this method is water and the hydrolysis process can be in acidic or basic media. The base catalyst enhances the formation of colloidal gel, whereas the acid catalyst leads to the formation of the polymeric gel. This method offers several advantages over other methods, including good homogeneity, low cost and high purity. The size of the nanoparticles depends on several parameters, such as the rate of hydrolysis and condensation, solution composition, pH, and temperature.

Published by Woodhead Publishing Limited, 2013

Fe_3O_4 nanoparticles were prepared by the gel-to-crystalline method using ferrous chloride under alkaline conditions at 80–100 °C (Figure 1.25). The mechanism for the formation of iron oxide nanoparticles starts by the formation of a metal hydroxide gel; this hydroxide gel forms a network in which the solvent is trapped. For the nanoparticle synthesis, a continuous influx of the solvents breaks the gel network, resulting in the formation of crystalline phase around 100 °C. The average crystallite size of the prepared nanoparticles was 11 nm with saturation magnetization of 390 e.m.u./cm^3 at 300 K (Ozkaya et al., 2009).

Xu et al. (2007) prepared pure Fe_3O_4 nanoparticles by heating $Fe(NO_3)_3$ in ethylene glycol at 40 °C for 2 h. After several drying steps, the gel was annealed under vacuum at 200–400 °C. It was concluded that as the annealing temperature changed, the phase of the magnetic nanoparticles

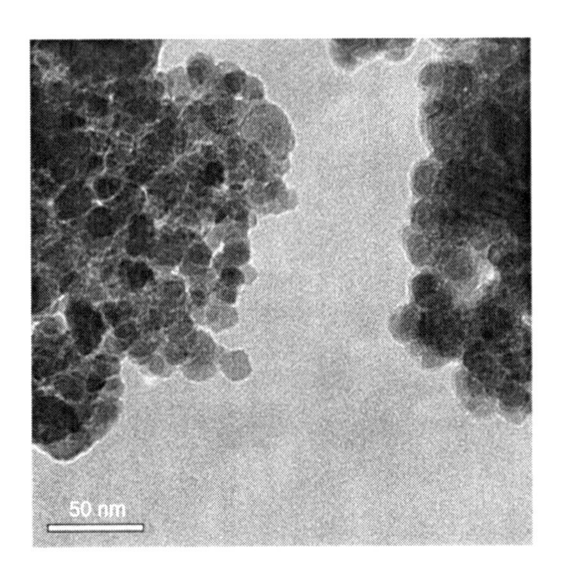

Figure 1.25 TEM image for Fe_3O_4 nanoparticles.

Source: Adapted with permission from Ozkaya et al. (2009).

and the value of M_s changed, e.g. the M_s values of Fe_3O_4 nanoparticles obtained at 200, 250 and 400 °C were 31, 47 and 60 e.m.u./g, respectively (Xu et al., 2007).

Electroprecipitation method

Fe_3O_4 nanoparticles have been prepared by electroprecipitation of $Fe(NO_3)_3.9H_2O$ in ethanol; the magnetite particles were collected on the cathode as black plates and then washed with ethanol followed by drying at room temperature. The mechanism for the formation of Fe_3O_4 nanoparticles by this method was suggested by Rodrigo's group, where iron nitrate is first reduced in water to form hydroxide ion, thus causing an increase in the pH and consequently formation of $Fe(OH)_3$ that is finally reduced to form Fe_3O_4 (Figure 1.26). In this

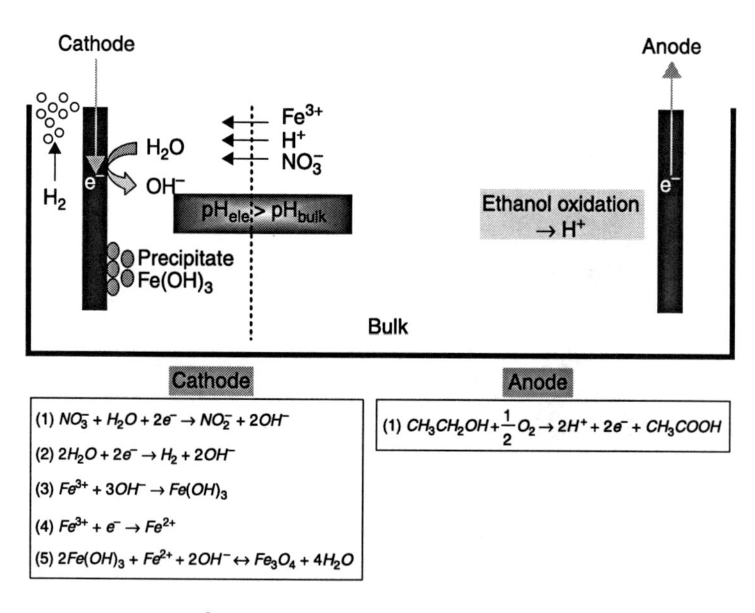

Figure 1.26 General scheme of the magnetite electroprecipitation process.

Source: Adapted with permission from Marques et al. (2008).

method the particle size can be tuned from 4.4 to 9 nm by adjusting the concentration of $Fe(NO_3)_3$ from 0.01 to 0.08 mol/l and adjusting the current density from 5 to 110 mA/cm^2 (Marques et al., 2008).

High-temperature decomposition of organic precursors

In this process, iron precursors are decomposed to yield improved samples with good particle size, good distribution and good crystallinity of the nanoparticles. Wu et al. (2009) have prepared Fe_3O_4 nanoparticles using ferric acetylacetonate $Fe(acac)_3$ and hydrazine under different reaction conditions such as hydrazine concentration, reaction temperature and reaction time. It was found that by increasing the concentration of hydrazine, reaction times and reaction temperature, the purity of Fe_3O_4 increased as well as the crystallinity and the particle size (Wu et al., 2009). The possible formation mechanism of Fe_3O_4 nanoparticles is proposed as shown in Eqs [1.11]–[1.13] (Figure 1.27):

$$N_2H_4 + H_2O \rightarrow N_2H_5^+ + OH^- \quad [1.11]$$

$$Fe(acac)_3 + 2OH^- + 2N_2H_5^+ \rightarrow FeO(OH) + 2N_2H_5acac + Hacac \quad [1.12]$$

$$12\ FeO(OH) + N_2H_4 \rightarrow 4Fe_3O_4 + N_2 + 8H_2O \quad [1.13]$$

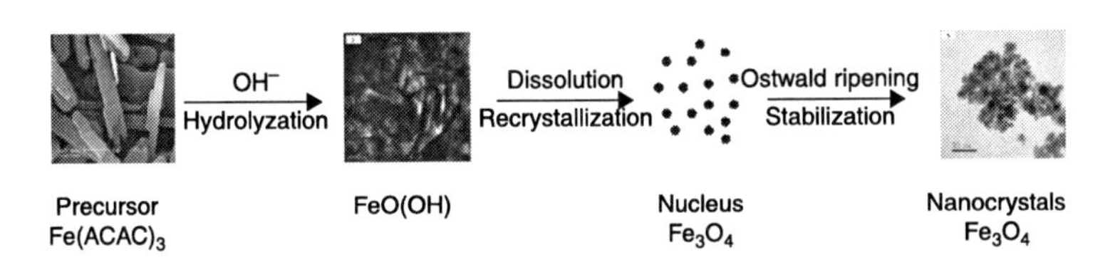

Figure 1.27 Schematic illustration of the transformation process for Fe_3O_4 nanocrystals.

Source: Adapted with permission from Wu et al. (2009).

Published by Woodhead Publishing Limited, 2013

Amara et al. (2009) synthesized magnetite nanoparticles by thermal decomposition of tri-iron dodecacarbonyl ($Fe_3(CO)_{12}$) in diethylene glycol diethylether as a continuous phase and oleic acid as a stabilizer; the particles were then annealed at high temperature (above 300 °C). The shape and size of the nanoparticles depend on the annealing temperature; the magnetic nanoparticles obtained at 300 °C have a spherical shape and crystallite size of 5.4 nm, whereas the particles obtained at 700 and 900 °C aggregate during annealing and the particle size increases with increasing annealing temperature (Figure 1.28). The M_s values at room temperature for the prepared nanoparticles were 41.7, 80 and 187 e.m.u./g for the nanoparticles prepared at 300, 700 and 900 °C, respectively. The high M_s value at 900 °C is due to the formation of Fe at that temperature by reduction of Fe_3O_4 with carbon as shown by Amara et al. (2009):

$$Fe_3O_4 + 2C \rightarrow 3Fe + 2CO_2 \quad [1.14]$$

Asuha et al. (2011) have reported the synthesis of Fe_3O_4 nanopowder via direct thermal decomposition of $[Fe(CON_2H_4)_6](NO_3)_3$. Similarly to Amara et al. (2009), they showed that as the reaction temperature increases, the average crystallite size and the saturation magnetization

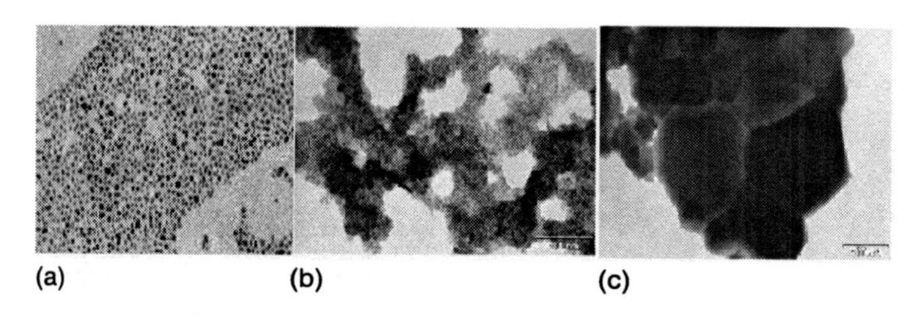

Figure 1.28 TEM micrographs of the nanoparticles produced by annealing at 300 (a), 700 (b) and 900 °C (c).

Source: Adapted with permission from Amara et al. (2009).

of the nanopowder increase. For example, the M_s values were 70.7, 79.4 and 89.1 e.m.u./g for the samples prepared at 200, 250 and 300°C, respectively (Asuha et al., 2011).

Flame synthesis of Fe_3O_4 nanoparticles

Magnetic nanoparticles have been produced by flame synthesis using coflow flame. This method is a simple and a more economical method in comparison to other methods. An iron pentacarbonyl precursor was exposed to high temperature to form iron oxide monomers by gas-phase chemical reaction. The monomers were then polymerized to give homogenous nucleation of 6- to 12-nm particles. The size and morphology of the prepared nanoparticles can be changed by changing the reaction parameters (Buyukhalipoglu and Morss Clyne, 2010).

Strobel and Pratsinis (2009) used the flame spray pyrolysis method (FSP) to prepare Fe_3O_4 nanoparticles from $Fe(CO)_5$ precursors (Figure 1.29). The average crystallite size of the prepared sample was 50 nm with M_s of 73 e.m.u./g.

Carbothermal reduction method

In this method carbon is used as reducing agent. Wang H et al. (2010) and Hu et al. (2011) separately have reacted pure Fe_2O_3 with glucose at high temperature. Glucose is the source of C and CO which reacts with pure Fe_2O_3 to form Fe_3O_4 nanoparticles as illustrated in Eqs [1.15] and [1.16]. The prepared Fe_3O_4 nanoparticles were ferromagnetic with M_s of 97.9 e.m.u./g (Wang H et al., 2010):

$$C + 3Fe_2O_3 \rightarrow 2Fe_3O_4 + CO \quad [1.15]$$

$$CO + 3Fe_2O_3 \rightarrow 2Fe_3O_4 + CO_2 \quad [1.16]$$

Published by Woodhead Publishing Limited, 2013

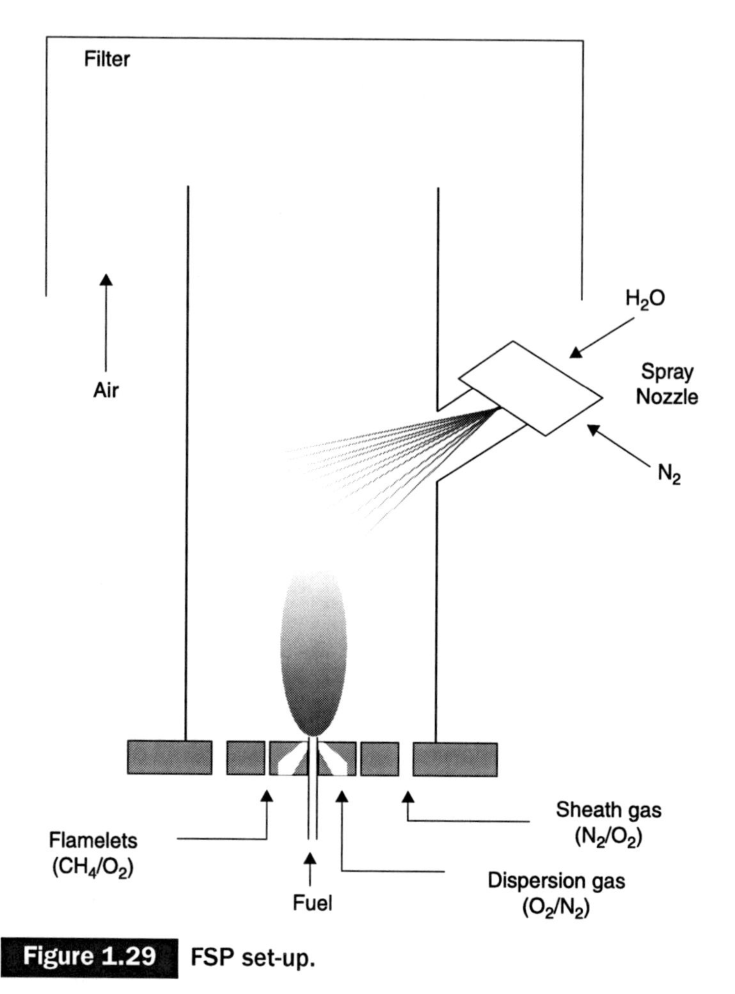

Figure 1.29 FSP set-up.

Source: Adapted with permission from Strobel and Pratsinis (2009).

Green synthesis of Fe_3O_4

Cai et al. (2010) synthesized Fe_3O_4 nanoparticles via soya bean sprouts (SBS) under ambient temperature, atmospheric and basic conditions. The basic idea for this method is that when soya bean sprouts are immersed in Fe^{3+} and Fe^{2+} solutions these ions are trapped on the wall of the SBS by electrostatic interactions where Fe_3O_4 nanoparticles would

Published by Woodhead Publishing Limited, 2013

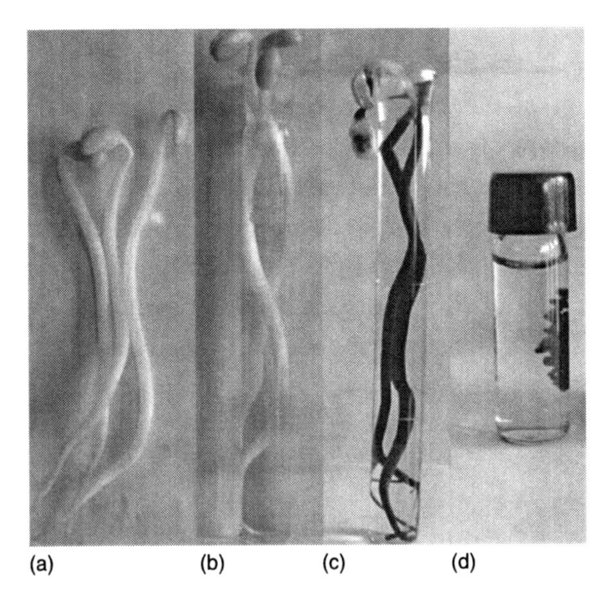

Figure 1.30 Photographs of SBS (a), SBS/Fe^{2+}/Fe^{3+} (b), SBS/Fe_3O_4 (c) and SBS/Fe_3O_4 fragments in a vial under an external magnetic field (d). The solutions are all pure water.

Source: Adapted with permission from Cai et al. (2010).

form via a coprecipitation process under basic conditions (Figure 1.30). The average diameter of the prepared nanoparticles was about 8 nm with saturation magnetization of 37.1 e.m.u./g.

Lu et al. (2011) reported the synthesis of Fe_3O_4 nanoparticles by stirring a mixture of glucose and ferric chloride at 80 °C; this mixture was then added into a solution of ammonia at 60 °C for 30 min. The mechanism for the formation of the particles occurs in two steps:

$$3Fe^{3+} + CH_2OH\text{–}(CHOH)_4\text{–}CHO + 2H_2O \xrightarrow{80C} 2Fe^{2+} + CH_2OH\text{–}(CHOH)_4\text{–}COOH + 2H^+ \quad [1.17]$$

Published by Woodhead Publishing Limited, 2013

$$Fe^{2+} + 2Fe^{3+} + 8OH^{-} \rightarrow Fe_3O_4 + 4H_2O \qquad [1.18]$$

Hai et al. (2010) have reported the synthesis of Fe_3O_4 nanoparticles from the corresponding α-Fe_2O_3 nanoparticles by reduction in trioctylamine (TOA) under high temperature. During the reaction large amounts of CO and CO_2 gases were released from the incomplete or complete combustion of organic substances in the reactor. The saturation magnetization of the nanoparticles was about 118 e.m.u./g Fe and the average particle size was about 15 nm (Hai et al., 2010).

Coating of magnetic nanoparticles

Magnetic nanoparticles, in particular iron oxide, exhibit unique physical, chemical, and magnetic properties, and therefore offer high potential for several biomedical applications such as cellular therapy (Cho et al., 2010), drug delivery (Lee et al., 2010), cancer treatment (Lv et al., 2008), etc. The aqueous dispersions of unprotected iron oxide nanoparticles are stable only in highly acidic or basic conditions. Therefore, surface protection and modification are essential for enhancing the stability and dispersibility of these particles in aqueous or organic solutions and increasing the biocompatibility of these nanoparticles. In addition, the protected layer can be attached by various bioactive molecules and thus promote the application of these nanoparticles for specific biomedical targets.

Coating methods

Several methods for the production of superparamagnetic composites have been reported, such as the deposition method and encapsulation of magnetic nanoparticles in polymeric or inorganic matrixes (Ulman, 1996). The surfaces of iron oxide nanoparticles can be modified through the creation of a few layers of organic polymer or inorganic metallic or oxide surfaces (e.g. silica (SiO_2) or titania (TiO_2)). Inorganic metallic SiO_2 is extensively used for the following reasons: (i) it is chemically inert, (ii) it is transparent and thus the chemical reaction can be monitored spectroscopically, (iii) it prevents coagulation of the magnetic particles during the chemical reaction, and (iv) it makes the surface enriched with silanol groups that can easily react with alcohols and silane coupling agents (Ulman, 1996). Many examples have been reported in the literature illustrating coating iron oxide nanoparticles with silica or other polymeric or bioactive molecules; some examples are given below.

Fe_3O_4/SiO_2 core–shell nanoparticles have been prepared by several methods, such as the sol–gel technique (Kim et al., 2005) and hydrothermal hydrolysis (Zhang E et al., 2008). In the sol–gel method, the coating thickness was about 4–5 nm. The latter method is the most common because it is a simple, easy controlled method and the synthesized γ-Fe_2O_3/SiO_2 nanoparticles are highly stable with good magnetic properties, whereas the former method requires complicated apparatus, complex procedures and special conditions. The average diameter of γ-Fe_2O_3/SiO_2 core–shell nanoparticles prepared by the hydrothermal method was about 30 nm. It was found that at 150 °C the particles obtained have a wide size distribution and the particles were aggregated; by increasing the temperature to 200 °C, uniform roundish nanoparticles were formed.

The thermal hydrolysis method involves a two-step mechanism: hydrolysis and condensation of silica alkoxide (tetraethylorthosilica (TEOS)) in an ethanol/ammonia mixture as illustrated in Eqs [1.19] and [1.20] (Lu et al., 2008). The formation mechanism of silica-coated nanoparticles is illustrated in Figure 1.31, where hydrolysis of TEOS leads to the formation of supersaturated silicic acid

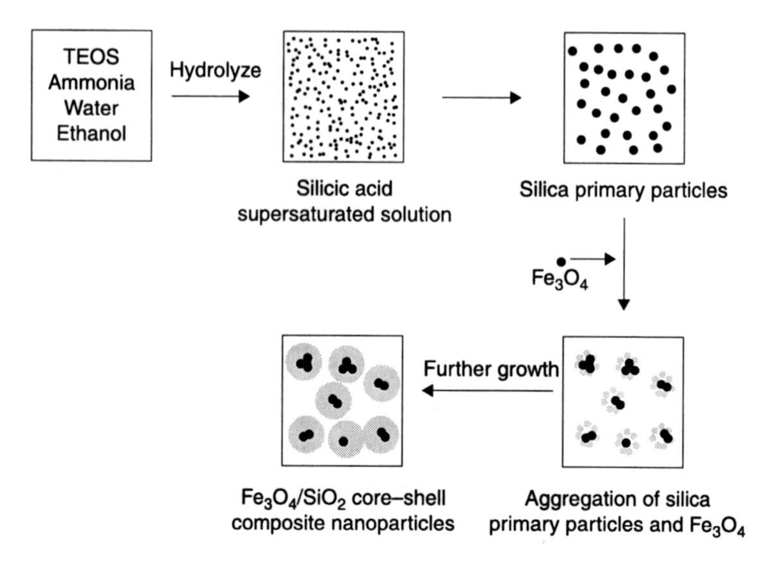

Figure 1.31 Schematic illustration of the mechanism of silica particle nucleation by aggregation of primary silica particles and synthetic process of Fe_3O_4/SiO_2 core–shell nanoparticles.

Source: Adapted with permission from Lu et al. (2008).

solution, which then condenses to small silica primary particles with a diameter of 5 nm. When Fe_3O_4 nanoparticles are added into the reaction solution, Fe_3O_4 nanoparticles aggregate with the silica particles to form Fe_3O_4/SiO_2 core–shell nanoparticles. It has been suggested that the magnetic particles should be added at an appropriate time during the hydrolysis and condensation of TEOS because the formed primary particles are essential to decrease the dipole–dipole interaction among the Fe_3O_4 nanoparticles, thus allowing the formation of Fe_3O_4/SiO_2 nanoparticles with a defined structure (Lu et al., 2008).

$$-\overset{|}{\underset{|}{Si}}-OR + H_2O \longrightarrow -\overset{|}{\underset{|}{Si}}-O^- + ROH + NH_4^+ \quad [1.19]$$

$$-\overset{|}{\underset{|}{Si}}-O^- + -\overset{|}{\underset{|}{Si}}-OR + NH_4^+ \rightarrow -\overset{|}{\underset{|}{Si}}-O-\overset{|}{\underset{|}{Si}}- - ROH + NH_4^+ \quad [1.20]$$

Wang et al. (2008) prepared α-Fe_2O_3/SiO_2 composites via hydrothermal hydrolysis of a mixture of $FeCl_3$ and PEG. The prepared nanoparticles were spherical with a diameter of about 50 nm. The thickness of the SiO_2 shell can be controlled by adjusting the concentration of TEOS. α-Fe_2O_3/SiO_2 composites can be transferred to Fe/SiO_2 composites by thermal reduction in H_2 gas. The prepared nanoparticles displayed weak ferromagnetism, whereas the reduced Fe/SiO_2 nanoparticles displayed a saturation magnetization of 32.7 e.m.u./g (Wang et al., 2008).

Nanoparticles have been coated with organic dyes or fluorophores as optical imaging agents and thus can be used in biomedical applications. However, recently lanthanide chelates are more favorable because, in comparison with organic dyes and quantum dots, they have sharp absorption, long lifetimes and high photostability. Zhiya's group synthesized multifunctional magnetic fluorescent nanoparticles consisting of a Fe_3O_4 core and a silica shell doped with terbium (Tb^{3+}) chelate (Figure 1.32). Fe_3O_4 nanoparticles were first prepared by a coprecipitation method of $FeCl_2$ and $FeCl_3$ precursors in citric acid under alkaline, thermal (80 °C) and inert conditions followed by coating with SiO_2 by using TEOS and a silane precursor containing an organic chromophore *p*-aminobenzoic acid (PABA) and a chelate (diethylenetriaminopentaacetic acid (DTPA)). The average crystallite size of the as-prepared nanoparticles was about 7 nm and increased to 52 nm after coating with silica. The modified Fe_3O_4 nanoparticles showed superparamagnetic properties with saturation magnetization of about 4.4 e.m.u./g (Ma et al., 2009).

Published by Woodhead Publishing Limited, 2013

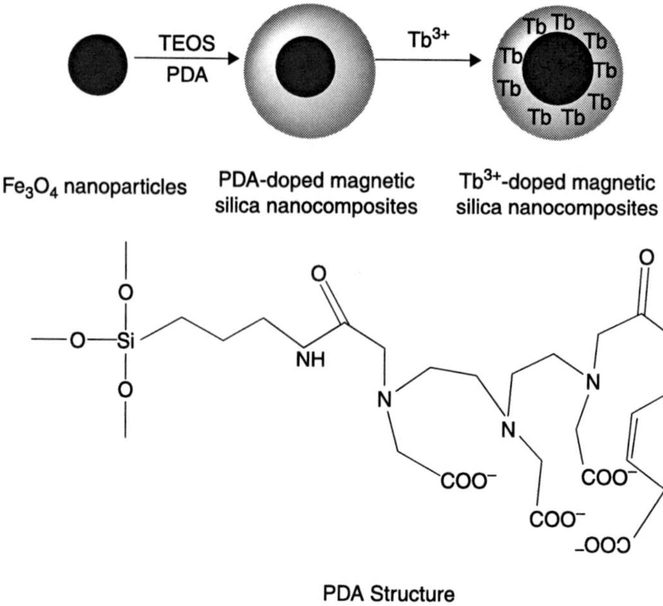

TEOS PDA Tb3+

Fe3O4 nanoparticles PDA-doped magnetic silica nanocomposites Tb3+-doped magnetic silica nanocomposites

PDA Structure

Figure 1.32 **Synthetic scheme for the multifunctional magnetic silica nanocomposites and the chemical structure of PDA silane.**

Source: Adapted with permission from Ma et al. (2009).

Chen T et al. (2011) reported the synthesis of organic/inorganic PNIPAm/Fe_3O_4 microgels (NIPAm = *N*-isopropylacrylamide as monomer). The PNIPAm were covalently cross-linked with surface-functionalized Fe_3O_4 nanoparticles. The cross-linked mechanism involves radical cross-linking polymerization of multiple C–C double bonds grafted on the surface of Fe_3O_4 nanoparticles, and the formation of covalent bonds between Fe_3O_4 nanoparticles and network chains. The average size of the as-prepared Fe_3O_4 nanoparticles was 13 ± 2 nm, whereas that for 3-(trimethyoxysilyl)propylmethacrylate (TMSPMA)/Fe_3O_4 nanoparticles was about 333 ± 11 nm in water and 162 ±

Published by Woodhead Publishing Limited, 2013

2 nm in acetone. This observation can be attributed to the fact that the TMSPMA layer inhibits the strong electrostatic interaction between Fe_3O_4 nanoparticles and thus prevents aggregation (Figure 1.33) (Chen et al., 2011).

Xu et al. (2009) reported the synthesis of α-Fe_2O_3/SiO_2 nanoparticles by the sol–gel method using three different raw iron materials, ferric citrate, ferric nitrate and ferric chloride, in TEOS and acidic media. When the amount of TEOS decreased the nanoparticles obtained were bigger in size with fine crystalline size and high saturation magnetization values (Figure 1.34).

Wong et al. (2007) reported the *in situ* synthesis of magnetic nanoparticles deposited as a shell onto a polymer (PNiPAM) core using the layer-by-layer (LbL) technique. The surface of

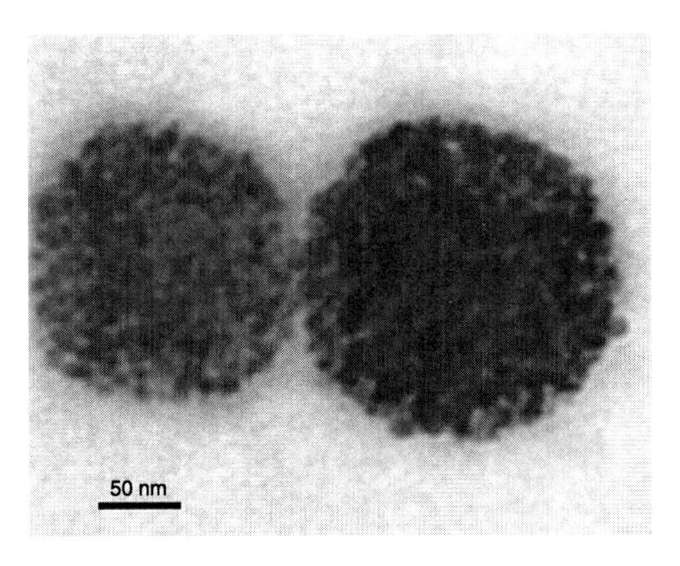

Figure 1.33 Typical TEM images of the PNIPAm/Fe_3O_4 hybrid microgels cross-linked with TMSPMA-modified Fe_3O_4 nanoparticles.

Source: Adapted with permission from Chen T et al. (2011).

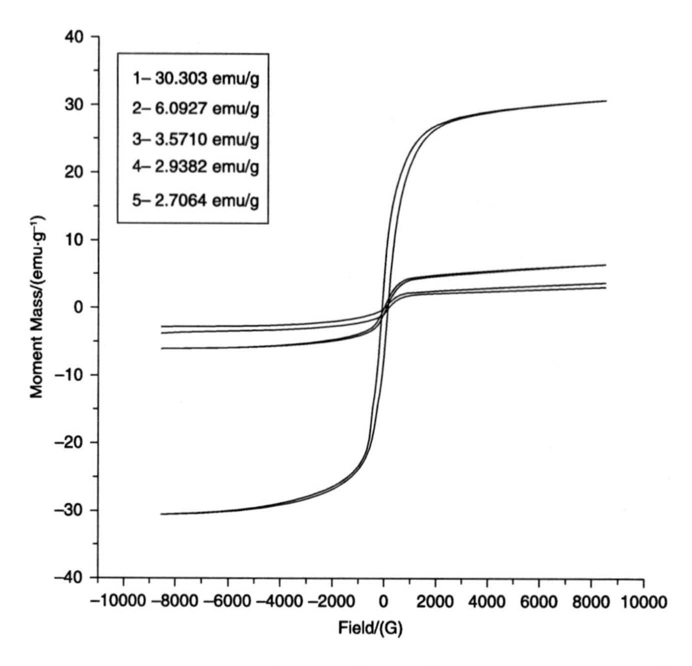

Figure 1.34 **Magnetization loop of precipitates with different amount of TEOS using ferric citrate as raw material. TEOS: 1, 2, 3, 4 and 5 ml.**

Source: Adapted with permission from Xu et al. (2009).

the PNiPAM polymer was modified with a polyelectrolyte shell to facilitate the deposition of the magnetic nanoparticles. Magnetic nanoparticles carrying a negative charge can be achieved by enclosing the magnetic nanoparticles in a negatively charged polymer such as polyacrylic acid (PAA). The synthesis started by the *in situ* preparation of PAA-modified Fe_3O_4 nanoparticles, in which an aqueous solution of a mixture of Fe^{3+} and Fe^{2+} was added to a mixture of PAA and NH_3 solution under inert conditions and ultrasonic radiation to obtain PAA magnetic nanoparticles with M_s of 45 e.m.u./g.

The PNiPAM core was synthesized via free radical emulsion polymerization and then the surface of the microgel was

Published by Woodhead Publishing Limited, 2013

modified by depositing one layer of positively charged polymer such as poly(diallyldimethylammonium chloride) (PDADMAC) to eventually form PDADMAC/PNiPAM microgels. Finally, the negatively charged PAA magnetic nanoparticles were deposited on the surface of the PDADMAC/PNiPAM microgels to form PNiPAM/PDADMAC/(PAA magnetic nanoparticles) with a hydrodynamic radius around 340 nm at 25 °C (Wong et al., 2007).

Magnetic nanoparticles have been applied to proteomics research. Matrix-assisted laser desorption/ionization time-of-flight mass spectroscopy (MALDI-ToF-MS) is a commonly used tool for peptide mapping and analysis. However, this tool is insufficient for the detection of low-concentration peptides or proteins because the MS signals of the trace peptides suffer strong interference from those of highly abundant proteins and contaminations present in the sample. Recently, magnetic nanomaterials have often been used as affinity probes for those peptides as their strong magnetic properties facilitate the identification of the nanomaterial target peptide/protein complexes from the sample solution. Chen H et al. (2010) reported the synthesis of $Fe_3O_4/SiO_2/$poly(methyl methacrylate) (PMMA) composite. The TEM analysis of the obtained composites showed spherical nanoparticles with an average diameter of 170 nm; each individual particle was coated with a uniform layer of SiO_2 shell with a thickness of about 35 nm and the thickness of the PMMA shell was about 20 nm. The saturation magnetization values were 49.5 and 36.7 e.m.u./g for Fe_3O_4/SiO_2 and Fe_3O_4/SiO_2/PMMA microspheres, respectively (Chen H et al., 2010).

Fe_3O_4/cysteine composites were prepared by the decomposition of iron pentacarbonyl ($Fe(CO)_6$) and cysteine under ultrasonic radiation. The average particle size of the nanoparticles increases as the concentration of the cysteine

Published by Woodhead Publishing Limited, 2013

increases. This can be attributed to the fact that excess cysteine creates sulfide bridges between two molecules of cysteine. The average crystallite size of the prepared Fe_3O_4 nanoparticles was about 30 nm and the thickness of the cysteine layer was about 10 nm. The saturation magnetization of the Fe_3O_4 nanoparticles was about 23 e.m.u./g and that for cysteine-capped Fe_3O_4 nanoparticles was about 10 e.m.u./g (Cohen et al., 2008).

Wang et al. (2006) reported the synthesis of Fe_3O_4/C nanocomposites by encapsulating Fe_3O_4 nanoparticles in carbon using a hydrothermal reaction. Glucose was used as a carbon source and to prevent oxidation of the Fe_3O_4 nanoparticles to Fe_2O_3. The average diameters of the prepared nanocomposites were in the range of 100–200 nm and the thickness of the light carbon shell was about 10 nm. The saturation magnetization values for the Fe_3O_4 nanoparticles and Fe_3O_4/C were 31.4 and 12.4 e.m.u./g, respectively.

Rashdan et al. (2010a) prepared SiO_2-coated Fe_3O_4 nanoparticles via a hydrothermal hydrolysis method by reacting Fe_3O_4 in a mixture of TEOS, ammonia and alcohol under ultrasonic radiation. The crystallite size of the Fe_3O_4 powder increased from 65 nm before coating to 85 nm after coating. In addition, the saturation magnetization values of uncoated Fe_3O_4 nanoparticles and Fe_3O_4/SiO_2 nanoparticles were about 75 and 60 e.m.u./g, respectively (Figure 1.35). This decrease in the saturation magnetization values can be attributed to the presence of non-magnetic SiO_2 molecules on the surface of the Fe_3O_4 nanoparticles (Rashdan et al., 2010a).

Magnetic nanoparticles that are coated with metals such as Co, Ni and Fe offer high magnetization values and maintain their superparamagnetism properties at larger particle size. Qiang et al. (2006) reported the synthesis of

Published by Woodhead Publishing Limited, 2013

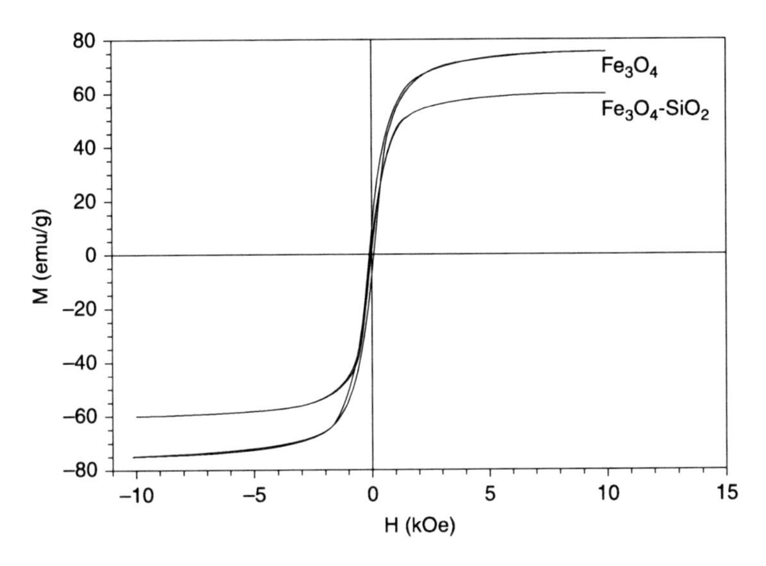

Figure 1.35 Hysteresis loop measurements of Fe_3O_4 before and after coating with SiO_2.

Source: Adapted with permission from Rashdan et al. (2010a).

Fe/Fe_3O_4 nanoparticles using a nanocluster deposition method, which gave Fe/Fe_3O_4 nanoparticles with a crystallite size less than 10 nm with a M_s of 80 e.m.u./g Fe.

Fe_3O_4 nanoparticles coated with ascorbic acid ($C_6H_6O_6$) were prepared by Xuan et al. (2007); the core nanoparticles were prepared via hydrothermal decomposition of ferric chloride in $NaNO_3$ aqueous solution and ascorbic acid. The average crystallite size of the as-prepared Fe_3O_4 nanoparticles was about 5.2 nm with a saturation magnetization of 5.2 e.m.u./g. This small value of M_s can be attributed to the small size of the Fe_3O_4 nanoparticles and the presence of $C_6H_6O_6$ on the surface of these particles (Xuan et al., 2007).

Wang et al. (2011) reported the synthesis of a magnetic hollow nanostructure composed of polystyrene (PS)/Fe_3O_4/SiO_2 nanocomposites. Fe_3O_4/SiO_2 nanoparticles were

Published by Woodhead Publishing Limited, 2013

prepared by conventional hydrothermal hydrolysis followed by mixing the positively charged PS molecules that are attracted to the negatively charged Fe_3O_4/SiO_2 nanoparticles through electrostatic interaction (Figure 1.36). Then these composites undergo calcination steps where magnetic hollow nanostructures with large cavities are obtained. Magnetic hollow nanoparticles are important in applications in drug loading and targeted drug delivery. Fe_3O_4 nanoparticles are spherical in shape with a particle size of 10–15 nm and the size of the PS nanosphere was about 200 nm. The average diameter and the shell thickness of

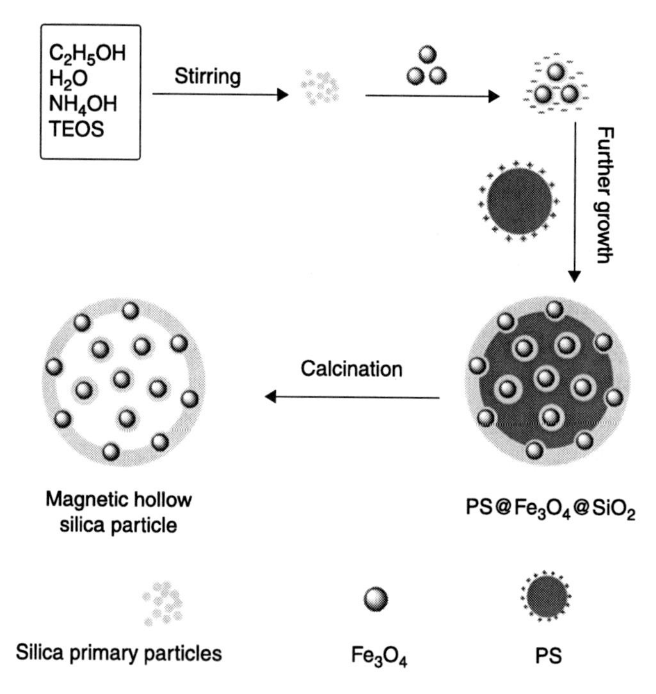

Figure 1.36 **Schematic showing the synthesis of raspberry-like magnetic hollow silica nanospheres.**

Source: Adapted with permission from Wang et al. (2011).

Published by Woodhead Publishing Limited, 2013

the obtained PS/Fe_3O_4/SiO_2 nanocomposites were 253 and 26 nm, respectively, with M_s of 7.84 e.m.u./g (Wang et al., 2011).

Fe_3O_4/C composite nanoparticles were synthesized using microwave energy and PS as a source of carbon. Microwave energy produces plasma with high heat to crack the organic polymer (PS) into atomic carbon that is absorbed by the magnetic nanoparticles to form graphitic nanoparticles (Hojati-Talemi et al., 2010).

Dumitrache et al. (2011) have also studied the synthesis of Fe/C core–shell nanoparticles via CO_2 laser pyrolysis starting with $Fe(CO)_5$ as the Fe precursor and C_2H_4 as the C source. Fe/C nanoparticles have been applied in the environment because the carbon shell protects Fe (zero-valence) from oxidation with atmospheric oxygen and helps to preserve the magnetic properties of Fe. The average crystallite size of the prepared samples increased with decreased C_2H_4 content and the saturation magnetization values increased when the iron concentration increased, e.g. when the Fe content was 39.4% the M_s was about 76.8 e.m.u./g, whereas it was 37.2 e.m.u./g for 10% Fe (Dumitrache et al., 2011).

Wang X et al. (2010) have reported the synthesis of Fe_3O_4/C composites via the solvothermal method at 500 °C using ferrocene ($Fe(C_5H_5)_2$) and carbon nanotubes (CNTs) as starting reagents in benzene. The obtained nanocomposites had a diameter in the range of 10–25 nm with a narrow size distribution and showed ferromagnetic behavior with saturation magnetization of 32.5 e.m.u./g.

Yu et al. (2011) prepared Fe_3O_4/SiO_2/TiO_2 (FST) composites where Fe_3O_4 nanoparticles were first prepared by a solvothermal synthesis of ferric chloride in PEG 2000, and then the particles were coated with layers of SiO_2 and TiO_2 (Figure 1.37). The saturation magnetization M_s of the FST nanocomposites was about 42.4 e.m.u./g.

Published by Woodhead Publishing Limited, 2013

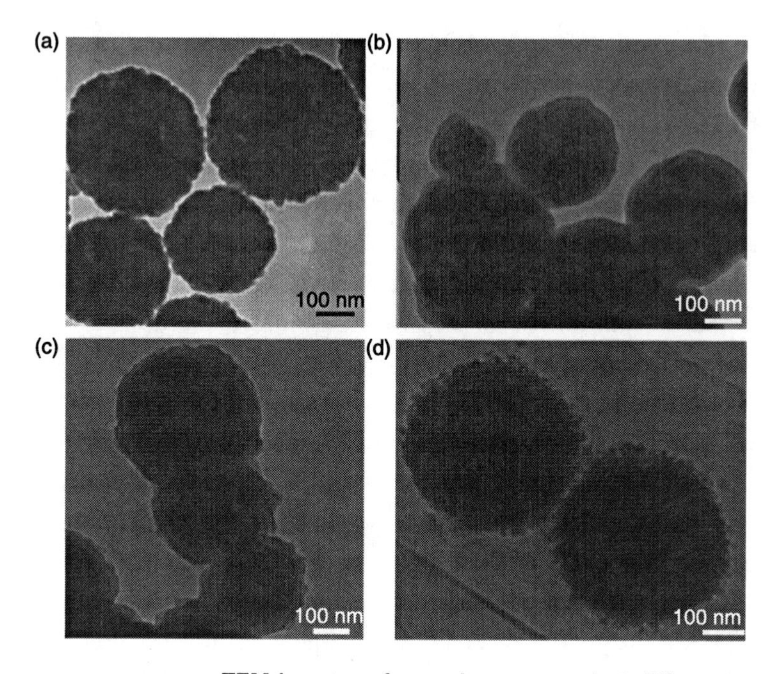

Figure 1.37 TEM images of samples prepared at different conditions: (a) Fe_3O_4 cores, (b) FS (Fe_3O_4/SiO_2), (c) FST ($Fe_3O_4/SiO_2/TiO_2$) and (d) FT (Fe_3O_4/TiO_2).

Source: Adapted with permission from Yu et al. (2011).

Chen L et al. (2010) synthesized Fe_3O_4/SiO_2 magnetic nanoparticles by dropping TEOS solution into a freshly prepared Fe_3O_4 nanoparticle solution (Figure 1.38). The prepared sample had a saturation magnetization of 68.6 e.m.u./g.

Zhang L-Y et al. (2010) prepared Fe_3O_4/chitosan nanoparticles in aqueous system via UV light irradiation. The reaction device is shown in Figure 1.39, where chitosan and Fe_3O_4 nanoparticles were mixed at pH 5.5, and then *N*,*N*-methylene-bis-acrylamide (MBA) and H_2O_2 were added, and the mixture irradiated with two 8-W UV lamps for 20 min. The mechanism for the formation of Fe_3O_4 is shown in Eqs [1.21]–[1.26]: Fe_3O_4 absorbs photons during

Published by Woodhead Publishing Limited, 2013

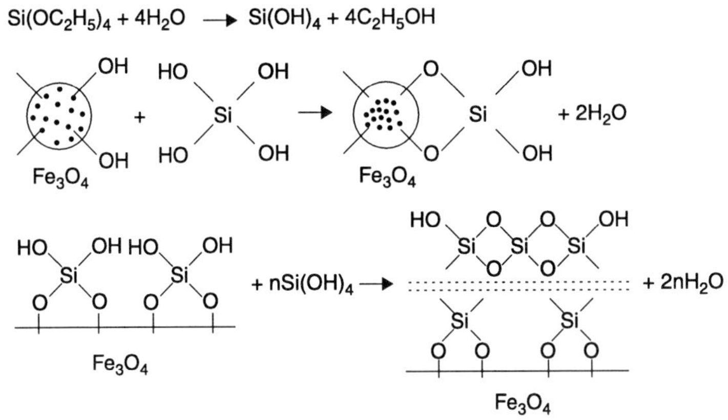

$$Si(OC_2H_5)_4 + 4H_2O \rightarrow Si(OH)_4 + 4C_2H_5OH$$

Figure 1.38 Formation mechanism of Fe_3O_4/SiO_2.

Source: Adapted with permission from Chen L et al. (2010).

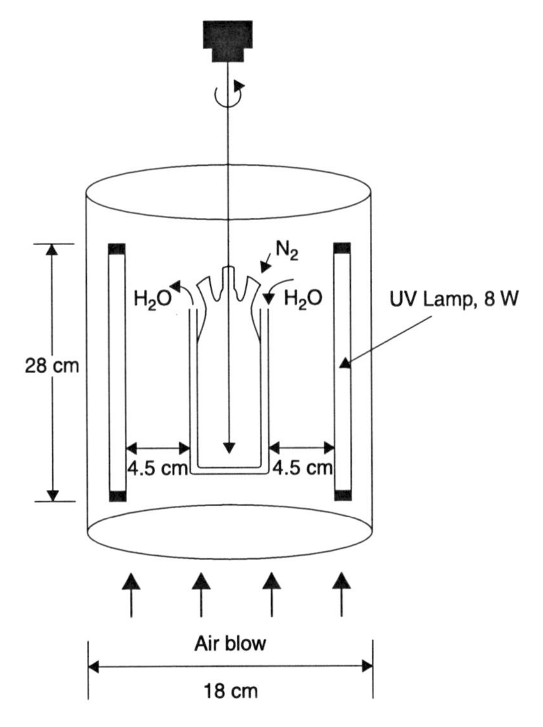

Figure 1.39 Schematic illustration of the photochemical reaction device.

Source: Adapted with permission from Zhang L-Y et al. (2010).

Published by Woodhead Publishing Limited, 2013

the photochemical process (Eq. [1.21]), and then chitosan molecules on the surface of Fe_3O_4/chitosan complex capture electrons and initiate the formation of chitosan free radicals (Eq. [1.22]). Fe_3O_4/chitosan free radicals can be initiated by other radicals such as $OH^{\cdot}$ or directly by UV light (Eqs [1.23] and [1.24]). Finally, chitosan chains were formed from the Fe_3O_4 nanoparticles via recombination of the chitosan free radicals and chitosan molecules might form a cross-linked structure on the Fe_3O_4 nanoparticle surface (Eq. [1.26]). The average diameters of uncoated Fe_3O_4 and Fe_3O_4/chitosan were 41 and 64 nm, respectively. The saturation magnetization (M_s) of the Fe_3O_4/chitosan nanoparticles was about 48.6 e.m.u./g, while that of the bare Fe_3O_4 nanoparticles was about 69.8 e.m.u./g (Zhang L-Y et al., 2010):

$$Fe_3O_4 \xrightarrow{hv} h^+_{VB} + e^- \qquad [1.21]$$

$$h^+_{VB} + Fe_3O_4/\text{chitosan} \rightarrow Fe_3O_4/\text{chitosan}^{\cdot} \qquad [1.22]$$

$$H_2O_2 \xrightarrow{hv} 2OH^{\cdot} \qquad [1.23]$$

$$OH^{\cdot} + Fe_3O_4/\text{chitosan} \rightarrow Fe_3O_4/\text{chitosan}^{\cdot} \qquad [1.24]$$

$$Fe_3O_4/\text{chitosan} \xrightarrow{hv} Fe_3O_4/\text{chitosan}^{\cdot} \qquad [1.25]$$

$$Fe_3O_4/\text{chitosan}^{\cdot} \rightarrow \text{MBA } Fe_3O_4/(\text{chitosan})_n \qquad [1.26]$$

C/Fe_3O_4 nanofibers were prepared by pyrolysis of ferrocene in supercritical CO_2 at 400 °C. CO_2 molecules react with ferrocene by substituting the cyclopentadienyl group and oxidizing Fe^{2+}, and producing amorphous carbon and hydrocarbons as shown in Eq. [1.27]. The diameter of the prepared nanofibers was 100 nm and that for the core iron was about 40 nm. The C/Fe_3O_4 exhibited ferromagnetic behavior with M_s of 27.5 e.m.u./g (Cao et al., 2007).

$$FeCp_2 + CO_2 \xrightarrow{400\,^{\circ}C} Fe_3O_4 + \text{a-C} + C_nH_m \qquad [1.27]$$

Published by Woodhead Publishing Limited, 2013

Iron oxide properties for biomedical application

Magnetic nanoparticles are perfect candidates for biomedical applications due to their high level of accumulation in target tissues, low toxicity and biophysical nature. For *in vivo* applications the magnetic particles must be coated with a biocompatible polymer during or after the synthesis process to prevent the formation of large aggregates and allow binding of drugs by covalent attachment or absorption on the particles. The small size (below 100 nm) of these particles is important in these kinds of applications due to the higher surface areas, low sedimentation rates and improved tissular diffusion. When magnetic nanoparticles are ferromagnetic/ superparamagnetic they can be manipulated by an external magnetic field and thus can be delivered to the targeted organs, where the attached biomolecules bound to the surface of these magnetic nanoparticles can be released.

Most applications of magnetic nanoparticles are based on: (i) controlling the magnetic field to position the magnetic nanoparticles in targeted organs or tissues, (ii) utilization of the magnetic moment of the magnetic nanoparticles as a disturbance of proton nuclear resonance, and (iii) loss of the magnetism of magnetic nanoparticles in colloids for heating. Applications of magnetic nanoparticles in biomedical areas require the use of a colloidal ferrofluid or magnetic colloids. The stability of any magnetic colloid depends on the balance between attractive (van der Waals and dipole–dipole) and repulsive (steric and electrostatic) forces between the particles and the supporting liquid. Therefore, to stabilize the suspended magnetic nanoparticles against these forces they are often coated with a shell of an appropriate material or surfactant such as oleic acid or alkylsilanes.

For *in vivo* applications the stability of the magnetic colloid must be granted in order to avoid embolism from agglomerates

Published by Woodhead Publishing Limited, 2013

within arteries, and thus in these cases biocompatibility is an additional requirement for the surfactant. Examples of such surfactants are dextran, PEG, citric acid, peptides and proteins. One of the challenges for applying nanoparticles in the human body is to extend the blood circulation time to allow these particles to accumulate in target tissues. The size, morphology, charge and surface chemistry of the nanoparticles determine their fate *in vivo* (Trehin et al., 2006).

For magnetic nanoparticles to be applied in biomedicine and drug delivery, the biomolecules may not bind to the magnetic nanoparticles without surface modification because the interaction between biomolecules and the magnetic nanoparticles is very weak. Therefore modification through organic linkers is commonly used, in particular those linkers that create an electrostatic interaction. For example, for magnetic nanoparticles to be applied in gene delivery, the particles must have a positive charge to bind negatively charged DNA molecules, whereas for drug delivery the positively charged magnetic nanoparticles will bind drug molecules that carry negative charge through carboxylic acid groups. When the drug/magnetic nanoparticle complex reaches the target organs, the drug molecules will be released in the presence of anions such as chloride or phosphate (McBain et al., 2008).

Petri-Fink et al. (2005) synthesized polyvinyl polymer (PVP)-coated Fe_3O_4 and its functionalized derivatives to test their interaction with human cancer cells. Four samples were prepared: Fe_3O_4/PVP, Fe_3O_4 (amino)/PVP, Fe_3O_4 (carboxy)/PVP and Fe_3O_4 (thiol)/PVP. The uncoated Fe_3O_4 nanoparticles were prepared by coprecipitation of ferric and ferrous chloride in ammonia, and had an average particle size of about 9 nm. The functionalized magnetic nanoparticles were obtained by mixing the bare Fe_3O_4 nanoparticles with different PVP molecules in acidic media. Prussian blue reaction was used to determine the ability of these PVP-functionalized nanoparticles to interact with human cells; none of the functionalized nanoparticles showed cytotoxicity except at high polymer concentration, and the human cells interacted with amino-PVP/Fe_3O_4 nanoparticles (Petri-Fink et al., 2005).

The modification of the nanoparticles' surface has a critical role in the blood half-life of particles such that positively charged particles do not specifically stick to cells. Papisov et al. have shown that the circulation times for cationic poly-L-lysine-coated magnetic nanoparticles were only 1–2 min compared with 2–3 h for bare particles. The negatively charged particles led to an increase in liver uptake. Therefore, it can be concluded that nanoparticle with neutral surface charge exhibit extended blood circulation times (Papisov et al., 1993; Chouly et al., 1996).

Dilnawaz et al. (2010) have used glyceryl monooleate (GMO) as a surfactant due to its bioadhesiveness and high viscosity, which increases the contact time at targeted tissues and thus provides sustained release of drug by slow diffusion. The best GMO/magnetic nanoparticle samples were prepared by stirring a mixture of Fe_3O_4 nanoparticles and GMO in basic conditions. The best GMO/magnetic nanoparticles obtained had a particle diameter around 144 nm, whereas the diameter of the bare magnetic nanoparticles was about 6–11 nm. For biocompatibility tests, the addition of GMO/magnetic nanoparticles to the tested cells resulted in rapid adsorption of the coated nanoparticles to the cell surfaces and during 48 h no growth inhibition was observed. In a separate test, changing the concentration of void nanoparticles showed no cytotoxicity. To test the ability of these nanoparticles to release the drug to the affected tissues the GMO/magnetic nanoparticles were

Published by Woodhead Publishing Limited, 2013

loaded with hydrophobic anticancer drugs such as paclitaxel and rapamycin, and the release study was carried out by estimating the amount of drug released from the nanoparticles under *in vitro* conditions. This experiment showed sustained release of drug up to more than 2 weeks, and this form of release is an essential requirement for cancer therapy (Dilnawaz et al., 2010).

Peng et al. (2011) functionalized Fe_3O_4/SiO_2 nanoparticles with a rhodamine-based fluorescent chemosensor for the detection of heavy metals such as Hg^{2+} in which *N*-(rhodamine-6G) lactam-ethylenediamine (Rho-en) is conjugated with the magnetic core–shell Fe_3O_4/SiO_2 nanoparticles. The preparation steps of Rho-Si molecules and attachment of these molecules to Fe_3O_4/SiO_2 nanoparticles are shown in Figure 1.40. The average particle size of the final product was about 50–60 nm with a diameter

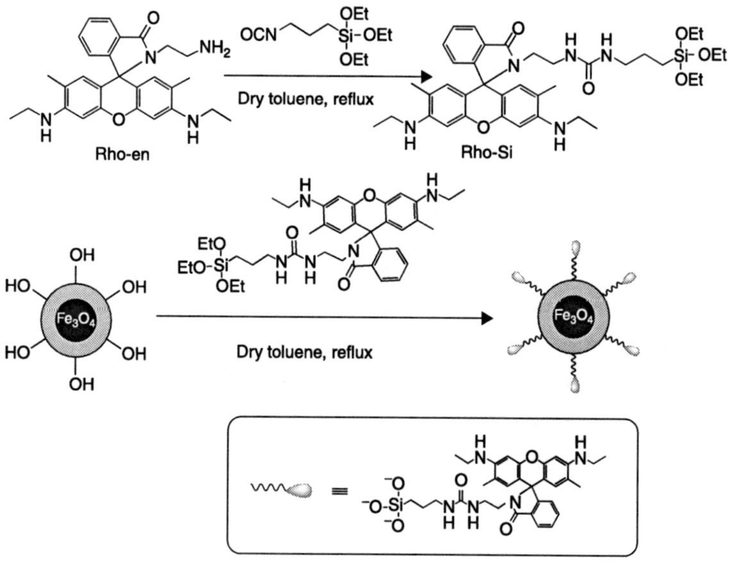

Figure 1.40 Synthesis of Rho-Si and Rho-Fe_3O_4/SiO_2.

Source: Adapted with permission from Peng et al. (2011).

Published by Woodhead Publishing Limited, 2013

of about 10 nm. The saturation magnetization (M_s) value of Rho-Fe_3O_4/SiO_2 was about 6.24×10^3 e.m.u./kg. When Hg^{2+} ions were added to Rho-Fe_3O_4/SiO_2 the fluorescence intensity was enhanced about 11-fold at 551 nm as a significant change in color from colorless to pink was observed (Figure 1.41) (Peng et al., 2011).

Ni et al. (2009) synthesized and characterized Fe_3O_4 magnetic nanoparticles, and studied their application as negative material for a lithium ion battery. The magnetic nanoparticles of Fe_3O_4 were prepared by heating an aqueous mixture of $(NH_4)_2Fe(SO_4)_2{\cdot}6H_2O$, hexamethylenetetramine and sodium sulfate at 90 °C for 24 h:

$$(CH_2)_6N_4 + 10H_2O \rightarrow 6HCHO + 4OH^- + 4[NH_4]^+ \quad [1.28]$$

$$(NH_4)_2Fe(SO_4)_2{\cdot}6H_2O \rightarrow Fe^{2+} + 2[NH_4]^+ + 2SO_4^{2-} + 6H_2O \quad [1.29]$$

$$Fe^{2+} + 2OH^- \rightarrow Fe(OH)_2 \quad [1.30]$$

$$4Fe(OH)_2 + O_2 \rightarrow 4FeOOH + 2H_2O \quad [1.31]$$

$$Fe(OH)_2 + 2FeOOH + 4O_2 \rightarrow Fe_3O_4 + 4H_2O \quad [1.32]$$

The average particle size of these magnetic nanoparticles was 160 nm. Conventional charge/discharge tests were

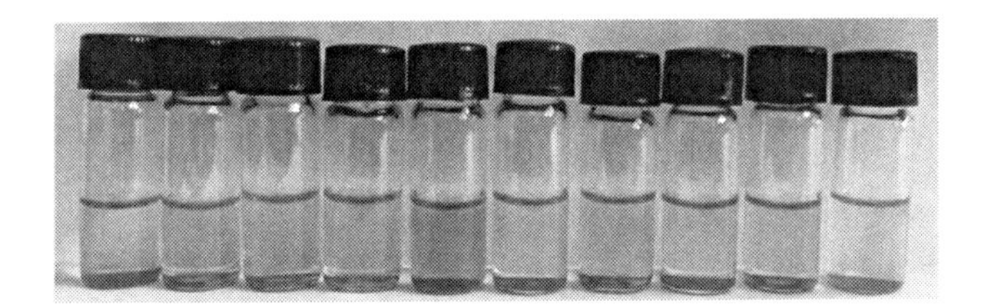

Figure 1.41 Color change of Rho-Fe_3O_4/SiO_2 in CH_3CN (0.3 g/l) after addition of 10 equiv. of metal ions. Left to right: 1, blank; 2, Ag; 3, Cd^{2+}; 4, Cu^{2+}; 5, Hg^{2+}; 6, Fe^{3+}; 7, Co^{2+}; 8, Cr^{3+}; 9, Ni^{2+}; 10, Zn^{2+}.

Source: Adapted with permission from Peng et al. (2011).

Published by Woodhead Publishing Limited, 2013

performed to study the electrochemical properties of the Fe_3O_4 and showed high initial discharge capacity of 1267 mAh/g at a current density of 0.1 mA/cm^2 (Ni et al., 2009).

Fe_3O_4 nanoparticles can be applied in the field of waste water treatment because these particles exhibit good adsorption efficiency due to higher surface area and greater active sites for interaction with metallic species. Panneerselvam et al. (2011) reported the preparation of Fe_3O_4 nanoparticles impregnated onto tea waste (Fe_3O_4/TW) as a low-cost adsorbent and its effectiveness in removing Ni ions from aqueous solution. The absorbent (Fe_3O_4/TW) particles were prepared by mixing tea waste with a solution of ferric and ferrous salts in basic solution and under inert atmospheric conditions. The obtained Fe_3O_4/TW absorbent was tested with a magnetic rod as shown in Figure 1.42 (Panneerselvam et al., 2011).

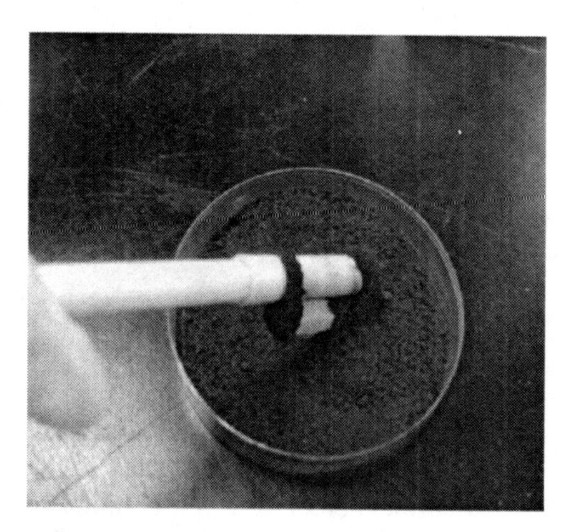

Figure 1.42 **Photograph Fe_3O_4 on a magnetic rod.**

Source: Adapted with permission from Panneerselvam et al. (2011).

Published by Woodhead Publishing Limited, 2013

The presence of Fe_3O_4 in Fe_3O_4/TW creates negative charges and thus attracts positively charged Ni(II) ions. The TW materials have insoluble cell walls with a fibrous content made up of cellulose-based structural proteins. The adsorption capacity was found to be 38.3 mg/g. It was found that the removal efficiency decreases from 99 to 87% by increasing the concentration of Ni(II) in solution from 50 to 100 mg/l (Panneerselvam et al., 2011).

Saiyed et al. (2007) studied the use of uncoated Fe_3O_4 nanoparticles as a support for the isolation of DNA fragments from agarose gel. The absence of a coated layer results in smaller particles providing a higher surface area for the adsorption. The average crystallite size of these nanoparticles was about 40 nm. Applying magnetic nanoparticles in DNA separation shows that DNA recovered from the agarose gel was greater than 80%, which is about 20% greater than that obtained by conventional phenol extraction and column methods, and the purified DNA is of a quality suitable for further manipulation (Saiyed et al., 2007).

The work reported by Tran et al. (2010b) aims to fabricate Fe_3O_4/curcumin (Cur) conjugates with a diameter below 500 nm, coated by chitosan or oleic acid, and then to use macrophages as a vehicle to carry these conjugates into tumors. Chitosan was chosen because it is an excellent biocompatible, biodegradable polymer with a high content of NH_2 groups, which ease the complexation reaction with metal ions in solution. Cur was used because it is non-toxic, autofluorescent and anticancerous. The uptake of Fe_3O_4/Cur could be visualized and monitored by fluorescent and magnetic imaging. The diameter was about 500 nm and the saturation magnetization of CSF/Cur was about 1.209 e.m.u./g. The uptake of CSF/Cur conjugates by cells *in vitro* has been studied by fluorescence microscopy (Figure 1.43).

Published by Woodhead Publishing Limited, 2013

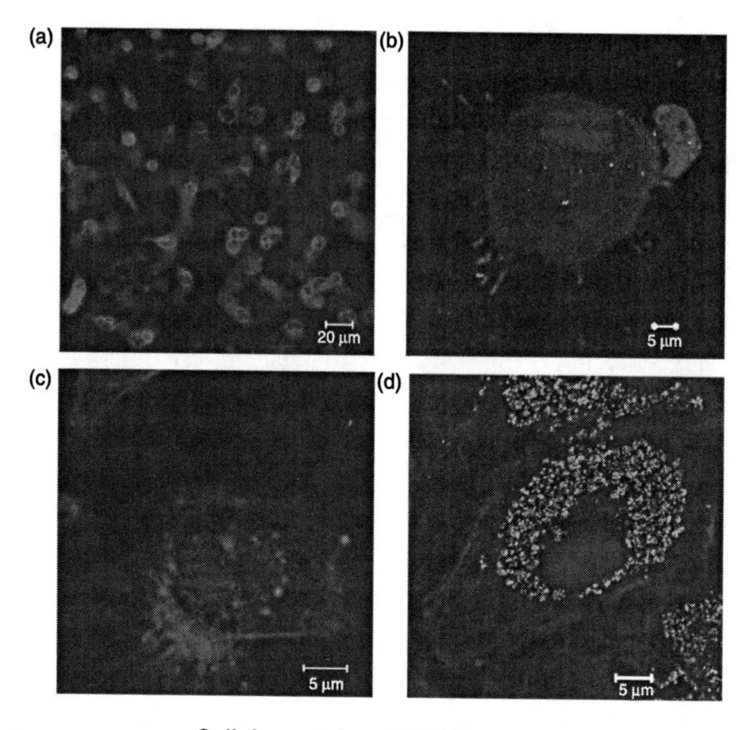

Figure 1.43 Cellular uptake of CSF/Cur and OLF/Cur conjugates by macrophages (CSF = chitosan-coated Fe_3O_4 fluid; OLF = oleic acid-coated Fe_3O_4 fluid). (a) Primary cultures of monocyte-derived macrophages stained for CD14 antigen (red). (b) Phagocytosis of CSF/Cur by human monocyte-derived macrophages. (c) Phagocytosis of CSF/Cur by mouse macrophages. (d) Phagocytosis of OLF/Cur by mouse macrophages. (Nanoparticle localization is visualized by autofluorescence of Cur).

Source: Adapted with permission from Tran et al. (2010b).

This study concluded that Fe_3O_4/Cur particles were efficiently internalized (Tran et al., 2010b).

Xu et al. (2011) prepared Fe_3O_4 baker's yeast biomass (FB) using glutaraldehyde as a cross-linking agent and this was

Published by Woodhead Publishing Limited, 2013

chemically treated with ethylenediaminetetraacetic dianhydride (EDTAD). EDTAD treated with bakers yeast biomass (FB) under heating in *N,N*-dimethylformamide (DMF) formed EFB particles. The mechanism of preparation and adsorption of metal ions on EFB is shown in Figure 1.44. The adsorption properties of EFB for Pb^{2+}, Cd^{2+} and Ca^{2+} were also investigated, and showed maximum adsorption capacity (88.16 mg/g for Pb^{2+} at pH 5.5, 40.72 mg/g for Cd^{2+} and 27.19 mg/g for Ca^{2+} at pH 6.0) was obtained at 10 °C (Xu et al., 2011).

This group has prepared chitosan-functionalized Fe_3O_4 magnetic nanoparticles and studied their application as MRI contrast agents. The obtained Fe_3O_4 nanoparticles were of spherical shape with average diameters of 17.12 ± 4.56 nm with a saturation magnetization of 57.4 e.m.u./g. Superparamagnetic Fe_3O_4 nanoparticles do not retain any magnetic moment and thus this indirectly helps to shorten the T_2 time and subsequently the image will appear dark as a result of the decrease of the signal detected. Accordingly, chitosan/Fe_3O_4 exhibits a bolstered enhancement of MRI

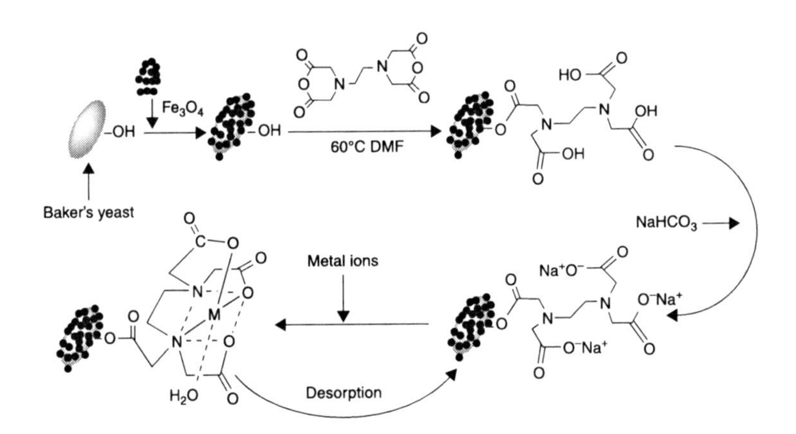

Figure 1.44 Preparation scheme of EFB and the adsorption mechanism of heavy metal ions on EFB.

Source: Adapted with permission from Xu et al. (2011).

contrast compared with the control phantom. Therefore, these nanoparticles can be utilized as a potential contrast agent for MRI (Haw et al., 2010).

1.2.4 *Natural and other types of nanoparticles*

Cormode at al. (2010) reported on the potential use of natural nanoparticles, which can be synthesized with quite precise size control and are potentially non-immunogenic and biodegradable, as contrast agents in existing medical imaging techniques, including lipoproteins, viruses and ferritin. For the case of lipoproteins this can be achieved via two mechanisms: (i) the contrast agent atoms can be attached to the protein constituent of the lipoprotein, such as unstable nuclei (e.g. ^{123}I for nuclear imaging techniques), chelated paramagnetic ions (i.e. gadolinium for MRI) and fluorophores (for fluorescence imaging techniques), or (ii) by loading the contrast agents or drugs in the hydrophobic core of lipoproteins: nanocrystals replacing the triglyceride and cholesterol ester core of high-density lipoprotein to create nanoparticles that are contrast agents for MRI, computed tomography or optical imaging, as well as the inclusion of paclitaxel in high density lipoproteins (HDL) so the particle acts as an anticancer therapeutic. It is known that viruses share the common structure of a shell composed of protein subunits that encloses either DNA or RNA, with a natural function to enter the cells of other organisms, produce copies of themselves, then leave to infect other cells. Moreover, large quantities of viruses can be synthesized using relatively straightforward methodology. In the past, the majority of research has focused on their roles as infectious agents, but more recently they are being used in novel materials, in electrode applications, as nanoreactors for enzymatic processes and as delivery agents for therapeutics, or

Published by Woodhead Publishing Limited, 2013

contrast-generating materials (Cormode et al., 2010). For example, the cowpea chlorotic mottle virus (CCMV) was the first virus to be adapted as an MRI contrast agent, where some Ca^{2+} ions (among the 180 metal-binding sites between its protein subunits) will be replaced by Gd^{3+} (Cormode et al., 2010). Moreover, viruses were modified using iron oxides and Au nanoparticles as well as quantum dots. Ferritin is known as a nanoparticle that stores and manages iron in the body, and its level represents a marker for diseases such as anemia, porphyria and hemochromatosis (Cormode et al., 2010). It contains an iron oxide core and hence can be used as a contrast agent for MRI. Alternatively, and similarly to the modification of viruses, the iron oxide core of ferritin has been replaced with a variety of materials such as uranium, platinum, quantum dots, etc.

Bennett et al. (2008) compared normal ferritin (NF) and cationized ferritin (CF) for the detection of basement membranes, matrices of proteins and proteoglycans that support epithelial and endothelial cells (Figure 1.45).

Curcumin (diferuloyl methane), known as a natural phytochemical, is derived from the roots of the *Curcuma longa* plant and has received considerable attention in many biomedical applications, including cancer prevention and cancer therapeutics, and has chemo/radiosensitizing properties in cancer cells (Yallapu et al., 2010). Previous studies show low systemic bioavailability and poor pharmacokinetics of curcumin, hence limiting the *in vivo* efficacy of curcumin, attributed mainly to the lipophilic characteristic: it was found that in patients treated with 10–12 g curcumin/day, only trace amounts of curcumin were found in blood (Yallapu et al., 2010). Yallapu et al. (2010) presented a very comprehensive investigation to develop a drug delivery system based on curcumin encapsulation in a poly(lactide-*co*-glycolic acid) (PLGA) nanoparticle, in order to improve the therapeutic efficacy of curcumin for cancer

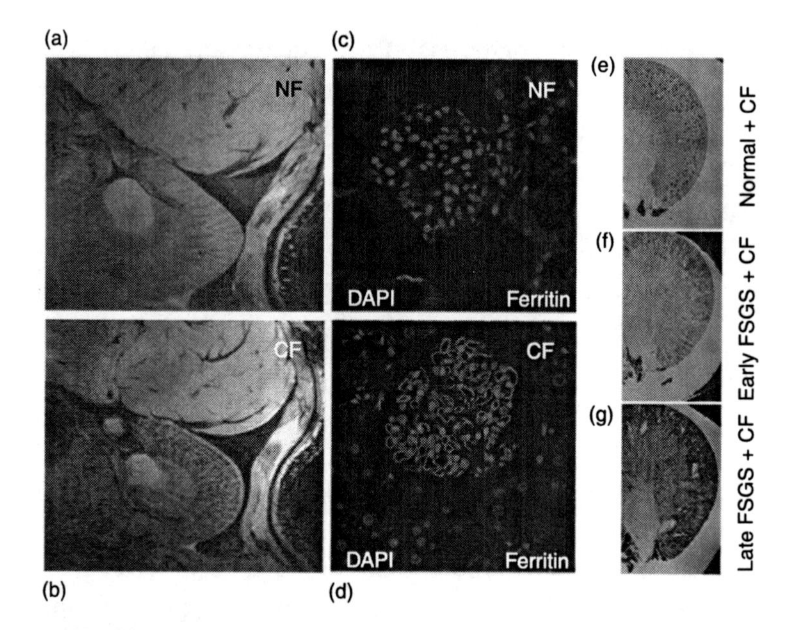

Figure 1.45 Detecting the basement membrane in kidney glomeruli. Magnetic resonance images of the kidney of a rat acquired 1.5 h after injection with (a) native (NF) and (b) cationic (CF) ferritin, with the speckled pattern of signal loss in (b) indicating detection of glomeruli. Confocal microscopy images of sections of kidney of a rat injected with (c) NF and (d) CF, with the cell nuclei stained with 4´, 6-diamidino-2-phenylindole (DAPI) and for ferritin. Magnetic resonance images of excised rat kidneys: (e) normal injected with CF, (f) early focal and segmental glomerulosclerosis (FSGS) injected with CF, and (g) late FSGS injected with CF.

Source: Adapted with permission from Bennett et al. (2008).

treatment. An optimized nanoparticle formulation of curcumin (nano-CUR6) exhibited superior cellular uptake, retention and release in cancer cells as well as a greater inhibitory effect on the growth of metastatic cancer cells compared with free curcumin (Figure 1.46).

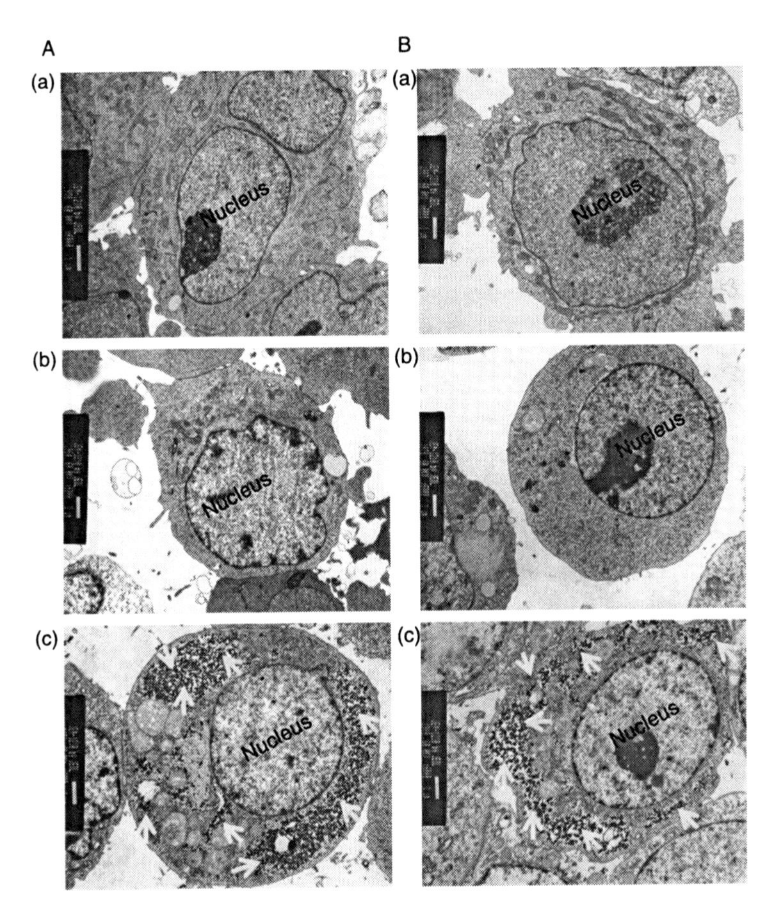

Figure 1.46 Cellular uptake of nano-CUR6 particles in cancer cells. Panels (a) and (b) represent TEM analysis of ovarian (A2780CP) and breast (MDA-MB-231) cancer cells, respectively. (a) Untreated cells, (b) curcumin-treated cells, and (c) nano-CUR6-treated cells. Arrows indicate the nano-CUR6 particle internalization area with a distinct contrast.

Source: Adapted with permission from Yallapu et al. (2010).

Published by Woodhead Publishing Limited, 2013

In vivo evaluation in terms of tissue distribution, time-dependent excretion profiles and tumor targeting ability of hydrophobically modified glycol chitosan (HGC) nanoparticles/encapsulated camptothecin (CPT) were carried out, as well as *in vitro* drug release and cytotoxicity against tumor cells (Min et al., 2008). It was reported that HGC nanoparticles inhibit the hydrolysis of lactone from CPT. It was also found that CPT/HGC showed improved performance compared with free CPT: longer circulation time in the blood, better targeting of drug to tumor tissue and substantial enhancement of antitumor activity.

In vivo biodistribution (with respect to liver, tumor and blood) of tritiated [^{3}H]tamoxifen (used as a radiomarker) loaded with 10 wt% poly(ethylene oxide)/modified poly(e-caprolactone) nanoparticles (PEO/PCL) with sizes ranging from 150 to 250 nm were analyzed in female mice, where tumor cells were injected prior to tests (Shenoy and Amiji, 2005). After accumulation in tumor, the nanoparticles release athymic encapsulated drug by diffusion and concurrent biodegradation. The results showed clearly that preferential and selective tumor targeting was achieved, even though a first accumulation within the liver was observed (26% could be recovered in tumor after 6 h post-injection).

A study was devoted to the treatment of liver cancer, which is a common lethal disease in Asia, using paclitaxel-loaded poly(γ-glutamic acid)/poly(lactide) nanoparticles. Paclitaxel is one of the most active anticancer drugs used in cancer chemotherapy (Liang et al., 2006). A high drug loading content concurrent with a high loading efficiency was obtained with a weight ratio of paclitaxel to block copolymer of 1/10. The antitumor efficacy studied in hepatoma tumor-bearing nude mice showed very effective targeting via asialoglycoprotein (ASGP) receptor-mediated recognition and this significantly reduced its size.

Published by Woodhead Publishing Limited, 2013

Fortina et al. (2007) presented a work on the applications of nanoparticles for diagnostics (assays can be divided into *in vitro*, e.g. diagnostic tests on blood serum, and *in vivo*, e.g. imaging of administered agents, applications) and therapeutics of colorectal cancer (CRC), which is the third most common neoplasm and the second leading cause of cancer-related mortality in the United States (Fortina et al., 2007). For example, HER2-specific IgG antibodies were conjugated at the surfaces of Au nanoshells using *ortho*-pyridyl-disulfide-*N*-hydroxysuccinimide PEG polymer. Normal colonic epithelial cells as well as primary CRC and metastatic tumors all express a unique surface-bound guanylyl cyclase C (GCC), which binds the diarrheagenic bacterial heat-stable peptide enterotoxin (ST). This makes GCC a potential target for metastatic tumor ablation using ST-bound nanoparticles in combination with thermal ablation with near-infrared (NIR) or radio frequency (RF) energy absorption (Fortina et al., 2007).

Monoclonal antibodies (mAbs) (used as homing agents) were attached either covalently or non-covalently at the surfaces of PLGA nanoparticles and then used as a delivery system for effective targeting of invasive epithelial breast tumor cells. This reduced side-effects caused by unspecific drug uptake into healthy tissues (Kocbek et al., 2007). Protein assay, surface plasmon resonance (SPR), flow cytometry and fluorescence immunostaining confirmed the presence of mAbs on nanoparticles in both cases. However, a binding assay using cell lysate revealed that the recognition properties were preserved only for nanoparticles with adsorbed mAbs (Kocbek et al., 2007).

A new, original and biocompatible targeting drug delivery system based on the high affinity of folic acid (FA) and folate receptor (FR), FA/PEG/P(HB–HO), where P(HB–HO) = poly(3-hydroxybutyrate-*co*-3-hydroxyoctanoate), was synthesized

Published by Woodhead Publishing Limited, 2013

(Zhang C et al., 2010). Doxorubicin (DOX) was adopted as a model anticancer drug, which is an effective and widely used anticancer agent in different cancers. The pharmacodynamics of DOX/FA/PEG/P(HB-HO) nanoparticles of an average size of 240 nm was also investigated by *in vitro* cellular uptake, *in vitro* cytotoxicity and *in vivo* antitumor activity. The results show that the DOX/FA/PEG/P(HB-HO) nanoparticles could focus on HeLa cells efficiently, and lead to a strong cytotoxicity due to the high affinity of FA and FR. *In vivo* antitumor activity showed a much better therapeutic efficacy in inhibiting tumor growth (Zhang C et al., 2010).

Juzenas et al. (2008) produced an important review on bioconjugation for the tracking and imaging of some selected quantum dots, as well as the possibility to use them as sensitizers for cancer therapies. (i) ZnS: ZnS doped with Mn^{2+} or Eu^{2+} cations produces fluorescent nanoparticles that can be used for both fluorescence and magnetic imaging; ZnS coated with mAbs, aptamers, folic acid or amino acid for specific targeting. (ii) Carbon dots (CDs), nano-scale carbon particles with simple surface passivation, exhibit strong photoluminescence, likely quantum confined due to the large surface-to-volume ratio. Additionally to their biocompatible and non-toxicity according to preliminary *in vivo* studies in mice, CDs have also been conjugated with biological and bioactive species (antibodies and molecules that target specific receptors) giving potential bioapplications, including optical bioimaging of cancer cells and tissues, early detection and therapy of breast cancers (functionalized with antibodies, they have been shown to effectively bind to breast cancer cells), etc. Finally, the use of quantum dots as photosensitizers and radiosensitizers for cancer therapy has also been presented (Juzenas et al., 2008).

Bharali and Mousa (2010) presented a comprehensive review on the recent progress in nanomedicine, including the

Published by Woodhead Publishing Limited, 2013

use of different nanoprobes for cancer detection and imaging as well as anticancer drug delivery. Some examples of the reported nano-scale systems based on chemotherapeutic agents (paclitaxel, cisplatin, DOX, fluorouracil, CPT and green tea and thyroid hormone) used for cancer therapy include:

(i) *In vivo* evaluation of the anticancer activity of a nanoparticulate paclitaxel formulation revealed a significant reduction in tumor volume in mice implanted with murine melanoma cells as compared with free paclitaxel.

(ii) A cisplatin carrier system comprised of inorganic calcium phosphate nanoparticles showed a cumulative release of cisplatin *in vitro* of about 70% after 20 days, but a slower release with decreasing crystallinity of the calcium phosphate nanoparticles was observed.

(iii) Encapsulation of DOX in nanoparticles resulted in reducing side-effects and an improvement of therapeutic efficacy in the treatment of solid tumors due to extended circulation time and accumulation at tumor sites: dextran-conjugated DOX (DEX–DOX) chitosan nanoparticles revealed enhanced antitumor effects against macrophage tumor xenografts in mice; in addition, an enhancement of tumor regression with an increase of the survival time was seen in treated animals as compared with DEX–DOX or free doxorubicin.

(iv) CPT and its derivatives exhibited superior anticancer activity, but their extreme lipophilic nature and the instability of the lactone ring limited their use. Hydrophobically modified HGC nanoparticles encapsulating CPT demonstrated a loading efficiency of around 80%, exhibited superior anticancer activity against human breast cancer xenografts in nude mice

Published by Woodhead Publishing Limited, 2013

and showed preferential accumulation in tumors with a drastic reduction of tumor growth as compared with free CPT.

It is known that angiogenesis, i.e. the formation of new capillaries from existing vasculature, is a crucial event for tumor growth, evasion and metastasis. Yu et al. (2010) developed a nanoparticulate drug delivery system decorated with peptide. Endothelial cell proliferation assay (*in vitro* cytotoxicity) and *in vitro* angiogenesis assay, *in vivo* pharmacokinetic study, *in vivo* tumor neovasculature targeting and paclitaxel-induced apoptosis in the tumor neovasculature endothelial cells and necrosis in tumor tissues studies show rapid, long-term and accurate *in vivo* tumor neovasculature targeting, as well as significant apoptosis of tumor neovasculature endothelial cells and necrosis of tumor tissues (Yu et al., 2010).

1.3 Toxicology

It is important to note that there are huge concerns about the environmental and health implications of nanotechnology, starting from the preparation and manipulation of nanomaterials (research laboratories and industrial manufacturing), technological applications as well as recycling. Also, the noticeable and fast growth of the nanotechnology industry worldwide has resulted in an important increase in discharges, and hence raises some difficulties in risk assessment and management of toxicity. However, the side-effects of nanoparticles on humans and the environment (ecotoxicology) are to be considered more seriously and urgently as well as the implementation of strict regulations. Very little is known about the mechanisms of

Published by Woodhead Publishing Limited, 2013

biological uptake and toxicity modes of action, about transport in and between environmental and biological compartments, and about the chemical behavior in the environment (Ju-Nam and Lead, 2008).

Ju-Nam and Lead (2008) presented an overview on the chemistry of some selected nanoparticles (carbon nanostructures such as nanotubes and fullerenes; metal oxides such as Fe_2O_3 and Fe_3O_4, ZnO, TiO_2, CeO_2; metals such as Au, Ag; etc.) and their behavior as well as toxicity in the natural aquatic environment. Previous studies had shown the potential impacts on a range of aquatic organisms with a lesser focus on terrestrial and other organisms, and their toxicity can be related to dissolution, surface properties or size (Ju-Nam and Lead, 2008). Moreover, it is questionable whether discharges are actually sufficient in volume or intensity to cause severe environmental problems, and current modeling studies suggest that risk is negligible for many nanoparticles (Ju-Nam and Lead, 2008).

More particularly, human toxicity associated with the use of nanoparticles during diagnosis and therapy should be taken more seriously. Lin et al. (2006) investigated the cytotoxicity of SiO_2 nanoparticles (15 and 46 nm) in human bronchoalveolar carcinoma-derived cells. They found that cell viability is reduced depending on the dose and time at 10–100 μg/ml dosage.

Barrena et al. (2009) reported that the use of nanoparticles in commercial products and industrial applications has increased greatly in recent years, although an understanding of the interaction mechanisms at the molecular level between nanoparticles and biological systems is largely lacking. Moreover, it is known that in some products, in particular skin creams and toothpastes, nanoparticles are in direct contact with the user's body or hence can enter the environment on a continual basis from the removal (e.g. by

Published by Woodhead Publishing Limited, 2013

washing) of such products or, even worse, a fatal accident during the production of engineered nanomaterials could release an important quantity of nanoparticles to the environment.

Moreover, Barrena et al. (2009) reported that scientists have also found ways of using nanomaterials in environmental remediation: dozens of sites under testing phase have already been injected with various nanomaterials, including polymers or TiO_2, long used to mineralize many undesired organic pollutants. Recently, iron nanoparticles were proposed as a low-cost technology for removing arsenic from drinking water. However, nanosized materials may not migrate through soils at rapid enough rates to be valuable in remediation and at the same time they may, in fact, become new environmental hazards themselves. For example, TiO_2 absorbs substantial UV radiation, yielding, in aqueous media, hydroxyl species. These species may cause substantial damage to DNA, resulting in additional environmental hazards (Barrena et al., 2009).

Metal-based nanoparticles, i.e. Fe_3O_4, Ag and Au nanoparticles, are commonly used in commercial nanoengineered materials such as antibacterial coatings, catalysts, in biomedicine or for personal care products (Barrena et al., 2009). Hence, Barrena et al. (2009) investigated their environmental risks and implications, phytotoxicity, and toxicity. The effects on plants and microorganisms of model nanoparticles were tested, including stable metal (Au, 10 nm mean diameter), a well-known bactericide (Ag, 2 nm mean diameter) and the widely used Fe_3O_4 (7 nm mean diameter). The toxicity of these nanoparticles was assayed using standard toxicity tests. Specifically, germination (cucumber and lettuce), bioluminescent (*Photobacterium phosphoreum*) and anaerobic toxicity tests were performed. Germination tests

Published by Woodhead Publishing Limited, 2013

were conducted at nanoparticle doses of 62, 100 and 116 μg/ml for Au, Ag and Fe_3O_4, respectively. The bioluminescent testing (*P. phosphoreum*) was conducted at doses of 28, 45 and 52 μg/ml for Au, Ag and Fe_3O_4, respectively. Finally, anaerobic tests were conducted at nanoparticle doses of 10, 16 and 18 μg/ml for Au, Ag and Fe_3O_4, respectively. According to Barrena et al. (2009), low or zero toxicity was observed for Au, Ag and Fe_3O_4 nanoparticles at the assayed concentrations. However, since nanoparticles must be accompanied by stabilizers, in some cases a positive or negative effect was observed due to the presence of the latter (e.g. TMAOH, sodium citrate and $NaBH_4$).

1.4 Conclusion

Several metals (mainly Au and Ag) and oxides (mainly Fe_3O_4) have been investigated at the nano-scale for biomedical applications, in particular cancer diagnosis and therapy. The advances are tremendous and the obtained results are very promising; however, much research work is still needed in terms of the treatment of other types of human diseases, and more particularly toxicity and environmental implications. It is important to mention that some natural nanoparticles have also been explored and the obtained results are very encouraging.

1.5 References

Akhavan O and Ghaderi E (2010), 'Self-accumulated Ag nanoparticles on mesoporous TiO_2 thin film with high bactericidal activities', *Surf. Coat. Technol.*, 204: 3676–3683.

Published by Woodhead Publishing Limited, 2013

Amara D, Felner I, Nowik I and Margel S (2009), 'Synthesis and characterization of Fe and Fe_3O_4 nanoparticles by thermal decomposition of triiron dodecacarbonyl', *Colloids Surf. A*, **339**: 106–110.

Aslam M, Schultz A, Sun T and Meade Dravid V P (2007), 'Synthesis of amine-stabilized aqueous colloidal iron oxide nanoparticles', *Crystal Growth Des.*, **7**: 471–475.

Asuha S, Suyala B, Siqintana X and Zhao S (2011), 'Direct synthesis of Fe_3O_4 nanopowder by thermal decomposition of Fe–urea complex and its properties', *J. Alloys Compounds*, **509**: 2870–2873.

Barrena R, Casals E, Colón J, Font X, Sánchez A et al. (2009), 'Evaluation of the ecotoxicity of model nanoparticles', *Chemosphere*, **75**: 850–857.

Bennett K M, Zhou H, Sumner J P, Dodd S J, Bouraoud N et al. (2008), 'MRI of the basement membrane using charged nanoparticles as contrast agents', *Magn. Reson. Med.*, **60**: 564–574.

Berciaud S, Cognet L, Blab G A and Lounis B (2004), 'Photothermal heterodyne imaging of individual nonfluorescent nanoclusters and nanocrystals', *Phys. Rev. Lett.*, **93**: 257402–257405.

Bharali D J and Mousa S A (2010), 'Emerging nanomedicines for early cancer detection and improved treatment: current perspective and future promise', *Pharmacol. Ther.*, **128**: 324–335.

Bhattacharya R and Mukherjee P (2008), 'Biological properties of "naked" metal nanoparticles', *Adv. Drug Deliv. Rev.*, **60**: 1289–1306.

Bohren C F and Huffman D R (1983), *Absorption and Scattering of Light by Small Particles*. New York: Wiley.

Bonoiu A C, Mahajan S D, Ding H, Roy I, Yong K T et al. (2009), 'Nanotechnology approach for drug addiction therapy: gene silencing using delivery of gold

Published by Woodhead Publishing Limited, 2013

nanorod–siRNA nanoplex in dopaminergic neurons', *Proc. Natl Acad. Sci. USA*, **106**: 5546–5550.

Boyer D, Tamarat P, Maali A, Lounis B and Orrit M (2002), 'Photothermal imaging of nanometer-sized metal particles among scatterers', *Science*, **297**: 1160–1163.

Brown K R, Fox A P and Natan M J (1996), 'Morphology-dependent electrochemistry of cytochrome *c* at Au colloid-modified SnO_2 electrodes', *J. Am. Chem. Soc.*, **118**: 1154–1157.

Burda C, Chen X, Narayanan R and El-Sayed M A (2005), 'Chemistry and properties of nanocrystals of different shapes', *Chem. Rev.*, **105**: 1025–1102.

Burygin G L, Khlebtsov B N, Shantrokha A N, Dykman L A, Bogatyrev V A et al. (2009), 'On the enhanced antibacterial activity of antibiotics mixed with gold nanoparticles', *Nanoscale Res. Lett.*, **4**: 794–801.

Buyukhalipoglu K and Morss Clyne A (2010), 'Controlled flame synthesis of α-Fe_2O_3 and Fe_3O_4 nanoparticles: effect of flame configuration, flame temperature, and additive loading', *J. Nanopart. Res.*, **12**: 1495–1508.

Byrne J D, Betancourt T and Brannon-Peppas L (2008), 'Active targeting schemes for nanoparticle systems in cancer therapeutics', *Adv. Drug Deliv. Rev.*, **60**: 1615–1626.

Cai Y, Shen Y, Xie A, Li S and Wanga X (2010), 'Green synthesis of soya bean sprouts-mediated superparamagnetic Fe_3O_4 nanoparticles', *J. Magn. Magn. Mater.*, **322**: 2938–2943.

Cao F, Chen C, Wang Q and Chen Q (2007), 'Synthesis of carbon–Fe_3O_4 coaxial nanofibres by pyrolysis of ferrocene in supercritical carbon dioxide', *Carbon*, **45**: 727–731.

Carralero V, Mena M L, Gonzalez-Cortes A, Yanez-Sedeno P and Pingarron J M (2006), 'Development of a high analytical performance tyrosinase biosensor based on a composite graphite–Teflon electrode modified with gold nanoparticles', *Biosens. Bioelectron.*, **22**: 730–735.

Chamakura K, Perez-Ballestero R, Luo Z, Bashir S and Liud J (2011), 'Comparison of bactericidal activities of silver nanoparticles with common chemical disinfectants', *Colloids Surf. B*, **84**: 88–96.

Chandran S P, Ghatak J, Satyam P V and Sastry M (2007), 'Interfacial deposition of Ag on Au seeds leading to $Au_{core}Ag_{shell}$ in organic media', *J. Colloid Interface Sci.*, **312**: 498–505.

Chen C C, Lin Y P, Wang C W, Tzeng H C, Wu C H et al. (2006), 'DNA–gold nanorod conjugates for remote control of localized gene expression by near infrared irradiation', *J. Am. Chem. Soc.*, **128**: 3709–3715.

Chen H M, Liu R-S and Tsai D P (2009), 'A versatile route to the controlled synthesis of gold nanostructures', *Cryst. Growth Des.*, **9**: 2079–2087.

Chen H, Deng C and Zhang X (2010), 'Synthesis of Fe_3O_4/SiO_2/PMMA core–shell–shell magnetic microspheres for highly efficient enrichment of peptides and proteins for MALDI-ToF MS analysis', *Angew. Chem. Int. Ed.*, **49**: 607–611.

Chen L, Xu Z, Dai H and Zhang S (2010), 'Facile synthesis and magnetic properties of monodisperse Fe_3O_4/silica nanocomposite microspheres with embedded structures via a direct solution-based route', *J. Alloys Compounds*, **497**: 221–227.

Chen L, Lin Z, Zhao C, Zheng Y, Zhou Y et al. (2011), 'Direct synthesis and characterization of mesoporous Fe_3O_4 through pyrolysis of ferric nitrate-ethylene glycol gel', *J. Alloys Compounds*, **509**: L1–L5.

Chen S H, Wu V C, Chuang Y C and Lin C S (2008), 'Using oligonucleotide-functionalized Au nanoparticles to

Published by Woodhead Publishing Limited, 2013

rapidly detect foodborne pathogens on a piezoelectric biosensor', *J. Microbiol. Methods*, **73**: 7–17.

Chen T, Cao Z, Guo X, Nie J, Xu J et al. (2011), 'Preparation and characterization of thermosensitive organic–inorganic hybrid microgels with functional Fe_3O_4 nanoparticles as crosslinker', *Polymer*, **52**: 172–179.

Chen Y-H, Tsai C-Y, Huang P-Y, Chang M-Y, Cheng P-C et al. (2007), 'Methotrexate conjugated to gold nanoparticles inhibits tumor growth in a syngeneic lung tumor model', *Mol. Pharm.*, **4**: 713–722.

Cheng Y, Samia A C, Meyers J D, Panagopoulos I, Fei B et al. (2008), 'Highly efficient drug delivery with gold nanoparticle vectors for *in vivo* photodynamic therapy of cancer', *J. Am. Chem. Soc.*, **130**: 10643–10647.

Chithrani B D, Ghazani A A and Chan W C W (2006), 'Determining the size and shape dependence of gold nanoparticle uptake into mammalian cells', *Nano Lett.*, **6**: 662–668.

Chiu W S, Radiman S, Abdullah Khiew P S, Huang N M and Abd-Shukor R (2007), 'One pot synthesis of monodisperse Fe_3O_4 nanocrystals by pyrolysis reaction of organometallic compound', *Mater. Chem. Phys.*, **106**: 231–235.

Cho H-S, Dong Z, Pauletti G M, Zhang J, Xu H et al. (2010), 'Fluorescent, superparamagnetic nanospheres for drug storage, targeting, and imaging: a multifunctional nanocarrier system for cancer diagnosis and treatment', *ACS Nano*, **4**: 5398–5404.

Cho K, Park J, Osaka T and Park S (2005), 'The study of antimicrobial activity and preservative effects of nanosilver ingredient', *Electrochim. Acta*, **51**: 956–960.

Choi C J, Dong X L and Kim B K (2001), 'Microstructure and magnetic properties of Fe nanoparticles synthesized by chemical vapor condensation', *Mater. Trans.*, **42**: 2046–2049.

Published by Woodhead Publishing Limited, 2013

Choi S-W, Kim W-S and Kim J-H (2003), 'Surface modification of functional nanoparticles for controlled drug delivery', *J. Dispers. Sci. Technol.*, **24**: 475–487.

Chouly C, Poulliquen D, Lucet I, Jeune J J and Jallet P (1996), 'Development of superparamagnetic nanoparticles for MRI: effect of particle size, charge and surface nature on biodistribution', *J. Microencapsul.*, **13**: 245–255.

Clark L C Jr and Lyons C (1962), 'Electrode systems for continuous monitoring in cardiovascular surgery', *Ann. NY Acad. Sci.*, **102**: 29–45.

Cohen H, Gedanken A and Zhong Z (2008), 'One-step synthesis and characterization of ultrastable and amorphous FeO colloids capped with cysteine molecules', *J. Phys. Chem. C*, **112**: 15429–15438.

Cormode D P, Jarzyna P A, Mulder W J M and Fayad Z A (2010), 'Modified natural nanoparticles as contrast agents for medical imaging', *Adv. Drug Deliv. Rev.*, **62**: 329–338.

Daniel M C and Astruc D (2004), 'Gold nanoparticles: assembly, supramolecular chemistry, quantum-size-related properties, and applications toward biology, catalysis, and nanotechnology', *Chem. Rev.*, **104**: 293–346.

Dickerson E B, Dreaden E C, Huang X, El-Sayed I H, Chu H et al. (2008), 'Gold nanorod assisted near-infrared plasmonic photothermal therapy (PPTT) of squamous cell carcinoma in mice', *Cancer Lett.*, **269**: 57–66.

Dilnawaz F, Singh A, Mohanty C and Sahoo S K (2010), 'Dual drug loaded super-paramagnetic iron oxide nanoparticles for targeted cancer therapy', *Biomaterials*, **31**: 3694–3706.

Dumitrache F, Morjan I, Fleaca C, Birjega R, Vasile E et al. (2011), 'Parametric studies on iron–carbon composite nanoparticles synthesized by laser pyrolysis for increased passivation and high iron content', *Appl. Surf. Sci.*, **257**: 5265–5269.

Elghanian R, Storhoff J J, Mucic R C, Letsinger R L and Mirkin C A (1997), 'Selective colorimetric detection of polynucleotides based on the distance-dependent optical properties of gold nanoparticles', *Science*, **277**: 1078–1081.

El-Sayed I H, Huang X and El-Sayed M A (2005), 'Surface plasmon resonance scattering and absorption of anti-EGFR antibody conjugated gold nanoparticles in cancer diagnostics: applications in oral cancer', *Nano Lett.*, **5**: 829–834.

El-Sayed I H, Huang X and El-Sayed M A (2006), 'Selective laser photo-thermal therapy of epithelial carcinoma using anti-EGFR antibody conjugated gold nanoparticles', *Cancer Lett.*, **239**: 129–135.

Faiyas A P A, Vinod E M, Joseph J, Ganesan R and Pandey R K (2010), 'Dependence of pH and surfactant effect in the synthesis of magnetite (Fe_3O_4) nanoparticles and its properties', *J. Magn. Magn. Mater.*, **322**: 400–404.

Felnerova D, Viret J-F, Reinhard G-K and Moser C (2004), 'Liposomes and virosomes as delivery systems for antigens, nucleic acids and drugs', *Curr. Opin. Biotechnol.*, **15**: 518–529.

Fortina P, Kricka L J, Graves D J, Park J, Hyslop T et al. (2007), 'Applications of nanoparticles to diagnostics and therapeutics in colorectal cancer', *Trends Biotechnol.*, **25**: 145–152.

Fu W, Shenoy D, Li J, Crasto C, Jones G, Dimarzio C, Sridhar S, and Aniji M (2005), 'Biomedical Applications of Gold Nanoparticles Functionalized Using Hetero-Bifunctional Poly(ethylene glycol) Spacer', *Mater. Res. Soc. Symp. Proc.*, **845**, AA5.4.1–AA5.4.6

Fukumori Y and Ichikawa H (2006), 'Nanoparticles for cancer therapy and diagnosis', *Adv. Powder Technol.*, **17**: 1–28.

Published by Woodhead Publishing Limited, 2013

Gao F, Yuan R, Chai Y, Chen S, Cao S and Tang M (2007), 'Amperometric hydrogen peroxide biosensor based on the immobilization of HRP on nano-Au/Thi/poly (*p*-aminobenzene sulfonic acid)-modified glassy carbon electrode', *J. Biochem. Biophys. Methods*, **70**: 407–413.

Geller R J, Chevalier R L and Spyker D A (1986), 'Acute amoxicillin nephrotoxicity following an overdose', *J. Toxicol. Clin. Toxicol.*, **24**: 175–182.

Ghosh P, Han G, De M, Kim C K and Rotello V M (2008), 'Gold nanoparticles in delivery applications', *Adv. Drug. Deliv. Rev.*, **60**: 1307–1315.

Gosselin R E (1956), 'A kinetic analysis with radioactive colloidal gold', *J. Gen. Physiol.*, **39**: 625–649.

Govorov A O, Zhang W, Skeini T, Richardson H, Lee J et al. (2006), 'Gold nanoparticle ensembles as heaters and actuators: melting and collective plasmon resonances', *Nanoscale Res. Lett.*, **1**: 84–90.

Goya G F, Grazú V and Ibarra M R (2008), 'Magnetic nanoparticles for cancer therapy', *Curr. Nanosci.*, **4**: 1–16.

Grabis J, Heidemane G and Rasmane D (2008), 'Preparation of Fe_3O_4 and γ-Fe_2O_3 nanoparticles by liquid and gas phase processes', *Mater. Sci.*, **14**: 292–295.

Gu H, Ho P L, Tong L, Wang L and Xu B (2003), 'Presenting vancomycin on nanoparticles to enhance antimicrobial activities', *Nano Lett.*, **3**: 1261–1263.

Gu Y-J, Cheng J, Lin C-C, Lam Y-W, Cheng S H et al. (2009), 'Nuclear penetration of surface functionalized gold nanoparticles', *Toxicol. Appl. Pharmacol.*, **237**: 196–204.

Haddad P S, Martins T M, Souza-Li L D, Li L M, Metze K et al. (2008), 'Structural and morphological investigation of magnetic nanoparticles based on iron oxides for biomedical applications', *Mater. Sci. Eng. C*, **28**: 489–494.

Hai H T, Kura H, Takahashi M and Ogawa T (2010), 'Facile synthesis of Fe_3O_4 nanoparticles by reduction phase

Published by Woodhead Publishing Limited, 2013

transformation from γ-Fe_2O_3 nanoparticles in organic solvent', *J. Colloid Interface Sci.*, **341**: 194–199.

Hainfeld J F, Slatkin D N, Focella T M and Smilowitz H M (2006), 'Gold nanoparticles: a new X-ray contrast agent', *Br. J. Radiol.*, **79**: 248–253.

Han G, Chari N S, Verma A, Hong R, Martin C T et al. (2005), 'Controlled recovery of the transcription of nanoparticle-bound DNA by intracellular concentrations of glutathione', *Bioconjug. Chem.*, **16**: 1356–1359.

Han G, Martin C T and Rotello V M (2006), 'Stability of gold nanoparticle-bound DNA toward biological, physical, and chemical agents', *Chem. Biol. Drug Des.*, **67**: 78–82.

Haw C Y, Mohamed F, Chia C H, Radiman S, Zakaria S et al. (2010), 'Hydrothermal synthesis of magnetite nanoparticles as MRI contrast agents', *Ceramics Int.*, **36**: 1417–1422.

He L, Musick M D, Nicewarner S R, Salinas F G, Benkovic S J et al. (2000), 'Colloidal Au-enhanced surface plasmon resonance for ultrasensitive detection of DNA hybridization', *J. Am. Chem. Soc.*, **122**: 9071–9077.

Hiergeist R, Andra W, Buske N, Hergt R, Hilger I et al. (1999), 'Application of magnetite ferrofluids for hyperthermia', *J. Magn. Magn. Mater.*, **201**: 420–422.

Hirsch L R, Stafford R J, Bankson J A, Sershen S R, Rivera B et al. (2003), 'Nanoshell-mediated near-infrared thermal therapy of tumors under magnetic resonance guidance', *Proc. Natl Acad. Sci. USA*, **100**: 13549–13554.

Hleb E Y, Hafner J H, Myers J N, Hanna E Y, Rostro B C et al. (2008), 'LANTCET: elimination of solid tumor cells with photothermal bubbles generated around clusters of gold nanoparticles', *Nanomedicine*, **3**: 647–667.

Hojati-Talemi P, Azadmanjiri J and Simon G P (2010), 'A simple microwave-based method for preparation of Fe_3O_4/carbon composite nanoparticles', *Mater. Lett.*, **64**: 1684–1687.

Published by Woodhead Publishing Limited, 2013

Hong R, Li J, Wang J and Li H (2007), 'Comparison of schemes for preparing magnetic Fe_3O_4 nanoparticles', *China Particuol.*, **5**: 186–191.

Hongqiu Z, Lin L, Ji T, Mingxing D and Long J (2001), 'Enhancement of the immobilization and discrimination of DNA probe on a biosensor using gold nanoparticles', *Chin. Sci. Bull.*, **46**: 1074–1077.

Hu M, Chen J, Li Z Y, Au L, Hartland G V et al. (2006), 'Gold nanostructures: engineering their plasmonic properties for biomedical applications', *Chem. Soc. Rev.*, **35**: 1084–1094.

Hu P, Zhang S, Wang H, Pan D, Tian J et al. (2011), 'Heat treatment effects on Fe_3O_4 nanoparticles structure and magnetic properties prepared by carbothermal reduction', *J. Alloys Compounds*, **509**: 2316–2319.

Huang X and El-Sayed M A (2010), 'Gold nanoparticles: optical properties and implementations in cancer diagnosis and photothermal therapy', *J. Adv. Res.*, **1**: 13–28.

Huang X, El-Sayed I H, Qian W and El-Sayed M A (2006a), 'Cancer cell imaging and photothermal therapy in the near-infrared region by using gold nanorods', *J. Am. Chem. Soc.*, **128**: 2115–2120.

Huang X, Jain P K, El-Sayed I H and El-Sayed M A (2006b), 'Determination of the minimum temperature required for selective photothermal destruction of cancer cells with the use of immunotargeted gold nanoparticles', *Photochem. Photobiol.*, **82**: 412–417.

Huang X, Qian W, El-Sayed I H and El-Sayed M A (2007a), 'The potential use of the enhanced nonlinear properties of gold nanospheres in photothermal cancer therapy', *Lasers Surg. Med.*, **39**: 747–753.

Huang X, Jain P K, El-Sayed I H and El-Sayed M A (2007b), 'Gold nanoparticles: interesting optical properties and recent applications in cancer diagnostics and therapy', *Nanomedicine*, **2**: 681–693.

Huang X, Jain P, El-Sayed I and El-Sayed M (2008), 'Plasmonic photothermal therapy (PPTT) using gold nanoparticles', *Lasers Med. Sci.*, **23**: 217–228.

Huff T B, Tong L, Zhao Y, Hansen M N, Cheng J X et al. (2007), 'Hyperthermic effects of gold nanorods on tumor cells', *Nanomedicine*, **2**: 125–132.

Iida H, Takayanagi K, Nakanishi T and Osaka T (2007), 'Synthesis of Fe_3O_4 nanoparticles with various sizes and magnetic properties by controlled hydrolysis', *J. Colloid Interface Sci.*, **314**: 274–280.

Jain K K (2003), 'Applications of nanobiotechnology in clinical diagnostics', *Clin. Chem.*, **53**: 2002–2009.

Jain P and Pradeep T (2005), 'Potential of silver nanoparticle-coated polyurethane foam as an antibacterial water filter', *Biotechnol. Bioeng.*, **90**: 59–63.

Jain P K, Eustis S and El-Sayed M A (2006a), 'Gold nanostructures: engineering their plasmonic properties for biomedical applications', *J. Phys. Chem. B*, **110**: 18243–18253.

Jain P K, Lee K S, El-Sayed I H and El-Sayed M A (2006b), 'Calculated absorption and scattering properties of gold nanoparticles of different size, shape, and composition: applications in biological imaging and biomedicine', *J. Phys. Chem. B*, **110**: 7238–7248.

Jain P K, El-Sayed I H and El-Sayed M A (2007), 'Au nanoparticles target cancer', *Nano Today*, **2**: 18–29.

Jennings T and Strouse G (2007), *Bio-Applications of Nanoparticles*. New York: Springer.

Ji X, Song X, Li J, Bai Y, Yang W and Peng X (2007), 'Size control of gold nanocrystals in citrate reduction: the third role of citrate', *J. Am. Chem. Soc.*, **129**: 13939–13948.

Published by Woodhead Publishing Limited, 2013

Jia J, Wang B, Wu A, Cheng G, Li Z and Dong S (2002), 'A method to construct a third-generation horseradish peroxidase biosensor: self-assembling gold nanoparticles to three-dimensional sol–gel network', *Anal. Chem.*, **74**: 2217–2223.

Jin R, Cao Y, Mirkin C A, Kelly K L, Schatz G C et al. (2001), 'Photoinduced conversion of silver nanospheres to nanoprisms', *Science*, **294**: 1901–1903.

Johannsen M, Gneveckow U, Thiesen B, Taymoorian K, Cho C H et al. (2007), 'Thermotherapy of prostate cancer using magnetic nanoparticles: feasibility, imaging, and three-dimensional temperature distribution', *Eur. Urol.*, **52**: 1653–1662.

Ju-Nam Y and Lead J R (2008), 'Manufactured nanoparticles: An overview of their chemistry, interactions and potential environmental implications', *Sci. Total Environ.*, **400**: 396–414.

Juzenas P, Chen W, Sun Y-P, Coelho M A N, Generalov R et al. (2008), 'Quantum dots and nanoparticles for photodynamic and radiation therapies of cancer', *Adv. Drug Deliv. Rev.*, **60**: 1600–1614.

Kateb B, Chiu K, Black K L, Yamamoto V, Khalsa B et al. (2011), 'Nanoplatforms for constructing new approaches to cancer treatment, imaging, and drug delivery: what should be the policy?', *NeuroImage*, **54**: S106–S124.

Katz E, Willner I and Wang J (2004), 'Electroanalytical and bioelectroanalytical systems based on metal and semiconductor nanoparticles', *Electroanalysis*, **16**: 19–44.

Kerker M (1969), *The Scattering of Light and other Electromagnetic Radiation*. New York: Academic Press.

Khlebtsov B, Zharov V, Melnikov A, Tuchin V and Khlebtsov N (2006), 'Optical amplification of photothermal therapy with gold nanoparticles and nanoclusters', *Nanotechnology*, **17**: 5167–5179.

Published by Woodhead Publishing Limited, 2013

Khlebtsov N G and Dykman L A (2010), 'Optical properties and biomedical applications of plasmonic nanoparticles', *J. Quant. Spectrosc. Radiat. Transf.*, **111**: 1–35.

Kim J-Y and Lee J-S (2009), 'Synthesis and thermally reversible assembly of DNA–gold nanoparticle cluster conjugates', *Nano Lett.*, **9**: 4564–4569.

Kim K, Huang S W, Ashkenazi S, O'Donnell M, Agarwal A et al. (2007), 'Photoacoustic imaging of early inflammatory response using gold nanorods', *Appl. Phys. Lett.*, **90**: 223901–223903.

Kim K D, Kim S S and Kim H T (2005), 'Formation and characterization of silica-coated magnetic nanoparticles by sol–gel method', *J. Ind. Eng. Chem.*, **11**: 584–589.

Kim P S, Djazayeri S and Zeineldin R (2011), 'Novel nanotechnology approaches to diagnosis and therapy of ovarian cancer', *Gynecol. Oncol.*, **120**: 393–403.

Klar T A (2007), in Nanophotonics with surface plasmons, in: Shalaev V and Kawata S (eds), *Gold Nanoparticles: Assembly, Supramolecular Chemistry, Quantum-Size-Related Properties, and Applications toward Biology, Catalysis, and Nanotechnology*, pp. 219–270. Amsterdam: Elsevier.

Knauera A, Thete A, Li S, Romanus H, Csáki A et al. (2011), 'Au/Ag/Au double shell nanoparticles with narrow size distribution obtained by continuous micro segmented flow synthesis', *Chem. Eng. J.*, **166**: 1164–1169.

Kocbek P, Obermajer N, Cegnar M, Kos J and Kristl J (2007), 'Targeting cancer cells using PLGA nanoparticles surface modified with monoclonal antibody', *J. Control. Release*, **120**: 18–26.

Kreibig U and Vollmer M (1995), *Optical Properties of Metal Clusters*. Berlin: Springer.

Kumar V S, Nagaraja B M, Shashikala V, Padmasri A H, Madhavendra S S et al. (2004), 'Highly efficient Ag/C

Published by Woodhead Publishing Limited, 2013

catalyst prepared by electro-chemical deposition method in controlling microorganisms in water', *J. Mol. Catal. A*, **223**: 313–319.

Lee J E, Lee N, Kim H, Kim J, Choi S H et al. (2010), 'Uniform mesoporous dye-doped silica nanoparticles decorated with multiple magnetite nanocrystals for simultaneous enhanced magnetic resonance imaging, fluorescence imaging, and drug delivery', *J. Am. Chem. Soc.*, **132**: 552–557.

Lee Y and Park T G (2011), 'Facile fabrication of branched gold nanoparticles by reductive hydroxyphenol derivatives', *Langmuir*, **27**: 2965–2971.

Li J A, Day D and Gu M (2008), 'Ultra-low energy threshold for cancer photothermal therapy using transferrin-conjugated gold nanorods', *Adv. Mater.*, **20**: 3866–3871.

Li L, Chu Y, Yang Liu Y and Wang D (2009), 'Solution-phase synthesis of single-crystalline Fe_3O_4 magnetic nanobelts', *J. Alloys Compounds*, **472**: 271–275.

Li W, Yuan R, Chai Y, Zhou L, Chen S and Li N (2008), 'Immobilization of horseradish peroxidase on chitosan/silica sol–gel hybrid membranes for the preparation of hydrogen peroxide biosensor', *J. Biochem. Biophys. Methods*, **70**: 830–837.

Li Y, Schluesener H J and Xu S (2010) 'Gold nanoparticle-based biosensors', *Gold Bull.*, **43**: 29–41.

Lian S, Wang E, Kang Z, Bai Y, Gao L et al. (2004), 'Synthesis of magnetite nanorods and porous hematite nanorods', *Solid State Commun.*, **129**: 485–490.

Liang H-F, Chen C-T, Chen S-C, Kulkarni A R, Chiu Y-L et al. (2006), 'Paclitaxel-loaded poly(γ-glutamic acid)–poly(lactide) nanoparticles as a targeted drug delivery system for the treatment of liver cancer', *Biomaterials*, **27**: 2051–2059.

Liao H and Hafner J H (2005), 'Gold nanorod bioconjugates', *Chem. Mater.*, **17**: 4636–4641.

Lin J, Qu W and Zhang S (2007), 'Disposable biosensor based on enzyme immobilized on Au–chitosan-modified indium tin oxide electrode with flow injection amperometric analysis', *Anal. Biochem.*, **360**: 288–293.

Lin L, Zhao H, Li J, Tang J, Duan M and Jiang L (2000), 'Study on colloidal Au enhanced DNA sensing by quartz crystal microbalance', *Biochem. Biophys. Res. Commun.*, 2000, **274**: 817–820.

Lin W, Huang Y-W, Zhou X-D and Ma Y (2006), '*In vitro* toxicity of silica nanoparticles in human lung cancer cells', *Toxicol. Appl. Pharmacol.*, **217**: 252–259.

Lin Y E, Vidic R D, Stout J E, McCartney C A and Yu V L (1998), 'Inactivation of *Mycobacterium avium* by copper and silver ions', *Water Res.*, **32**: 1997–2000.

Link S and El-Sayed M A (1999), 'Size and temperature dependence of the plasmon absorption of colloidal gold nanoparticles', *J. Phys. Chem. B*, **103**: 4212–4217.

Liu H L, Hou P, Zhang W X, Kim Y K and Wu J H (2010), 'Synthesis of monosized core–shell Fe_3O_4/Au multifunctional nanoparticles by PVP-assisted nanoemulsion process', *Colloids Surf. A*, **356**: 21–27.

Liu S, Peng L, Yang X, Wu Y and He L (2008), 'Electrochemistry of cytochrome P450 enzyme on nanoparticle-containing membrane-coated electrode and its applications for drug sensing', *Anal. Biochem.*, 375: 209–216.

Liu X, Lloyd M C, Fedorenko I V, Bapat P, Zhukov T et al. (2008), 'Enhanced imaging and accelerated photothermalysis of A549 human lung cancer cells by gold nanospheres', *Nanomedicine*, 3: 617–626.

Liu Z D, Li Y F, Ling J and Huang C Z (2009), 'A localized surface plasmon resonance light-scattering assay of mercury (II) on the basis of Hg^{2+}–DNA complex induced aggregation of gold nanoparticles', *Environ. Sci. Technol.*, **43**: 5022–5027.

Published by Woodhead Publishing Limited, 2013

Lok C-N, Ho C-M, Chen R, He Q-Y, Yu W-Y et al. (2006), 'Proteomic analysis of the mode of antibacterial action of silver nanoparticles', *J. Proteome Res.*, **5**: 916–924.

Loo C, Lin A, Hirsch L, Lee M H, Barton J et al. (2004), 'Nanoshell-enabled photonics-based imaging and therapy of cancer', *Technol. Cancer Res. Treat.*, **3**: 33–40.

Loo C, Lowery A, Halas N, West J and Drezek R (2005), 'Immunotargeted nanoshells for integrated cancer imaging and therapy', *Nano Lett.*, **5**: 709–711.

Lowery A R, Gobin A M, Day E S, Halas N J and West J L (2006), 'Immunonanoshells for targeted photothermal ablation of tumor cells', *Int. J. Nanomed.*, **1**: 149–154.

Lu W, Shen Y, Xie A and Zhang W (2011), 'Green synthesis and characterization of superparamagnetic Fe_3O_4 nanoparticles', *J. Magn. Magn. Mater.*, **322**: 1828–1833.

Lu Z, Dai J, Song X, Wang G and Yang W (2008), 'Facile synthesis of Fe_3O_4/SiO_2 composite nanoparticles from primary silica particles', *Colloids Surf. A*, **317**: 450–456.

Lv G, He F, Wang X, Gao F, Zhang G, Wang T et al. (2008), 'Novel nanocomposite of nano Fe_3O_4 and polylactide nanofibers for application in drug uptake and induction of cell death of leukemia cancer cells', *Langmuir*, **24**: 2151–2156.

Ma Z, Dosev D, Nichkova M, Dumas R K, Gee S J et al. (2009), 'Synthesis and characterization of multifunctional silica core–shell nanocomposites with magnetic and fluorescent functionalities', *J. Magn. Magn. Mater.*, **321**: 1368–1371.

Mallidi S, Larson T, Aaron J, Sokolov K and Emelianov S (2007), 'Molecular specific optoacoustic imaging with plasmonic nanoparticles', *Opt. Express*, **15**: 6583–6588.

Mariko U, Mariko H-S, Kingo U and Yasuhide N (2005), 'Photo-control of the polyplexes formation between DNA

Published by Woodhead Publishing Limited, 2013

and photo-cation generatable water-soluble polymers', *Curr. Drug Deliv.*, **2**: 207–214.

Marques R F C, Garcia C, Lecante P, Ribeiro S J L, Noe L et al. (2008), 'Electro-precipitation of Fe_3O_4 nanoparticles in ethanol', *J. Magn. Magn. Mater.*, **320**: 2311–2315.

McBain S C, Yiu H H and Dobson J (2008), 'Magnetic nanoparticles for gene and drug delivery', *Int. J. Nanomed.*, **3**: 169–180.

McIntosh C M, Esposito E A, Boal A K, Simard J M, Martin C T et al. (2001), 'Inhibition of DNA transcription using cationic mixed monolayer protected gold clusters', *J. Am. Chem. Soc.*, **123**: 7626–7629.

Mie G (1908), 'A contribution to the optics of turbid media, especially colloidal metallic suspensions', *Ann. Phys.*, **25**: 377–445.

Min K H, Park K, Kim Y-S, Bae S M, Lee S et al. (2008), 'Hydrophobically modified glycol chitosan nanoparticles-encapsulated camptothecin enhance the drug stability and tumor targeting in cancer therapy', *J. Control. Release*, **127**: 208–218.

Mirkin C A, Letsinger R L, Mucic R C and Storhoff J J (1996), 'A DNA-based method for rationally assembling nanoparticles into macroscopic materials', *Nature*, **382**: 607–609.

Moller R and Fritzsche W (2007), 'Metal nanoparticle-based detection for DNA analysis', *Curr. Pharm. Biotechnol.*, **8**: 274–285.

Murphy C J, Sau T K, Gole A M, Orendorff C J, Gao J et al. (2005), 'Anisotropic metal nanoparticles: synthesis, assembly, and optical applications', *J. Phys. Chem. B*, **109**: 13857–13870.

Murphy C J, Gole A M, Hunyadi S E and Orendorff C J (2006), 'One-dimensional colloidal gold and silver nanostructures', *Inorg. Chem.*, **45**: 7544–7554.

Published by Woodhead Publishing Limited, 2013

Nam J M, Stoeva S I and Mirkin C A (2004), 'Bio-bar-code-based DNA detection with PCR-like sensitivity', *J. Am. Chem. Soc.*, **126**: 5932–5933.

Naveenraj S, Anandan S, Kathiravan A, Renganathan R and Ashokkumar M (2010), 'The interaction of sonochemically synthesized gold nanoparticles with serum albumins', *J. Pharm. Biomed. Anal.*, **53**: 804–810.

Ni S, Wang X, Zhou G, Yang F, Wang J et al. (2009), 'Hydrothermal synthesis of Fe_3O_4 nanoparticles and its application in lithium ion battery', *Mater. Lett.*, **63**: 2701–2703.

Niidome T, Nakashima K, Takahashi H and Niidome Y (2004), 'Preparation of primary amine-modified gold nanoparticles and their transfection ability into cultivated cells', *Chem. Commun.*, **17**: 1978–1979.

Niidome T, Yamagata M, Okamoto Y, Akiyama Y, Takahashi H et al. (2006), 'PEG-modified gold nanorods with a stealth character for *in vivo* applications', *J. Controlled Rel.*, **114**: 343–347.

Niidome Y, Niidome T, Yamada S, Horiguchi Y, Takahashi H et al. (2006), 'Pulsed-laser induced fragmentation and dissociation of DNA immobilized on gold nanoparticles', *Mol. Cryst. Liq. Cryst.*, **445**: 201/[491]–206/[496].

Njagi J and Andreescu S (2007), 'Stable enzyme biosensors based on chemically synthesized Au–polypyrrole nanocomposites', *Biosens. Bioelectron.*, **23**: 168–175.

Ozkaya T, Toprak M S, Baykal A, Kavas H, Koseoglu Y et al. (2009), 'Synthesis of Fe_3O_4 nanoparticles at 100 °C and its magnetic characterization', *J. Alloys Compounds*, **472**: 18–23.

Paciotti G F, Kingston D G I and Tamarkin L (2006), 'Colloidal gold nanoparticles: a novel nanoparticle platform for developing multifunctional tumor-targeted drug delivery vectors', *Drug Dev. Res.*, **67**: 47–54.

Published by Woodhead Publishing Limited, 2013

Pang L, Li J, Jiang J, Shen G and Yu R (2006), 'DNA point mutation detection based on DNA ligase reaction and nano-Au amplification: a piezoelectric approach', *Anal. Biochem.*, **358**: 99–103.

Pankhurst Q A, Connolly J, Jones S K and Dobson J (2003), 'Applications of magnetic nanoparticles in biomedicine', *Appl. Phys.*, **36**: R167–R181.

Panneerselvam P, Morad N and Tan K A (2011), 'Magnetic nanoparticles (Fe_3O_4) impregnated onto tea waste for the removal of nickel (II) from aqueous solution', *J. Hazard. Mater.*, **186**: 160–168.

Papavassiliou G C (1979), 'Optical properties of small inorganic and organic metal particles', *Prog. Solid State Chem.*, **12**: 185–271.

Papisov M I, Bogdanov A, Schaffer B, Nossiff N, Shen T et al. (1993), 'Colloidal magnetic-resonance contrast agents-effect of particle surface on biodistribution', *J. Magn. Magn. Mater.*, **122**: 383–386.

Peng X, Wang Y, Tang X and Liu W (2011), 'Functionalized magnetic core–shell Fe_3O_4/SiO_2 nanoparticles as selectivity-enhanced chemosensor for Hg(II)', *Dyes Pigments*, **91**: 26–32.

Petri-Fink A, Chastellain M, Juillerat-Jeanneret L, Ferrari A and Hofmann H (2005), 'Development of functionalized superparamagnetic iron oxide nanoparticles for interaction with human cancer cells', *Biomaterials*, **26**: 2685–2694.

Pissuwan D, Niidome T, Michael B. Cortie M B (2011), 'The forthcoming applications of gold nanoparticles in drug and gene delivery systems', *Journal of Controlled Release*, **149**, 65–71.

Pissuwan D, Valenzuela SM and Cortie MB (2006), 'Therapeutic possibilities of plasmonically heated gold nanoparticles', *Trends Biotechnol.*, **24**: 62–67.

Published by Woodhead Publishing Limited, 2013

Pissuwan D, Valenzuela S M and Cortie M B (2008), 'Prospects for gold nanorod particles in diagnostic and therapeutic applications', *Biotechnol. Genet. Eng. Rev.*, **25**: 93–112.

Pitsillides C M, Joe E K, Wei X, Anderson R R, and Lin C P (2003), 'Selective cell targeting with light-absorbing microparticles and nanoparticles', *Biophys. J.*, **84**: 4023–4032.

Polte J, Erler R, Thnemann A F, Sokolov S, Ahner T T et al. (2010), 'Nucleation and growth of gold nanoparticles studied via *in situ* small angle X-ray scattering at millisecond time resolution', *J. Am. Chem. Soc.*, **132**: 1296–1301.

Porter A E, Muller K, Skepper J, Midgley P and Welland M (2006), 'Uptake of C60 by human monocyte macrophages, its localization and implications for toxicity: studied by high resolution electron microscopy and electron tomography', *Acta Biomater.*, **2**: 409–419.

Pustovalov V K, Smetannikov A S and Zharov V P (2008), 'Photothermal and accompanied phenomena of selective nanophotothermolysis with gold nanoparticles and laser pulses', *Laser Phys. Lett.*, **5**: 775–792.

Qiang Y, Antomy J, Sharma A, Nutting J, Sikes D and Meyer D (2006), 'Iron/iron oxide core–shell nanoclusters for biomedical applications', *J. Nanopart. Res.*, **8**: 489–496.

Rashdan S, Bououdina M and Al-Saie A (2010a), 'Synthesis, characterization of SiO_2 and TiO_2 coated Fe_3O_4 nanoparticles for biomedical applications', *Int. J. Mater. Eng. Innovat.*, **1**: 426–435.

Rashdan S, Bououdina M, Al-Saie A, Ghanem E, Bin-Thani A et al. (2010b), 'Synthesis, crystal structure and magnetic properties of iron oxide nanoparticles for biomedical applications', *Int. J. Nanopart.*, **3**: 220–228.

Published by Woodhead Publishing Limited, 2013

Rena L and Chow G M (2003), 'NIR-sensitive Au–Au_2S nanoparticles for drug delivery', *Mater. Sci. Eng. C*, **23**: 113–116.

Rosi N L and Mirkin C A (2005), 'Nanostructures in biodiagnostics', *Chem. Rev.*, **105**: 1547–1562.

Roth J (1996), 'The silver anniversary of gold: 25 years of the colloidal gold marker system for immunocytochemistry and histochemistry', *Histochem. Cell Biol.*, **106**: 1–8.

Roy K, Mao H-Q, Huanhg S-K and Leong K-W (1999), 'Oral gene delivery with chitosan–DNA nanoparticles generates immunologic protection in a murine model of peanut allergy', *Nat. Med.*, **5**: 387–391.

Ruparelia J P, Chatterjee A K, Duttagupta S P and Mukherji S (2008), 'Strain specificity in antimicrobial activity of silver and copper nanoparticles', *Acta Biomater.*, **4**: 707–716.

Sadeghi B, Jamali M, Kia Sh, Amininia A and Ghafari S (2010), 'Synthesis and characterization of silver nanoparticles for antibacterial activity', *Int. J. Nano. Dimen.*, **1**: 119–124.

Saha B, Bhattacharya J, Mukherjee A, Ghosh A K, Santra C R et al. (2007), '*In vitro* structural and functional evaluation of gold nanoparticles conjugated antibiotics', *Nanoscale Res. Lett.*, **2**: 614–622.

Saiyed Z M, Parasramka M, Telang S D and Ramchand C N (2007), 'Extraction of DNA from agarose gel using magnetic nanoparticles (magnetite or Fe_3O_4)', *Anal. Biochem.*, **363**: 288–290.

Sanpui P, Pandey S B, Ghosh S S and Chattopadhyay A (2008), 'Green fluorescent protein for *in situ* synthesis of highly uniform Au nanoparticles and monitoring protein denaturation', *J. Colloid Interface Sci.*, **326**: 129–137.

Sardar R, Heap T B and Shumaker-Parry J S (2007), 'Versatile solid phase synthesis of gold nanoparticle dimers using an asymmetric functionalization approach', *J. Am. Chem. Soc.*, **129**: 5356–5357.

Sathishkumar M, Sneha K, Won S W, Cho C-W, Kim S et al. (2009), 'Cinnamon zeylanicum bark extract and powder mediated green synthesis of nano-crystalline silver particles and its bactericidal activity', *Colloids Surf. B*, **73**: 332–338.

Shenhar R, Norsten T B and Rotello V M (2005), 'Polymer-mediated nanoparticle assembly: structural control and applications', *Adv. Mater.*, **17**: 657–669.

Shenoy D B and Amiji M M (2005), 'Poly(ethylene oxide)-modified poly(epsilon-caprolactone) nanoparticles for targeted delivery of tamoxifen in breast cancer', *Int. J. Pharmac.*, **293**: 261–270.

Shumyantseva V V, Carrara S, Bavastrello V, Riley D J, Bulko T V et al. (2005), 'Direct electron transfer between cytochrome P450scc and gold nanoparticles on screen-printed rhodium–graphite electrodes', *Biosens. Bioelectron.*, **21**: 217–222.

Sokolov K, Aaron J, Hsu B, Nida D, Gillenwater A, Follen M et al. (2003a), 'Optical systems for *in vivo* molecular imaging of cancer', *Technol. Cancer Res. Treat.*, **2**: 491–504.

Sokolov K, Follen M, Aaron J, Pavlova I, Malpica A, Lotan R et al. (2003b), 'Real-time vital optical imaging of precancer using anti-epidermal growth factor receptor antibodies conjugated to gold nanoparticles', *Cancer Res.*, **63**: 1999–2004.

Sondi I and Salopek-Sondi B (2004), 'Silver nanoparticles as antimicrobial agent: a case study on *E. coli* as a model for Gram-negative bacteria', *J. Colloid. Interface Sci.*, **275**: 177–182.

Song C, Zhao G, Zhang P and Rosi N L (2010), 'Expeditious synthesis and assembly of sub-100 nm hollow spherical gold nanoparticle superstructures', *J. Am. Chem. Soc.*, **132**: 14033–14035.

Published by Woodhead Publishing Limited, 2013

Sonnichsen C, Franzl T, Wilk T, von Plessen G and Feldmann J (2002), 'Plasmon resonances in large noble-metal clusters', *New J. Phys.*, **4**: 93.1–93.8.

Sperling R A, Gil P R, Zhang F, Zanella M and Parak W J (2008), 'Biological applications of gold nanoparticles', *Chem. Soc. Rev.*, **37**, 1896–1908.

Spuch-Calvar M, Pérez-Juste J and Liz-Marzán L M (2007), 'Hematite spindles with optical functionalities: Growth of gold nanoshells and assembly of gold nanorods', *J. Colloid Interface Sci.*, **310**: 297–301.

Strobel R and Pratsinis S E (2009), 'Direct synthesis of maghemite, magnetite and wustite nanoparticles by flame spray pyrolysis', *Adv. Powder Technol.*, **20**: 190–194.

Sun S and Zeng H (2002), 'Size-controlled synthesis of magnetite nanoparticles', *J. Am. Chem. Soc.*, **124**: 8204–8205.

Sun S, Zeng H, Robinson D B, Raoux S, Rice P M et al. (2004), 'Monodisperse MFe_2O_4 (M = Fe, Co, Mn) nanoparticles', *J. Am. Chem. Soc*, **126**: 273–279.

Takahashi H, Niidome Y and Yamada S (2005), 'Controlled release of plasmid DNA from gold nanorods induced by pulsed near-infrared light', *Chem. Commun.*, **17**: 2247–2249.

Tang T, Krysmann M J and Hamley I W (2008), '*In situ* formation of gold nanoparticles with a thermoresponsive block copolymer corona', *Colloids Surf. A*, **317**: 764–767.

Tangkuaram T, Ponchio C, Kangkasomboon T, Katikawong P and Veerasai W (2007), 'Design and development of a highly stable hydrogen peroxide biosensor on screen printed carbon electrode based on horseradish peroxidase bound with gold nanoparticles in the matrix of chitosan', *Biosens. Bioelectron.*, **22**: 2071–2080.

Tartaj P, Morales P M, Veintemillas-Verdaguer S, Gonnzalez-Carreño T and Serna C J (2003), 'The preparation of magnetic nanoparticles for applications in biomedicine', *J. Phys. D*, **36**: R182–R197.

Tavakoli A, Sohrabi M and Kargari A (2007), 'A review of methods for synthesis of nanostructured metals with emphasis on iron compounds', *Chem. Papers*, **61**: 151–170.

Teja A S and Koh P-Y (2009), 'Synthesis, properties, and applications of magnetic iron oxide nanoparticles', *Prog. Crystal Growth Character. Mater.*, **55**: 22–45.

Thirumurugan G and Dhanaraju M D (2011), 'Novel biogenic metal nanoparticles for pharmaceutical applications', *Adv. Sci. Lett.*, **4**: 339–348.

Tirelli N (2006), '(Bio)Responsive nanoparticles', *Curr. Opin. Colloid Interface Sci.*, **11**: 210–216.

Tran H V, Tran L D, Ba C T, Vu H D, Nguyen T N et al. (2010a), 'Synthesis, characterization, antibacterial and antiproliferative activities of monodisperse chitosan-based silver nanoparticles', *Colloids Surf. A*, **360**: 32–40.

Tran L D, Hoang N M, Mai T T, Tran H V, Nguyen N T et al. (2010b), 'Nanosized magnetofluorescent Fe_3O_4–curcumin conjugate for multimodal monitoring and drug targeting', *Colloids Surf. A* **371**: 104–112.

Trehin R, Figueiredo J L, Pittet M J, Weissleder R, Josephson L et al. (2006), 'Fluorescent nanoparticles uptake for brain tumor visualization', *Neoplasia*, **8**: 302–311.

Ulman A (1996), 'Formation and structure of self-assembled monolayers', *Chem. Rev.*, **96**: 1533–1554.

Vo-Dinh T and Cullum B (2000), 'Biosensors and biochips: advances in biological and medical diagnostics', *Fresenius J. Anal. Chem.*, **366**: 540–551.

Wang C, Yan J, Cui X and Wang H (2011), 'Synthesis of raspberry-like monodisperse magnetic hollow hybrid nanospheres by coating polystyrene template with Fe_3O_4/SiO_2 particles', *J. Colloid Interface Sci.*, **354**: 94–99.

Published by Woodhead Publishing Limited, 2013

Wang H, Hu P, Pan D, Tian J, Zhang S et al. (2010), 'Carbothermal reduction method for Fe_3O_4 powder synthesis', *J. Alloys Compounds*, **502**: 338–340.

Wang J, Polsky R and Xu D (2001), 'Silver-enhanced colloidal gold electrochemical stripping detection of DNA hybridization', *Langmuir*, **17**: 5739–5741.

Wang J, Xu D and Polsky R (2002), 'Magnetically-induced solid-state electrochemical detection of DNA hybridization', *J. Am. Chem. Soc.*, **124**: 4208–4209.

Wang S, Cao H, Gu F, Li C and Huang G (2008), 'Synthesis and magnetic properties of iron/silica core–shell nanostructures', *J. Alloys Compounds*, **457**: 560–564.

Wang X, Zhao Z, Qu J, Wang Z and Qiu J (2010), 'Fabrication and characterization of magnetic Fe_3O_4–CNT composites', *J. Phys. Chem. Solids*, **71**: 673–676.

Wang Z, Guo H, Yu Y and He N (2006), 'Synthesis and characterization of a novel magnetic carrier with its composition of Fe_3O_4/Carbon using hydrothermal reaction', *J. Magn. Magn. Mater.*, **302**: 397–404.

Wei F, Dinesh S, Jane L, Curtis C, Graham J et al. (2005), 'Biomedical applications of gold nanoparticles functionalized using hetero-bifunctional poly(ethylene glycol) spacer', *Mater. Res. Soc. Symp. Proc.*, **845**: AA5.4.1–AA5.4.6.

Weissleder R (2001), 'A clearer vision for *in vivo* imaging', *Nat. Biotechnol.*, **19**: 316.

Weizmann Y, Patolsky F and Willner I (2001), 'Amplified detection of DNA and analysis of single base mismatches by the catalyzed deposition of gold on Au-nanoparticles', *Analyst*, **126**: 1502–1504.

Wijaya A, Schaffer S B, Pallares I G and Hamad-Schifferli K (2008), 'Selective release of multiple DNA oligonucleotides from gold nanorods', *ACS Nano*, **3**: 80–86.

Williams D N, Ehrman S H and Holoman T R P (2006), 'Evaluation of the microbial growth response to inorganic nanoparticles', *J. Nanobiotechnol.*, **4**: 1–8.

Willner B, Katz E and Willner I (2006), 'Electrical contacting of redox proteins by nanotechnological means', *Curr. Opin. Biotechnol.*, **17**: 589–596.

Willner I, Patolsky F, Weizmann Y and Willner B (2002), 'Amplified detection of single-base mismatches in DNA using microgravimetric quartz crystal microbalance transduction', *Talanta*, **56**: 847–856.

Wong B, Yoda S and Howdle S M (2007), 'The preparation of gold nanoparticle composites using supercritical carbon dioxide', *J. Supercrit. Fluids*, **42**: 282–287.

Wong J. E, Gahawar A. K, Müller-Schulte D, Bahadur D and Richtering W (2007), 'Layer-by layer assembly of a magnetic nanoparticle shell on a thermoresponsive microgel core', *J. Magn. Magn. Mater.*, **311**: 219–223.

Wu X, Tang J, Zhang Y and Wang H (2009), 'Low temperature synthesis of Fe_3O_4 nanocrystals by hydrothermal decomposition of a metallorganic molecular precursor', *Mater. Sci. Eng. B* **157**: 81–86.

Xiao Y, Patolsky F, Katz E, Hainfeld J F and Willner I (2003), 'Plugging into enzymes: nanowiring of redox enzymes by a gold nanoparticle', *Science*, **299**: 1877–1881.

Xu J, Yang H, Fu W, Du K, Sui Y et al. (2007), 'Preparation and magnetic properties of magnetite nanoparticles by sol–gel method', *J. Magn. Magn. Mater.*, **309**: 307–311.

Xu M, Zhang Y, Zhang Z, Shen Y, Zhao M and Pan G (2011), 'Study on the adsorption of Ca^{2+}, Cd^{2+} and Pb^{2+} by magnetic Fe_3O_4 yeast treated with EDTA dianhydride', *Chem. Eng. J.*, **168**: 737–745.

Xu Q, Mao C, Liu N N, Zhu J J and Sheng J (2006), 'Direct electrochemistry of horseradish peroxidase based on

Published by Woodhead Publishing Limited, 2013

biocompatible carboxymethyl chitosan–gold nanoparticle nanocomposite', *Biosens. Bioelectron.*, **22**: 768–773.

Xu X, Wang J, Yang C, Wu H and Yang F (2009), 'Sol–gel formation of γ-Fe_2O_3/SiO_2 nanoparticles: Effects of different iron raw material', *J. Alloys Compounds*, **468**: 414–420.

Xuan S, Hao L, Jiang W, Gong X, Hu Y et al. (2007), 'Preparation of water-soluble magnetic nanocrystals through hydrothermal approach', *J. Magn. Magn. Mater.*, **308**: 210–213.

Xue M H, Xu Q, Zhou M and Zhu J J (2006), 'In situ immobilization of glucose oxidase in chitosan–gold nanoparticle hybrid film on Prussian Blue modified electrode for high-sensitivity glucose detection', *Electrochem. Commun.*, **8**: 1468–1474.

Yallapu M M, Gupta B K, Jaggi M and Chauhan S C (2010), 'Fabrication of curcumin encapsulated PLGA nanoparticles for improved therapeutic effects in metastatic cancer cells', *J. Colloid Interface Sci.*, **351**: 19–29.

Yan A, Liu X, Qiu G, Wu H, Yi R et al. (2008), 'Solvothermal synthesis and characterization of size-controlled Fe_3O_4 nanoparticles', *J. Alloys Compounds*, **458**: 487–491.

Yan H, Zhang J, You C, Song Z, Yu B et al. (2009), 'Influence of different synthesis conditions on properties of Fe_3O_4 nanoparticles', *Mater. Chem. Phys.*, **113**: 46–52.

Yang G, Yuan R and Chai Y Q (2008), 'A high-sensitive amperometric hydrogen peroxide biosensor based on the immobilization of hemoglobin on gold colloid/L-cysteine/gold colloid/nanoparticles Pt–chitosan composite film-modified platinum disk electrode', *Colloids Surf. B*, **61**: 93–100.

Yang X, Skrabalak S E, Li Z-Y, Xia Y and Wang L V (2007a), 'Photoacoustic tomography of a rat cerebral cortex *in*

Published by Woodhead Publishing Limited, 2013

vivo with Au nanocages as an optical contrast agent', *Nano Lett.*, **7**: 3798–3802.

Yang X, Wang Q, Wang K, Tan W and Li H (2007b), 'Enhanced surface plasmon resonance with the modified catalytic growth of Au nanoparticles', *Biosens. Bioelectron.*, **22**: 1106–1110.

Yangde Z, Zhaowu Z, Weihua Z, Xingyan L, Zhenfa L et al. (2008), 'The roles of hydrochloric acid and polyethylene glycol in magnetic fluids', *J. Magn. Magn. Mater.*, **320**: 1328–1334.

Yao Z-F, Huanga K-L, Liu S-Q, Song X-Z, Li Y-H et al. (2011), 'A novel method to prepare gold-nanoparticle-modified nanowires and their spectrum study', *Chem. Eng. J.*, **166**: 378–383.

Yu A, Liang Z, Cho J and Caruso F (2003), 'Nanostructured electrochemical sensor based on dense gold nanoparticle films', *Nano Lett.*, **3**: 1203–1207.

Yu D-H, Lu Q, Xie J, Fang C and Chen H-Z (2010), 'Peptide-conjugated biodegradable nanoparticles as a carrier to target paclitaxel to tumor neovasculature', *Biomaterials*, **31**: 2278–2292.

Yu X, Liu S and Yu J (2011), 'Superparamagnetic γ-Fe_2O_3/SiO_2/TiO_2 composite microspheres with superior photocatalytic properties', *Appl. Catal. B*, **104**: 12–20.

Yuanbi Z, Zumin Q and Jiaying H (2008), 'Preparation and analysis of Fe_3O_4 magnetic nanoparticles used as targeted-drug carriers', *Chin. J. Chem. Eng.*, **16**: 451–455.

Zhang C, Zhao L-Q, Dong Y-F, Zhang X-Y, Lin J et al. (2010), 'Folate-mediated poly(3-hydroxybutyrate-*co*-3-hydroxyoctanoate) nanoparticles for targeting drug delivery', *Eur. J. Pharm. Biopharm.*, **76**: 10–16.

Zhang D, Tong Z, Li S, Zhang X and Ying A (2008), 'Fabrication and characterization of hollow Fe_3O_4 nanospheres in a microemulsion', *Mater. Lett.*, **62**: 4053–4055.

Published by Woodhead Publishing Limited, 2013

Zhang E, Tang Y, Peng K, Guo C and Zhang Y (2008), 'Synthesis and magnetic properties of γ-Fe_2O_3/SiO_2 core–shell nanoparticles under hydrothermal conditions', *Solid State Commun.*, **148**: 496–500.

Zhang L, Jiang X, Wang E and Dong S (2005), 'Attachment of gold nanoparticles to glassy carbon electrode and its application for the direct electrochemistry and electrocatalytic behavior of hemoglobin', *Biosens. Bioelectron.*, **21**: 337–345.

Zhang L, Yuan R, Chai Y and Li X (2007), 'Investigation of the electrochemical and electrocatalytic behavior of positively charged gold nanoparticle and L-cysteine film on an Au electrode', *Anal. Chem. Acta*, **596**: 99–105.

Zhang L-Y, Zhu X-J, Sun H-W, Chi G-R, Xu J-X et al. (2010), 'Control synthesis of magnetic Fe_3O_4–chitosan nanoparticles under UV irradiation in aqueous system', *Curr. Appl. Phys.*, **10**: 828–833.

Zhang P, Chu A Y-C, Sham T-K, Yao Y and Lee S-T (2009), 'Chemical synthesis and structural studies of thiol-capped gold nanoparticles', *Can. J. Chem.*, **87**: 335–340.

Zhao D-L, Zeng X-W, Xia Q-S and Tang J-T (2009), 'Preparation and coercivity and saturation magnetization dependence of inductive heating property of Fe_3O_4 nanoparticles in an altering current magnetic field for localized hyperthermia', *J. Alloys Compounds*, **469**: 215–218.

Zhao H Q, Lin L, Li J R, Tang J A, Duan M X et al. (2001), 'DNA biosensor with high sensitivity amplified by gold nanoparticles', *J. Nanopart. Res.*, **3**: 321–323.

Zhao J, Henkens R W, Stonehuerner J, O'Daly J P and Crumbliss A L (1992), 'Direct electron transfer at horseradish peroxidase-colloidal gold modified electrodes', *J. Electroanal. Chem.*, **327**: 109–119.

Zharov V P, Galitovsky V and Viegas M (2003), 'Photothermal detection of local thermal effects during

Published by Woodhead Publishing Limited, 2013

selective nanophotothermolysis', *Appl. Phys. Lett.*, **83**: 4897–4899.

Zharov V P, Galitovskaya E and Viegas M (2004), 'Photothermal guidance for selective photothermolysis with nanoparticles', *Proc SPIE*, **5319**: 291–300.

Zharov V P, Galitovskaya E N, Johnson C and Kelly T (2005a), 'Synergistic enhancement of selective nanophotothermolysis with gold nanoclusters: potential for cancer therapy', *Lasers Surg. Med.*, **37**: 219–226.

Zharov V P, Kim J W, Curiel D T and Everts M (2005b), 'Self-assembling nanoclusters in living systems: application for integrated photothermal nanodiagnostics and nanotherapy', *Nanomedicine*, **1**: 326–345.

Zheng Y Y, Wang X B, Shang L, Li C R, Cui C et al. (2010), 'Fabrication of shape controlled Fe_3O_4 nanostructure', *Mater. Character.*, **61**: 489–492.

Zhou X C, O'Shea S J and Li S F Y (2000), 'Amplified microgravimetric gene sensor using Au nanoparticle modified oligonucleotides', *Chem. Commun.*, **11**: 953–954.

Zhu S Y, Zhang L L, Yu Q, Wang T Z, Chen J et al. (2010), 'Facile synthesis of a novel dendritic nanostructure of Fe_3O_4–Au nanorods', *Mater. Sci. Eng. B*, **175**: 172–175.

Published by Woodhead Publishing Limited, 2013

2

Synergism effects during friction and fretting corrosion experiments – focusing on biomaterials used as orthopedic implants

J. Geringer, Ecole Nationale Supérieure des Mines de Saint-Etienne, France and Penn State University, USA, M. T. Mathew and M. A. Wimmer, Department of Orthopedics, Rush University Medical Center, USA and D. D. Macdonald, Penn State University, USA

DOI: 10.1533/9780857092205.133

Abstract: This chapter is focused on the specific phenomenon of wear (friction and fretting) and corrosion related to orthopedic implants. Both fields are closely linked through mechanical (wear) and chemical (corrosion) factors, and by mutual synergism. After defining differences between wear corrosion and fretting corrosion, we focus our attention on the synergism that exists between mechanical wear and corrosion. Careful characterization of synergistic effects has proved to be the key factor in determining the rates of tribological degradation of metals

Published by Woodhead Publishing Limited, 2013

and alloys. Indeed, an insulating material, such as poly(methylmethacrylate) (PMMA), which is not susceptible to corrosion, is subjected to mechanical damage during wear or fretting. However, in the case of a metal fretting against a soft material like PMMA, the surface does not suffer purely mechanical degradation, as it is too hard and its mechanical properties (Young's modulus, yield strength, etc.) are far superior to those of PMMA. Thus, metals suffer degradation under these circumstances when in contact with an aqueous solution, because of the *conjoint* action of corrosion and mechanics. Thus, this chapter is mainly focused on describing wear and fretting in a corrosive medium, their differences, and determining the effects of corrosion, mechanics and the synergistic interactions between them.

Key words: biomaterial, tribo-corrosion, fretting corrosion, wear corrosion, hip implant.

2.1 Introduction

2.1.1 Orthopedic implants: key issues

The first attempt to treat the misalignment, i.e. osteoclasis (surgical fracture of a bone in order to correct a deformity) and mal-united femoral fracture, in which a previous fracture did not heal correctly, was performed in the sixteenth century (Jakob et al., 2008). In the first quarter of the 1800s, the first hemiarthroplasty (replacement of the femoral head instead of the complete hip joint) was performed for restoring hip joints (Barton, 1827). Since the sixteenth century, significant progress has been made in hip arthroplasty (total hip replacement). Nowadays, hip arthroplasty is a common procedure. In 2007, the number of arthroplasties performed

Published by Woodhead Publishing Limited, 2013

in France was about 120 000 (Postel et al., 1985). Finally, it was 140 000 in 2011 (Holtzwarth et al., 2012). The increase in the number of arthroplasties is general around the world, especially in developed countries. From an economic perspective, fretting corrosion (wear under small displacements (microns)) is one of the main problems resulting in the aseptic loosening of hip prosthesis (*http://www.600bn.com/?tag=orthopedic-implants*). In the United States, orthopedic implants, especially hip implants, are a US$3-billion business, with more than 250 000 being performed each year (Bozic et al., 2009). One in every 30 Americans is walking with a hip prosthesis (*http://www.600bn.com/?tag=orthopedic-implants*). In Europe, the market for hip implants is close to that in the United States, i.e. US$3–4 billion (*http://www.jofdf.org/article.php3?id_article=709*). Metal-on-metal (MoM) bearings for total hip replacement have regained attractiveness due to low volumetric wear, good postoperative stability and design flexibility with reduced bone loss (Bozic et al., 2009). However, detrimental effects of the released metal ions on the local tissues and remote organs have been reported (Jacobs et al., 2006). There is a problem related to the size of debris, but no detrimental effects occur with metallic ions and/or oxide particles, due to dissolution of the metal, as the result of the tribo-corrosion process. In order to investigate tribological (mechanical) and corrosive (electrochemical) challenges using a single set-up, the area of 'tribo-corrosion' has recently made its appearance (Mischler, 2008) as an important field of research and clinical medicine, especially for MoM couples, which are the most implanted material(s) for hip implants in the United States.

Arthroplasty is dedicated to curing weakness of femoral bone resulting from injuries, cancer pathologies, etc. Significant

Published by Woodhead Publishing Limited, 2013

progress has been made in orthopedics and more advanced methods are available to reconstruct a hip joint. As human life expectancy increases, people desire to remain mobile to much greater ages than was previously the case in order to live a normal life. Moreover, the mortality rate of people over 70 years of age due to bone fractures is up to 30% (Simon, 2005). Thus, it is necessary to improve the performance of replacement hip joints. Over the next few years, the use of artificial hip joints will likely increase significantly, and this kind of surgery will become an important clinical management issue in orthopedics, patient health and health policy (Amstutz et al., 1982, 1992; Aspenberg et al., 1992; Andrew et al., 1996).

The cost of hip replacement ranges from US$5000 (for the less complicated surgical operations) to US$15 000 (second surgical operation with rehabilitation), and even more than that if significant infection occurs, post-operative psychological problems develop and/or rehabilitation is complicated. It is for these reasons that lifetime orthopedic implants are a huge issue in health policy, where a 'lifetime orthopedic implant' is one that lasts for the life of the patient. This chapter is dedicated to a review of the performance of lifetime biomaterials, especially of hip implants.

2.1.2 Short historical introduction to hip implants

This section is dedicated to the first 150 years of hip implant evolution. Table 2.1 summarizes some of the major developments in arthroplasty from 1826 to 1973. This is not an exhaustive compilation, but some key points, according to the authors' opinions, are highlighted.

Published by Woodhead Publishing Limited, 2013

Table 2.1 **Advances in hip prosthesis evolution from the 1800s to 1970s.**

Year		Author
1822	Pseudarthrosis	R. White (Hallab et al., 2004)
1827	Pseudarthrosis	J. Barton (Hallab et al., 2004)
1890	Femoral head of ivory	T. Gluck (Gluck, 1890)
1913	Resurfacing of natural joint	J. B. Murphy (Murphy, 1913)
1923	'Molded arthroplasty' using hollow hemisphere made of glass, Pyrex®	M. N. Smith-Petersen (Hallab et al., 2004)
1938	Vitallium® , i.e. Co–Cr alloy	M. N. Smith-Petersen (Schmalzried et al., 2007)
1938	Use of metal on metal, stainless steel	P. Wiles (Wiles, 1958)
1938	Use of PMMA for femoral stem	J. Judet, France (Pramanik et al., 2005)
1938	Fixation using 'fast-setting dental acrylic'	E. J. Haboush (Pramanik et al., 2005)
1939	Femoral head and long-stemmed prosthesis, hemiarthroplasty, without a cup	F. R. Thompson and A. T. Moore (Pramanik et al., 2005)
1949	Total hip prosthesis	Judet brothers (Judet and Judet, 1949)
1951	Metal–metal implants, stainless steel and Co–Cr later	McKee and Ferrar (McKee, 1982)
1958	Total hip replacement Teflon® cup	Sir J. Charnley (Charnley, 1979; McKee, 1982)
1962	Low friction arthroplasty	Sir J. Charnley (Charnley, 1979)
1970	Alumina–alumina total hip arthroplasty	P. Boutin (Boutin, 1972)

Published by Woodhead Publishing Limited, 2013

The first hip joint amputation reported in literature was in 1806 by Dr. Brashear (Brashear, 1853). At the beginning of these surgical procedures, the main aim was to replace the joint, especially for young patients, not only for amputation. White and Barton were the first surgeons who attempted restoration of the mobility of a defective hip joint (Barton, 1827; Hallab et al., 2004). Barton was also the first to highlight that motion prevents fusion of the bone (immobile patient) and later leads to the death of the patient.

Thus, inter-positioning of membranes between the femoral head and acetabulum (pelvis bone) cavity was a strategy for restoring the joint. However, surgical successes were not complete, because of problems of biocompatibility when soft tissues from pigs, for instance, were used for interposition between head and acetabulum.

The first hemiarthroplasty of the hip joint was practiced by Gluck in 1890 (Gluck, 1890). The prosthetic femoral head was manufactured from ivory and its work was classified as being the 'artistic work' of a carpenter or sculptor; however, no following patients were available (Gomez and Morcuende, 2005).

Smith-Petersen tried different materials for the cup arthroplasty, such as glass, Pyrex®, viscaloid (celluloid derivative), Bakelite® and Vitallium® (Co–Cr alloy), after discussing the issues with his dentist. Five hundred Vitallium® moulds, for hip resurfacing (Simpson and Villar, 2010), were implanted with good clinical results (Schmalzried et al., 2007).

Dr Wiles was the first surgeon to use MoM assemblies, e.g. made from stainless steel. He performed the first hip arthroplasty. The femoral head was fixed onto a metallic nail and the cup was screwed onto the acetabulum. One of his patients exhibited a prosthesis lifetime of 13 years (Wiles, 1958).

Published by Woodhead Publishing Limited, 2013

From 1938, significant progress in hip prosthesis development was observed (Pramanik et al., 2005). Judet was the first to use an acrylic material for replacing hip surfaces (Judet and Judet, 1949). This material triggered no specific inflammation of the surrounding tissues. However, the acrylic element failed because of problems in the manufacturing process under large mechanical articulations. The material was satisfactory in terms of biocompatibility, but its failure resulted from inadequate mechanical properties.

Thus, Haboush suggested using another acrylic material, poly(methylmethacrylate) (PMMA), as the bone cement for inserting the metallic femoral stem into the bone. PMMA was considered to be an adhesive material (Pramanik et al., 2005).

After World War II, progress was again promoted in the field of arthroplasty. In 1949, the Judet brothers implanted a short prosthesis made of PMMA; however, failure occurred due to the accumulation of wear debris and inflammation (Judet and Judet, 1949). They suggested generalizing the stemmed prosthesis and it was successful for the next generation of orthopedic surgeons. Modern arthroplasty was initiated by McKee and Farrar, and later by Sir John Charnley. After a first attempt in 1940, McKee and Farrar implanted, in 1948 and reported in 1951, the first total hip prosthesis. Two prostheses were fabricated from stainless steel and they triggered pain after just a few months. However, in one case Co–Cr alloy was employed with significant success with 3 years of satisfactory performance (McKee, 1982). The design of the prosthesis was in the form of a screw. Instead of screws, later ideas were focused on the use of adhesives or cements for maintaining the implanted elements. The solution came from dentists, because they were using cement for fixing teeth in the jawbone. This idea was implemented with significant success. Initially, some investigations were carried out on the biocompatibility with respect to human cells and

Published by Woodhead Publishing Limited, 2013

animal subjects (Henrichsen et al., 1952; Spence, 1954; Wiltse, 1957). The bone cement was used for anchoring the metallic stem in the femoral bone; it also acted as a sealing agent. Thus, Sir Charnley compared two series, i.e. with and without bone cement, and the one with bone cement yielded better results (McKee, 1982). Another concern was the evolution of frictional forces between the head and the cup. After using a Teflon® cup against metal and finding the generation of a large amount of debris, ultra-high-molecular-weight polyethylene (UHMWPE) was introduced to reduce wear debris generation during friction and micro-motion (Charnley, 1979). The gold standard in the form of metal-on-polymer (MoP) was born for hip arthroplasty and all couples of materials, i.e. MoM and ceramic-on-ceramic (CoC), were compared with this couple. Close to this gold standard, the CoC couple was developed by Boutin (Boutin, 1972; Boutin et al., 1988), i.e. alumina against alumina. Figure 2.1 shows a

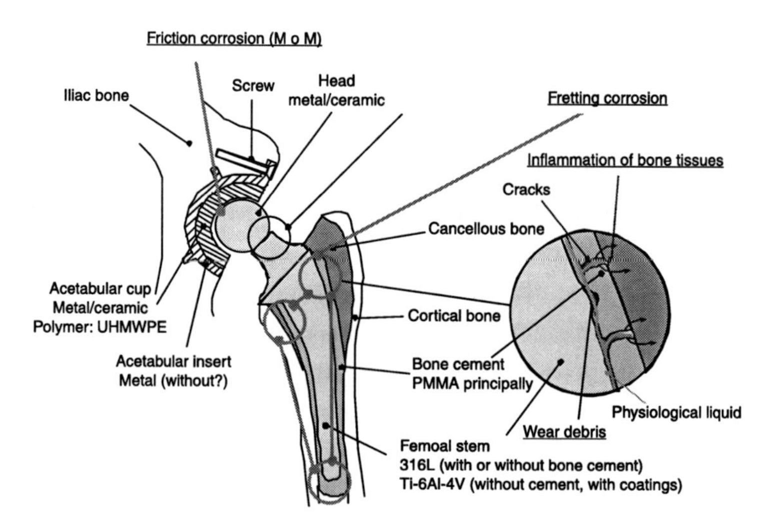

Figure 2.1 Hip implant where wear corrosion (identified as 'friction corrosion' in the figure) and fretting corrosion occur.

Published by Woodhead Publishing Limited, 2013

hip implant in the place of a natural joint. Couples of various materials were described, and the locations where wear corrosion and fretting corrosion occur were identified. When debris is produced, by fretting or wear, inflammation of bone tissues commonly occurs, because of interactions between foreign materials, debris and biological parts, i.e. cells (especially osteoblasts and osteoclasts), tissues and ligaments.

After 15 years of field-testing and follow-up analyses, the CoC couples demonstrated the lowest wear rates, but ongoing investigations continue to be made to increase the fracture toughness of ceramic materials – the Achilles' heel of CoC.

This historical review reveals the significant effect that anchoring the stem in the femoral bone has on implant performance. Alternatively, spray deposition of alumina on the femoral stem for promoting cell/protein adherence and bone integration has been explored. Some investigations were carried out for optimizing the alumina deposit on femoral stems. Rieu et al. promoted this spray and they described the best parameters of ceramic plasma-sprayed coatings for improving the bone fixation (Lopez and Rieu, 1990; Rieu, 1993; Carrerot et al., 1996). Alumina possesses a mineral structure that facilitates bone formation. The key point is the attachment of bone cells on the femoral stem or the external surface of the metal-backing. Designs, shapes and materials were optimized for the best lifetimes of the implants. However, anchoring of the implants, especially femoral stems, depends on cell adhesion on this coating or on bone cement. After the surgical operation, by a few weeks, sealing is commonly observed between the bone and bone cement or alumina coating. This step is completed when patients do not walk. Problems occur when the patient walks, subjecting the implant to a cyclical stress. Indeed, the mechanical properties between bone, bone cement (Wan

Published by Woodhead Publishing Limited, 2013

et al., 1999) and the metal implant or ceramic deposit are hugely different from one implant technology to another. For instance, Young's modulus is approximately 200 GPa for metallic alloys and ceramics, and around 20 (cortical bone) to 2 (cancellous bone) GPa for the bone. One might suggest that deformation of bone is definitely different in one implant than in another under the same stress. Commonly, this phenomenon is called 'stress shielding'. The metallic implant shields stresses that should be imposed on bone cells for improving the process of bone regeneration. Thus, adhesion of bone cells as osteoblasts is not sufficient in implants subjected to micro-motion (Rubin et al., 1993). The primary issue to be considered for effective use of these lightweight materials is to tailor the material and the processes to the parts of the implant structure. Typically, a sheet is used to create two- and (simpler) three-dimensional shapes such as hoods, deck lids and body panels. More complex three-dimensional forms with reinforcing webs are more commonly created from castings. In the selection of the fabrication method, cost and functionality must be analyzed to create both an efficient and a cost-effective solution. Under certain conditions, an assembly created from multiple stamped parts welded together will be the most effective; under other conditions, a single large-scale casting that integrates multiple features may be optimum.

2.1.3 Wear corrosion and fretting corrosion damage on retrieval implants

As described in the previous subsection, displacements occur between the femoral stem and bone after implantation. Thus, this motion between two materials in contact can be divided into two ranges: micro-motions will be characterized as 'fretting corrosion' and larger motions as 'wear corrosion'. A complete definition of these phenomena will be presented in Section 2.2.

Bone remodeling, i.e. regeneration of bone, is efficient when deformation is applied on the bone due to stress transfer between an implant and bone (Niinimaki et al., 1995; Joshi et al., 2000; Niinomi and Nakai, 2011). Prosthesis design is a relevant factor for improving bone remodeling (Boyle and Kim, 2011). However, differences in mechanical properties cannot be neglected between the implant and bone. Thus, debonding is promoted between these materials in contact. The bone cement between the femoral stem and the bone could act as a bumper (cushion effect), but it is not sufficient for promoting bone remodeling. Debonding involves first fretting and wear, and then debris generation. The debris is inorganic and metallic material, and it can reach bone tissues (Langlais, 1993). In addition, the presence of debris disturbs cells' activity, i.e. the interaction between osteoblasts and osteoclasts. At the end of this process, implant retrieval occurs and hence another surgical operation is required ('reintervention') (Waterhouse, 1982; Kovacs et al., 1997). After retrieval, oxide debris is sometimes located on the femoral stem (Zhang et al., 2009) due to fretting corrosion between the stem and bone cement or bone. Moreover, corrosion products can be deposited between the head and the neck due to fretting corrosion (Pellier et al., 2011).

Commonly, fretting occurs when reciprocal displacement is lower than 100 μm and wear occurs for higher displacements. Concerning hip implants, if wear occurs (a few millimeters) between the femoral stem and bone, the motion of the hip implant should produce pain in patients. Consequently, wear degradation is not usual for the assembly of femoral stem bone cement or bone. However, between the head and cup, the amplitude of the displacement could be higher than 100 μm. According to ISO 14242-1:2002

(Implants for surgery – Wear of total hip-joint prostheses – Part 1: Loading and displacement parameters for wear-testing machines and corresponding environmental conditions for test), motions due to angular displacements are higher than a few hundred micrometers. For MoP assemblies, the metallic head is subjected to degradation even though the counterpart UHMWPE is a soft ('smooth') material compared with the metal. The repeated cycles of loading involve the creation of micro-grooves on the metallic head (Oliveira et al., 2011) and especially plastic deformation. For another type of couple (head and cup) with MoM contact, the surfaces in contact are subjected to wear due to relative displacements. Moreover, when small amounts of debris are dispersed in the surrounding physiological fluid and tissues adjacent to the joint, cobalt ions and other metallic ions are also released due to wear and corrosion of the metal component (Yan et al., 2009). Fretting and/or wear promote depassivation of metallic materials, rupturing the passive film due to wear, and corrosion is triggered in usually passive metals. Thus, in the case of all implants, including MoP and MoM, debris (ions and particles) is the link between implants and tissue response that is known as inflammation, and later leads to aseptic loosening of implant. Fretting and wear result in depassivation of the metal, i.e. destroying a passive film that is only a few nanometers thick (Fischmeister and Roll, 1984; Wegrelius et al., 1999; Nicic and Macdonald, 2008; Heuer et al., 2011; Macdonald, 2011). The thickness depends on the medium and the materials; however, in a saline solution, it is found that the passive oxide film is 3–5 nm on a typical stainless steel. Mechanical wear or fretting promotes destruction of the passive film and consequently promotes corrosion. The role of the passive film is essential in determining the degradation of passive metals and alloys, including stainless steels or any metallic

Published by Woodhead Publishing Limited, 2013

alloy due to tribo-corrosion (Mischler et al., 1999). The details of the mechanisms of degradation are complex. Some questions still exist as to the mechanistic details, because it is difficult to differentiate wear mechanisms and corrosion kinetics. Corrosion kinetics could be accelerated due to mechanical wear, but the other way is also possible, i.e. corrosion might accelerate wear. In particular, for biomedical applications, this synergistic interaction between wear and corrosion is relevant and some investigations are in progress to better understand the role of synergism in bioimplant systems (hip implants and dental implants) (Mathew et al., 2009). Following this, the relevant points about this synergism will be described, because of the significant impact on the degradation process.

2.2 Wear corrosion and fretting corrosion: theoretical background

This section will present a summary of the theoretical background related to wear corrosion and fretting corrosion. Both topics are related to the topic of tribo-corrosion. Wood (2010) attempted to provide an overview of this research area. As previously mentioned, the formation and removal of the passive film is a key aspect of the metal's behavior during the tribo-corrosion process and more generally the lifetime of metals (Macdonald, 1999). The tribo-corrosion process in orthopedic implants needs to be discussed in terms of the specific couple of interest – MoP, MoM or CoC.

The CoC couple is considered as a no-wear couple if we consider the hip walking simulator tests. The wear rate is 500 times lower than that for MoP couples and 50 times lower than that for MoM couples (Essner et al., 2005). The usual wear tests, i.e. continuous, are not significant for discriminating

Published by Woodhead Publishing Limited, 2013

ceramic materials. Best experimental procedures for wear tests of CoC couples are related to shock. This result is related to the comparison between *in vivo* and *in vitro* explanted ceramic implants. Some studies highlight such observations through the comparison between retrieval implants and worn implants involved in specific shock devices with micro-separation (Nevelos et al., 2000, 2001; Stewart et al., 2003; Clarke et al., 2009). Recently, some results were provided from a specific device for which the micro-separation is controlled. The applied normal force on the head-cup assembly could reach 9000 N, under the most severe conditions, and the micro-separation up to 1.3 mm (Uribe et al., 2012). The wear stripes are similar to those highlighted on retrieval implants. Finally, the CoC couple is worn by the shock mechanism in order to reproduce the *in vivo* retrieval implant. This typical mechanism of wear will not be detailed in the following test. Notwithstanding, this mechanism should be interesting to study experimentally and theoretically during the next investigations for MoP and MoM couples.

Thus, in this section, we will address fretting corrosion and wear corrosion without micro-separation.

2.2.1 Mechanical and electrochemical parameters for studying tribo-corrosion

The mechanical parameters that apply during tribo-corrosion experiments have been well described by many authors for a long time. In the 1880s, Hertz (Hertz, 1882) defined contact mechanics through an experimental investigation. Furthermore, a particular emphasis on this field was provided by Greenwood and Williamson (1966), Johnson (1985) and Hills et al. (1993).

From a purely mechanical point of view of tribo-corrosion, it is necessary to define the basics of contact mechanics. The

Published by Woodhead Publishing Limited, 2013

mechanical properties of both materials (solid) in contact (Young's modulus, Poisson's ratio), can be summarized in terms of six relevant mechanical values:

- The relative displacement between both solids in contact.
- The normal load, F_n, i.e. load applied during wear between materials in contact.
- The tangential load, F_t, i.e. load perpendicular to the normal load.
- The friction coefficient, $\mu = F_t/F_n$.
- The dissipated energy during wear, $E = \int F_t dl$.
- The contact width, $2a$.

These mechanical parameters make it possible to understand the tribo-corrosion phenomenon. The principal physical phenomenon is the dissipated energy during wear. This energy is mechanically related to destruction of the passive film. Energy dissipation is also linked to the corrosive behavior of metals, by transferring the mechanical energy to chemical processes. It is worth noting that the chemical energy comes from the oxidation–reduction reactions, i.e. oxidation of the metal and reduction of water (or hydronium ion).

Secondly, the electrochemical parameters are related to two different conditions: the open circuit potential (OCP) can be measured between a reference electrode, such as the standard calomel electrode (SCE), and the investigated metal sample. This device is the simplest one, since it involves only two electrodes. However, the input impedance of the voltmeter is a key issue, because the voltage-measuring device should, ideally, not draw any current and hence should be as high as possible (typically 10^{10}–10^{12} ohms). The second type of experiment employs an imposed potential, using a three-electrode device – a reference electrode, the sample (working electrode) and a counter electrode that is commonly platinum wire. In this

Published by Woodhead Publishing Limited, 2013

configuration the potential between the working electrode and the reference electrode is controlled by a potentiostat, which automatically controls the current between the working electrode and the counter electrode, so as to maintain the control function (the desired potential between the working electrode and the reference electrode). The main goal of this kind of experiment is to measure the current density and then to calculate the metal mass loss by applying the well-known Faraday law (Macdonald, 1999). Thus, the current density can be related to the rates of chemical reactions that occur during metal dissolution. A more detailed description of electrochemical measurements is described elsewhere, to which the reader is referred (Mischler, 2008). Electrochemical impedance spectroscopy (EIS) is capable of providing detailed information on the phenomena related to tribo-corrosion and has been used to great effect for this purpose by the present authors (Geringer and Macdonald, 2012). The power of EIS lies in the fact that it is a frequency domain technique that is capable of probing electrochemical phenomena over a wide range of relaxation times in a single experiment (Macdonald and McKubre, 1982). Pellier et al. (2011) shows that decreasing the OCP during wear and/or fretting is entirely related to the decrease of the polarization resistance due to destruction of the passive film. Another point is the evolution of the pseudo-capacitance of the metallic sample under tribo-corrosion exposure, and some investigations are in progress on this topic (Geringer et al., 2010).

2.2.2 Fretting corrosion and wear corrosion mechanisms: similarities and differences

A review of the literature reveals that some of the published works focus on defining and describing fretting corrosion mechanisms (Waterhouse, 1982; Geringer et al., 2005,

Published by Woodhead Publishing Limited, 2013

2006), while others concentrate on defining and describing wear corrosion mechanisms (Celis et al., 2006; Geringer et al., 2009). The essential features of these degradation mechanisms and a comparison between both types of tribo-corrosion processes have been summarized by one of the present authors (Geringer et al., 2011).

Both phenomena reside within the realm of tribo-corrosion (Wood, 2010). As the result of abrasion, even if one of the materials is smooth, the protective oxide layer is destroyed and the corrosion of the metal component of the couple occurs at an accelerated rate. The relevant differentiating feature is the relative displacement between both materials in contact. If $e < 1$, as defined by $e = D/a$, where D is the relative displacement and a is the half contact width, a confined zone exists during the tribological experiment, resulting in classical fretting corrosion. On the other hand, if $e > 1$, the process is defined as 'wear corrosion'. This means that in the case of $e < 1$, in the confined zone, the passive film is not rebuilt and the corrosion of the metal is continuously enhanced during the wear tests. On the contrary, during sliding wear, the oxide film is rebuilt because part of the worn surface is exposed to the bulk solution without the presence of the slide. As noted elsewhere (Geringer et al., 2005), the wear rate of stainless steel against a soft ('smooth') material, such as PMMA, is three times higher than that of the smooth material, i.e. the polymer. It is worth noting that the isolation of the metal from ground is a key point in the experimental investigations. This condition is crucial for ensuring that the current density produced by destruction of the passive film is only due to friction and not due to current leakage from electrical ground, for example.

Thus, differences between the phenomena of fretting corrosion and wear corrosion reflect the relative impact of corrosion and mechanical wear. However, as noted above,

Published by Woodhead Publishing Limited, 2013

corrosion and wear act synergistically, and a comprehensive model for tribo-corrosion must accurately capture these synergistic relationships, as described below.

2.3 Synergism between mechanical and corrosive degradation

2.3.1 Definitions of synergism terms

Synergism in the tribo-corrosion field has been investigated since the 1980s. If one considers stainless steel, Type 316L, for example, under pure wear conditions against a polymer, under dry conditions, mechanical wear is virtually non-existent. On the other hand, if one considers the corrosion rate of stainless steel, under pure corrosion conditions (i.e., in the absence of wear), it is close to 0.1 μm/year. Accordingly, the loss of material is, again, virtually non-existent. However, under cojoint conditions of corrosion and mechanical wear, the observed corrosion rate is greatly enhanced over that of corrosion or wear alone. In order to accurately define this synergistic mechanism, some theoretical points were developed. The first step in this approach is due to the studies in the mining industry concerning the abrasive/corrosive wear of stainless steel (Allen et al., 1981). The paradox described previously was studied: while stainless steel is resistant against corrosion (moreover, it is expensive compared with ferritic steels), its wear rate is greatly enhanced in abrasion corrosion conditions, due to the presence of particles. Later, a theoretical approach toward describing synergism was developed by Watson et al. (1995a, b). Thus, a general theoretical approach for the modeling of erosion corrosion, abrasion corrosion and wear corrosion was suggested and tested in many experimental cases (Stack, 2002; Jiang et al., 2002; Jiang and Stack, 2006;

Stack and Chi, 2003; Stack and Pungwiwat, 2004; Stack et al., 2005; Stack and Abd El Badia, 2008; Srinivasa et al., 2008; Mathew et al., 2008a; Stack and Abdelrahman, 2010).

As we emphasize above, the passive layer is responsible for the kinetic stability of a reactive metal in contact with a corrosive medium, particularly its defect structure and resistance to dissolution and mechanical disruption. The properties of the corrosive medium, including its composition (concentration of ions and proteins, etc.), are also essential in understanding the wear of metals. The total wear volume is the sum of the mechanical wear, the corrosive wear and the enhanced corrosion wear due to mechanics and the enhanced mechanical wear due to corrosion (the synergistic terms). The formula for the total wear volume is:

$$W = W_c + W_m + (\Delta W_{cm} + \Delta W_{mc}) \qquad [2.1]$$

where:
W: total wear volume
W_c: wear volume due to corrosion
W_m: wear volume due to mechanics
ΔW_{cm}: synergistic wear volume, corrosion enhancing wear due to mechanical factors
ΔW_{mc}: synergistic wear volume, mechanics enhancing wear due to corrosion

The different terms have been defined as (Stack et al., 2010; Mathew et al., 2008a, 2010):

$$K_{wc} = K_{co} + K_{wo} + (\Delta K_c + \Delta K_w) \qquad [2.2]$$

The terms have the same definitions as those of Eq. [2.1]:

$K_{co} = W_c$: pure corrosive wear
$K_{wc} = W_m$: pure tribology
$\Delta K_c = \Delta W_{mc}$
$\Delta K_w = \Delta W_{cm}$

Published by Woodhead Publishing Limited, 2013

These equations highlight the synergistic terms. Thus, one can define S, the synergistic term, as:

$$S = W - (W_c + W_m) \text{ or } S = K_{wc} - (K_{co} + K_{wc}) \qquad [2.3]$$

Load and the velocity of sliding are commonly the most relevant mechanical parameters that can be readily controlled in experimental investigations. Applied potential of the metallic sample is also most relevant, because it is the primary variable controlling the electrochemistry of the system and hence corrosion. Moreover, the electrochemistry of the system is intimately linked to the concentrations of species in solution: ions, molecules, dissolved gas, etc. Owing to their impact on the electrochemistry, these species have an important influence on degradation due to corrosion.

Many fields are concerned with tribo-corrosion phenomena, such as the nuclear, so finally, specific attention was given to this topic because many issues, such as health policy, are concerned with this scientific phenomenon. This section identifies and quantifies the importance of synergistic effects under fretting corrosion and wear corrosion conditions in the orthopedic field with biomaterials used for hip prostheses (Stack et al., 2010).

2.3.2 Methodology for studying synergistic effects

First of all, for calculating all of the terms in Eq. [2.1], a specific methodology has to be established. Before running a tribo-corrosion experiment, the cleaning process (i.e. preparation of the specimen prior to testing) has to be investigated carefully under smooth surface conditions. W, the total wear volume, is related to a worn sample after a wear or fretting test. The wear volume is always calculated at

Published by Woodhead Publishing Limited, 2013

the end of the test by profilometry. However, the third body (e.g. debris) has to be removed; it is the reason why the surface finish has to be maintained while removing the debris and in order to ensure no additional grooving of the worn surface. Thus, the cleaning process after testing might have an influence if it is too harsh. Especially for tests in solution, W_m has to be measured under conditions where the corrosive wear, i.e. dissolution of metal, is not allowed by controlling the applied potential (Pellier et al., 2011). W_c is calculated under pure corrosive conditions, i.e. without any wear. However, it is worth noting that one should wonder if samples have to be in contact or the surface of the metallic surface should be free. The authors chose to maintain the samples in contact in order to be as close as possible to the wear case. The synergistic term that could be calculated is W_{mc}, i.e. the effect of mechanics on the corrosive wear. Indeed, without wear (or fretting) there is a background current. Most of the time it is cathodic and for studying synergistic mechanisms it is better that this current should be close to 0. Indeed, if the current due to the applied potential is positive, the contribution of wear (or fretting) will not be measurable. The current that is produced by wear is deduced by the difference between the current monitored during wear (or fretting) and the background current described previously, without wear. Figure 2.2 highlights the additional current produced during wear.

$$\Delta W_{mc} = \sum_{\Delta t} \frac{\delta I * \Delta t * M}{n * F * d} \tag{2.4}$$

where $\delta I = I_{\text{measured}} - I_{\text{background}}$, $\Delta t = 0.5$ s is the interval of time between each point, $M = 56.4$ g/mol is the molecular weight, $n = 2$ is the number of electrons involved in the anodic process, $F = 96\,485$ C/mol is the Faraday constant and $d = 8$ g/cm^3 is the density.

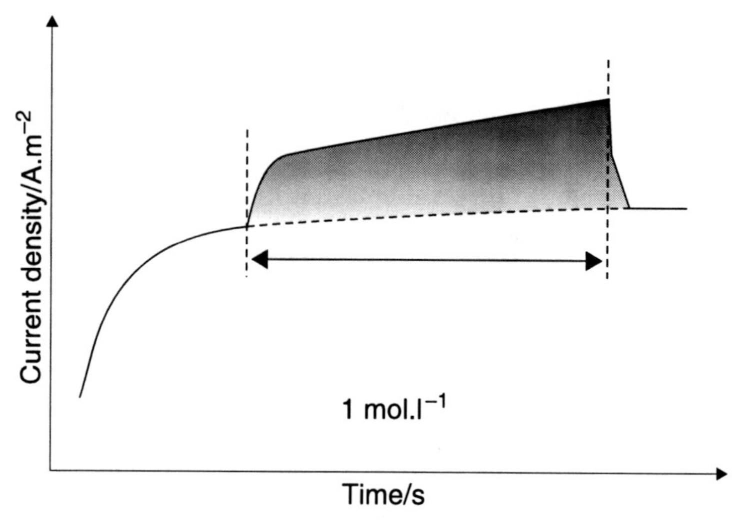

Figure 2.2 Current density according to time. Colored zone is related to the current produced during wear; 1 mol/l is related to NaCl concentration.

Finally, the term ΔW_{cm} is deduced by subtraction of all known terms. From this point, it is possible to know during a tribo-corrosion process if mechanics promotes the corrosion or inversely.

In the following sections, two case studies are presented. The first is related to fretting corrosion of metal (316L stainless steel) and polymer that should simulate the contact between materials; PMMA was chosen because of its very close mechanical properties to those of bone or bone cement. The second reason for this choice is related to the electrical insulation of PMMA. It allows studying only corrosion of metal without any disturbance and complications about the electrical contact with the counter sample. The third reason is the transparency of PMMA. Using a camera on the top of the device it is possible to record live degradations, showing gaseous release and generation of debris during the fretting corrosion process. The second case

Published by Woodhead Publishing Limited, 2013

will be related to Co–Cr–Mo alloy against ceramic material under conditions of wear corrosion with high amplitudes of displacement. The common point with the previous case is that one material is metallic and the second one is insulating. For electrochemical measurements, it is better to focus our attention on one material from the electrical point of view.

2.4 Fretting corrosion: synergism

2.4.1 *Case study*

As mentioned before, fretting corrosion is wear under small displacement. One of the biggest challenges for understanding this specific kind of degradation is knowing the part of mechanics and the part of corrosion.

First of all, the experimental device in the case of fretting is a key point for investigating fretting corrosion experiments. Figure 2.3 shows the mechanical assembly. The bumper is dedicated to a 'smoother' response of the electromagnetic motor, especially when the sliding direction changes (when the 316L stainless steel sample passes through a null velocity). Particular attention was paid to the threshold displacement between partial slip and gross slip. This point is discussed in Pellier et al. (2011). It is worth noting that between two fretting corrosion devices the compliance, i.e. elastic deformation, is the same in solution. Thus, results should be compared between both devices. Undoubtedly fretting corrosion is the physical origin of metal degradation and the reproducibility of tests was checked, i.e. following if compliance according to time is constant. The point was to check if there was any discrepancy of the compliance vs. time. If one was highlighted, the

Published by Woodhead Publishing Limited, 2013

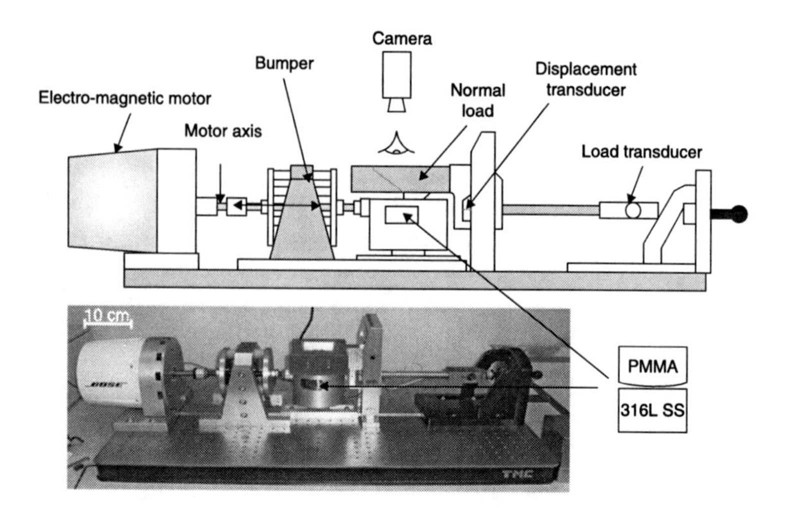

Figure 2.3 Fretting corrosion device.

Source: Geringer et al. (2012).

mechanical assembly was checked. The normal load was 127.5 N between samples in contact. Figure 2.4 shows the evolution of the friction coefficient, μ, and the energistic criterion, A:

$$A = \frac{E_d}{E_{tot}}$$

Fouvry et al. (1997) defined and used this energy-based criterion for defining the threshold between partial slip and gross slip. When $A > 0.2$, gross slip occurs with a spherical contact. From the theoretical point of view (because of no discontinuity in the contact area), 0.2 is demonstrated for a spherical contact, i.e. plane against sphere. However, a cylindrical contact highlights discontinuity at the boundary of the contact area (rectangular area); thus stresses mapping shows this kind of discontinuity. Thus, using the criterion of 0.2 is not permitted from a mathematical point of view for a

Published by Woodhead Publishing Limited, 2013

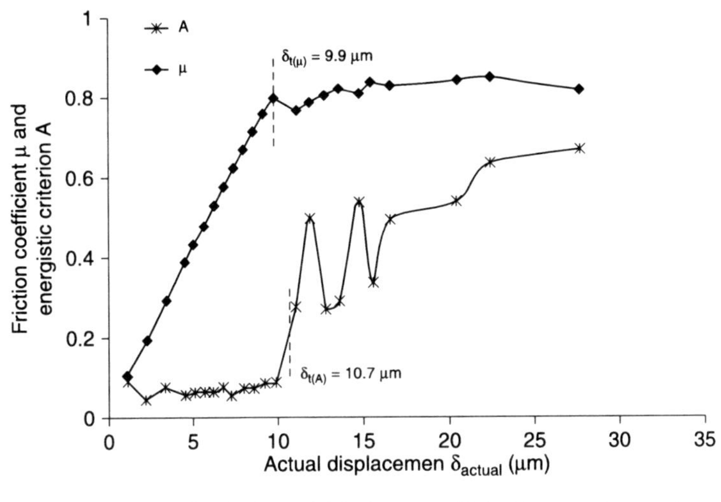

Figure 2.4 **Evolution of friction coefficient, μ, and energy-based criterion, A, according to the actual displacement, δ_{actual} (μm).**

cylinder–plane contact. It has, however, been demonstrated (Geringer et al., 2006) that this criterion of 0.2 is the right one for this contact from the experimental point of view. Figure 2.4 shows the evolution of μ, friction coefficient, and A, the energy-based criterion, for a cylinder–plane contact under 127.5 N, from an imposed actual displacement of 1–30 μm. A threshold displacement is highlighted around 10 μm. It means that, under this value, slip is partial and, over this value, the fretting regime is gross slip. The experimental value was ±40 μm, i.e. gross slip regime.

From the electrochemical point of view, the stainless steel sample is inserted in an electrochemical device. Parstat 2263 is the electrochemical potentiostat with floating mass. This point is relevant because current leakage during fretting has to be avoided. A three-electrode set up was used, at applied potential:

Published by Woodhead Publishing Limited, 2013

- Working electrode: the stainless steel sample.
- Counter electrode: circular wire of platinum having a diameter of about 60 mm.
- Reference electrode: SCE, $E = +246$ mV(SHE) at $T = 22$ °C.

Positioning of the counter electrode was always the same for all experiments. Indeed, from the electrical point of view, it allows one to fix the ohmic drop for all experiments.

Two electrochemical conditions were considered (Table 2.2). The OCP conditions are as close as possible to the *in vivo* conditions, i.e. metallic stem of the hip prosthesis in solution. Unfortunately, OCP does not allow monitoring of current density. It is the reason why experiments were carried out at an applied potential, –400 mV(SCE), close to

Table 2.2 **Electrochemical measurement steps for each electrochemical conditions: OCP or cathodic applied potentials (E = −400 or −800 mV(SCE))**

Electrochemical conditions	OCP	Applied potential: −400 or −800 mV(SCE)
1	Cathodic polarization: −1 V(SCE), 5 min	
2	Without fretting: 1 h + EIS	Without fretting: 10 min + EIS
3	With fretting: 4 h + 10 EIS, each 20 min during the experiment	
4	Without fretting: 14 h + 2 EIS after fretting stop and 1 EIS after 14 h	Without fretting: 10 min + 2 EIS after fretting stop
5	No experiment	Without fretting: 14 h OCP measurement and 1 EIS after 14 h

Published by Woodhead Publishing Limited, 2013

the values of OCP, and –800 mV(SCE) for studying 'pure mechanical' degradation in solution, i.e. preventing the corrosive wear of stainless steel. Thus, the current density should be monitored and EIS can be practiced: ±10 mV around the applied potential (AC amplitude), from 10^5 to 0.1–0.01 Hz, with measurement of 10 points per decade.

The experimental protocol was described in Pellier et al. (2011). Table 2.1 was dedicated to describing the electrochemical steps for practicing EIS investigations. Thus, it is necessary to ensure that the system is linear, stable and causal; constraints that are imposed by linear systems theory (LST) (Macdonald et al., 1986). The first step of the protocol is dedicated to producing a reproducible initial state. The second is dedicated to producing well-defined electrochemical conditions. The third is dedicated specifically to the fretting corrosion tests, which last for a duration of 4 h, i.e. 14 400 s. The fourth step is related to stabilizing the system just after fretting corrosion has been completed. It is worth noting that, under an applied potential, a fifth step was practiced in order to characterize the electrochemical conditions. This step will not be considered further in this chapter.

Four solutions were studied: from 10^{-3} to 1 mol/l, by steps of 10. Each solution could contain 0, 1 or 20 g/l.

Thus, from mechanical and electrochemical topics, under fretting corrosion, the influence of chlorides and albumin concentration should be studied for understanding the synergism effect between mechanics and corrosion on stainless steel. This point will be particularly focused on in the following subsection.

2.4.2 Results of synergism studies

Figure 2.5(a) presents results concerning the impact of mechanical wear on total wear. According to the ionic

Published by Woodhead Publishing Limited, 2013

strength, the part of the mechanical wear decreases. Thus, the corrosion process prevails over the mechanical (wear) process. Figure 2.5(b and c) presents the contribution of the synergistic terms on the wear process. First, the effect of corrosion on the mechanical wear is examined. There is a discontinuity of this ratio for an ionic strength of 0.154 mol/l, i.e. for Ringer's solution (constituted by 147 mmol/l Na^{+}, 3.4 mmol/l K^{+}, 2.0 mmol/l Ca^{2+}, 150.7 mmol/l Cl^{-} and 1.8 mmol/l HCO_3^{-}). This solution contains numerous ions and the effect on corrosion of stainless steel is very complex, compared with a 1:1 electrolyte solution containing only NaCl. It is the reason why the effect of this usual solution in the field of biology, for example, will not be described in the following. In Figure 2.5(b), at 0 and 1 g/l, a slight decrease of the impact of corrosion on the mechanical wear is noted. However, for 20 g/l of albumin, the trend is the opposite. Consequently, the mechanical wear rate of 316L, enhanced by corrosion, is increased by approximately 80% in the presence of albumin. This point is relevant in relation to the synergistic approach. When the ionic strength increases, corrosion is not directly promoted; however, the corrosive degradation promotes mechanical degradation, which is dominant. In Figure 2.5(c), the graph shows clearly that albumin protects the stainless steel surface against degradation due to fretting corrosion.

Moreover, it is worth noting that a small quantity of protein decreases the corrosive wear enhanced by corrosion. The same point, that is one highlighted in Figure 2.5(b), should be: 0.1 mol/l is a threshold concentration. The wear volume increases from 0.1 to 1 mol/l of NaCl. However, the ratio between ΔW_{mc} and W is constant from 0.1 mol/l. The same point is highlighted in Figure 2.5(c).

Published by Woodhead Publishing Limited, 2013

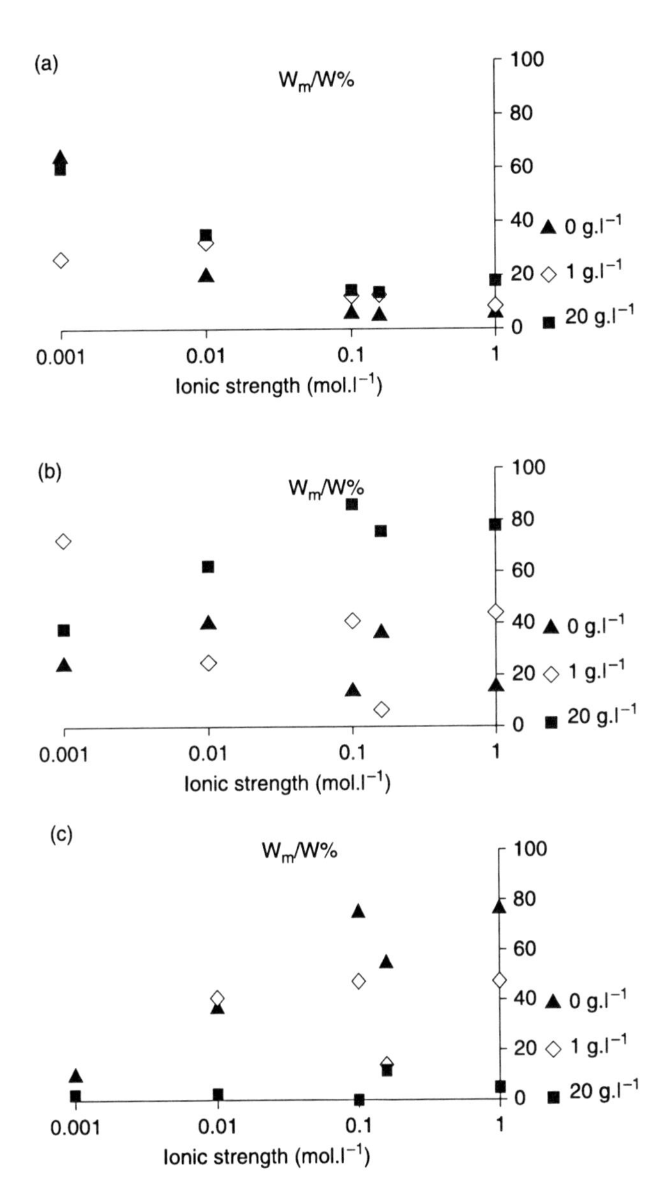

Figure 2.5 Percentages of synergisms: (a) W_m/W, ratio of mechanical wear to total wear, (b) $\Delta W_{cm}/W$, ratio of the synergistic term, mechanical wear enhanced by corrosion, and (c) $\Delta W_{mc}/W$, ratio of the synergistic term, corrosive wear enhanced by mechanics.

Published by Woodhead Publishing Limited, 2013

2.4.3 Discussion and conclusions

From the above, we see that albumin inhibits the corrosive wear of Type 316L stainless steel. Figure 2.6 shows the total wear volume for different ionic strengths of the solution and for different protein concentrations. The protein concentration of 20 g/l inhibits total wear by a factor of approximately 2 as compared with the condition without albumin. In media that are as close as possible to the actual physiological fluid, i.e. with protein, the role of corrosion on the mechanical wear is a key issue with stainless steel 316L. Thus, proteins are expected to have an important impact on the lifetime of implants made of stainless steel. The principal method of improving the durability of a metallic implant might involve, for example, the grafting of proteins onto the surface. This concept should be relevant for the development of the next generation of hip implants. Moreover, studying

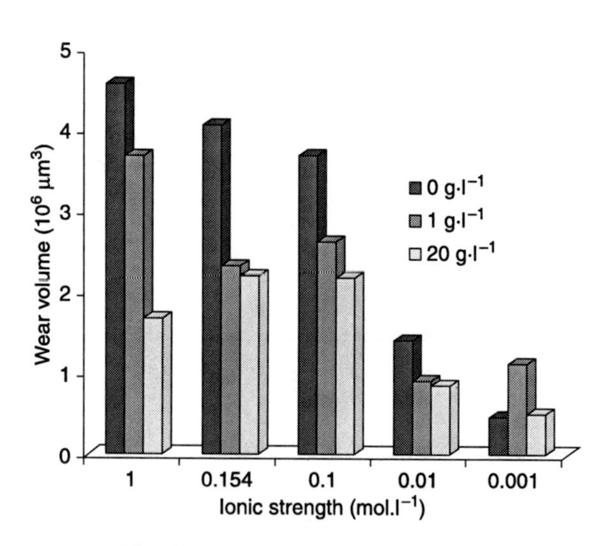

Figure 2.6 Total wear volumes of stainless steel 316L according to ionic strength and albumin concentrations.

Published by Woodhead Publishing Limited, 2013

different alloys under fretting corrosion conditions is the only way of defining the wear mechanisms. Selecting metallic alloys on the basis of this kind of test (under fretting corrosion degradation conditions) will be an important issue in the future. Indeed, wear is intimately related to hip degradation, for example.

The next section is dedicated to the study of wear corrosion of metals constituting hip implants, recognizing the synergistic effects.

2.5 Wear corrosion: synergism

2.5.1 Case study

Another type of hip implants is MoM. This couple of materials is dedicated to the joint of the head and cup for a hip prosthesis (Figure 2.1). First of all, one sample involved in the contact has to be electrically isolated – using the same methodology described previously for the experimental device. It is the reason why a MoM couple is impossible to study from this point of view. Thus, a combination of insulating material and metal has to be investigated. Figure 2.7 described the tribo-corrosion apparatus for studying the contact between a ceramic head (alumina) and metallic sample, Co–Cr–Mo. A test system with a pin-on-ball configuration has been constructed to mimic the contact conditions in femoral joint MoM.

2.5.2 Materials and methods

The tribological pair consisted of a flat Co–Cr–Mo cylindrical disc of 12 mm diameter (surface roughness $R_a = 9.4 \pm 2.6$ nm, exposed area 1.0 cm^2) that articulated against a ceramic ball

Published by Woodhead Publishing Limited, 2013

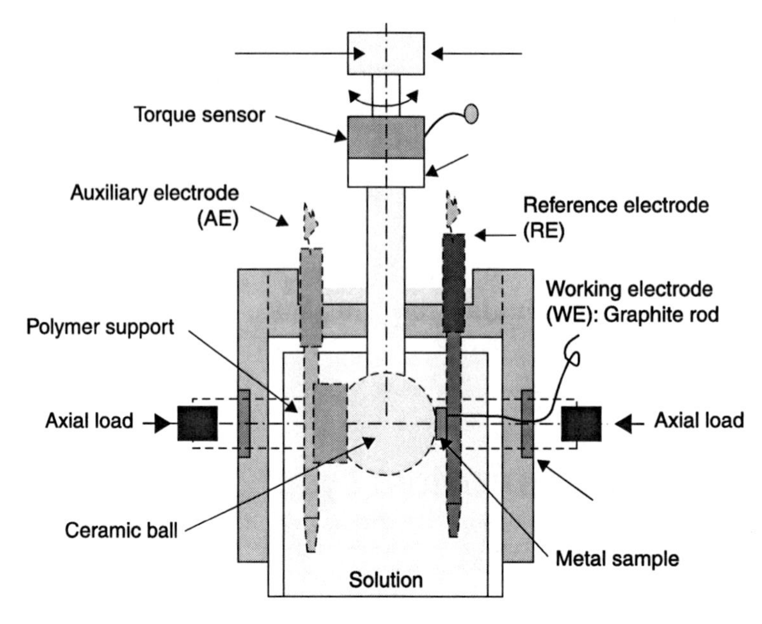

Figure 2.7 Schematic diagram of the apparatus for studying tribo-corrosion between a ceramic ball and a metal component.

of 28 mm diameter with a 16 N contact load (Hertzian stress: 350 MPa) and ±15° of rotation at 1 Hz. The testing sequence was defined specifically according to this kind of experiment. Table 2.3 describes all of the steps. One aim is to identify the role of proteins in modifying tribo-corrosion processes in the T1 (2.4% NaCl solution) and T2 (bovine calf serum (BCS) 30%) steps. From the initial potentiodynamic tests, E_{corr} was determined to be –0.32 V (v. SCE). Thus, the imposed potential was equal to E_{corr} and the current was monitored during tribo-corrosion tests. Furthermore, three steps were dedicated to the study of synergism between corrosion and wear. In order to analyze synergistic effects of corrosion and wear, a pure corrosion test (i.e. no movement, T3) was conducted for 100 000 s (corresponding to 100 000 cycles)

Published by Woodhead Publishing Limited, 2013

Table 2.3 Methodology of wear corrosion tests

Aims	Tests	Solution	Cycles	Corrosion conditions
Protein effect	T1	2.4% NaCl	1000	Potentiostatic
Protein effect	T2	BCS	1000	Potentiostatic
Synergism	T3, K_{co}, pure corrosion	BCS	100 000	Potentiostatic
Synergism	T4, K_{wo}, pure mechanics	BCS	100 000	Potentiostatic/ cathodic
Synergism	T5, K_{wc}, total	BCS	100 000	Potentiostatic

under potentiostatic conditions at the corrosion potential (E_{corr}). Subsequently, two tribo-corrosion tests (T4 and T5) were conducted under potentiostatic conditions at other potentials. Thus, cathodic polarization at a potential of –0.9 V (E vs. SCE) was maintained for T4. The T5 test was conducted again at the free corrosion potential (E_{corr}). The total wear volume loss was evaluated based on the Co, Cr and Mo content in the medium using inductive coupled plasma mass spectrometry (ICP-MS), as well as by wear scar profilometry.

2.5.3 Results from experiments on synergism

The evolution of the current for the tribo-corrosion of Co–Cr–Mo alloy in 2.4 wt% NaCl solution vs. BCS solution is shown for five cycles in Figure 2.8. The value of current is 10 times lower in BCS compared with 2.4% NaCl solution, indicating less corrosion in BCS. Proteins clearly protect the Co–Cr–Mo alloy sample against wear corrosion

Published by Woodhead Publishing Limited, 2013

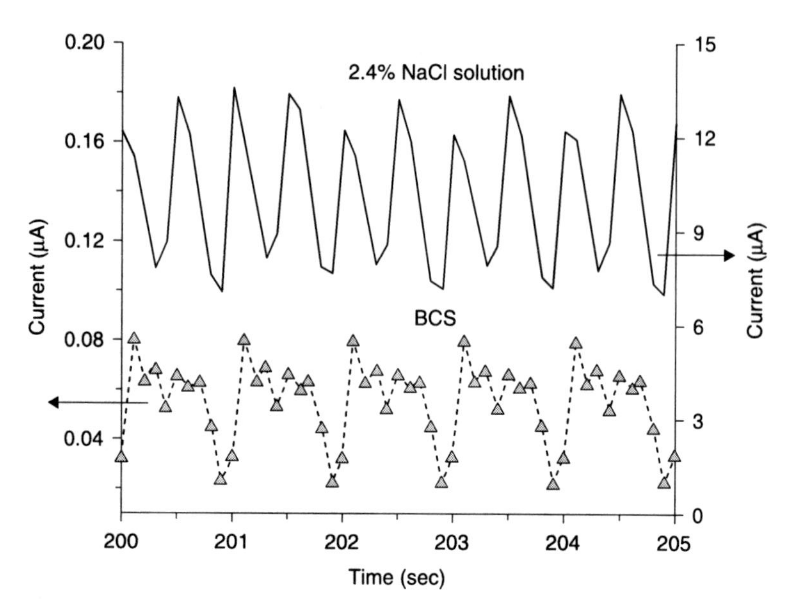

Figure 2.8 Monitored current at the applied potential corresponding to the OCP for Co–Cr–Mo alloy in 2.4% NaCl and BCS (30 g/l) solutions under tribo-corrosion conditions. Current decay during the plateau of wear.

degradation. Figure 2.9 displays the weight loss distribution (from wear scar profilometry and total metal ions released in the solution, as determined by ICP-MS) for the three conditions, i.e. pure corrosion (K_{co}), pure tribology (K_{wo}) and tribo-corrosion (K_{wc}). Both the metal content and the profilometric wear estimations correlate satisfactorily ($R^2 = 0.85$).

2.5.4 Discussion and conclusions

The total wear volume, K_{wc}, is much higher than the sum of pure corrosion, K_{co}, and the tribological (pure wear) components, K_{wo}. Hence, the synergistic component (S) can

Published by Woodhead Publishing Limited, 2013

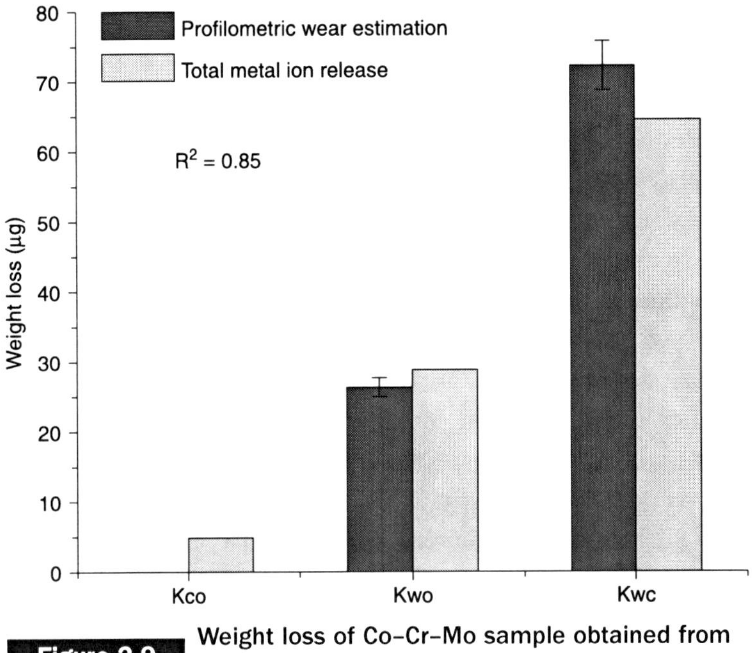

Figure 2.9 Weight loss of Co–Cr–Mo sample obtained from profilometry and by measuring the total amount of metal ions in solution after tribological tests; K_{co}: T3 step; K_{wc}: T4 step; K_{wc}: T5 step.

be estimated by using relation [2.3] (Yan et al., 2007; Mathew et al., 2008a; Wimmer et al., 2010). The synergistic component (Figure 2.10a) could be the result of the intermittent variations of the corrosion kinetics (Figure 2.8), which might eventually accelerate the overall wear mechanisms. Hence, the interplay of wear and corrosion mechanisms has a huge impact (58%) on the overall material loss. Figure 2.8 illustrates the role of protein in the tribo-corrosion process. The low value of the current and the difference in the current pattern during each tribological cycle in BCS compared with the NaCl solution show that the surface chemistry is significantly altered. It is also observed that repassivation and depassivation kinetics (in each cycle) are closely related to the tribological events or articulations. Moreover, protein plays a significant role in determining the current decay, as indicated by the asterisk in Figure 2.8 of the tribo-activated surface (Mathew et al., 2008b). These observations are in agreement with earlier reports that complex synergistic interactions with proteins might assist in the formation of a tribo-chemical reaction layer on the articulating surfaces (Wimmer et al., 2010), which will improve MoM implant performance. A better understanding of the dominant tribo-corrosive interactions is required to further improve MoM wear *in vivo*. From these results, fretting corrosion promotes synergistic effects during tribo-corrosion (Figure 2.10). This fact should be relevant in choosing modular junctions for hip prostheses in terms of the specific materials and material combinations employed. As fretting involves the most synergistic contributions in tribo-corrosion processes, this approach should be very useful for studying future material couples involved in hip implants and in other fields, such as structural materials in nuclear and/or more generally industrial environments where tribo-corrosion is an important issue.

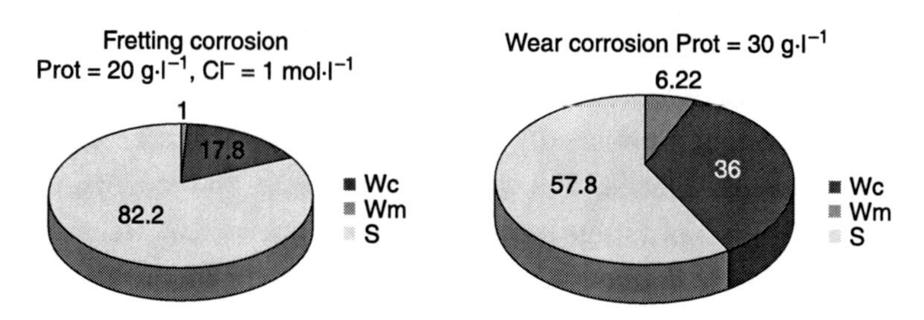

Figure 2.10 (a) Fretting corrosion between 316L and PMMA under 20 g/l. (b) Wear corrosion between Co–Cr–Mo and alumina; percentage of W_c, pure corrosion; W_m, pure mechanical wear; S, synergistic term.

Published by Woodhead Publishing Limited, 2013

2.6 Conclusions and future trends

Problems related to tribo-corrosion and focused on hip implants have been described and discussed according to various types of materials. We have focused our attention on metal degradation, as this degrades hip prosthesis performance. Thus, fretting corrosion degradation between Type 316L stainless steel and PMMA (for simulating bone and/or bone cement) has been described with a focus on the influence of chloride ions and proteins on the synergistic interaction between wear and corrosion. Experimental results from specific experiments show that albumin protects 316L stainless steel against fretting corrosion degradation. The second case study was related to wear corrosion of Co–Cr–Mo against ceramic material, i.e. pure alumina. The same conclusion as that for fretting corrosion can be drawn for wear corrosion, even though the mechanical conditions (contact pressure, etc.) and the materials properties were different between the fretting corrosion and wear corrosion tests. Evidently, the OCP and the current density at applied potentials are different between both tribological conditions. However, the synergistic approach yields insight into the behavior of materials subjected to tribology processes. Between fretting and wear corrosion, the contribution of the synergistic term to the total wear volume is higher for fretting corrosion than for wear corrosion. With regard to the mechanisms of wear, synergy is more prominent in the case of fretting, especially in the case of contact between a hard material, such as a metal, and a smooth material, like a polymer. By describing and quantifying the contribution of the synergistic term to materials degradation, this allows one to obtain information on the tribological process. From these two case studies, i.e. fretting corrosion and wear corrosion, a methodology was defined for better

Published by Woodhead Publishing Limited, 2013

exploring mechanisms, including both corrosion and mechanical aspects, occurring during tribology in liquid media, especially for metals in aqueous solution. This approach should be used for studying wear of metallic material subjected to wear/fretting in solution. From the experimental point of view, these new experimental tools are available and are readily implemented. The experimental information gleaned from these new tools will surely have an enormous impact on defining the physico-electrochemical processes involved and ultimately in the modeling of mechanisms. Thus, purely corrosion models and purely mechanical models are clearly obsolete, and attention must now be focused on describing and predicting the synergism that exists between corrosion and mechanical wear. Toward that end, this type of modeling is in progress by adapting the point defect model (Macdonald, 2011) for the growth and breakdown of passive films on metal surfaces in describing pure corrosion to the case of fretting corrosion. The importance of the PDM in this regard is that the model incorporates both electrochemical and mechanical wear effects, and hence provides the required theoretical basis for further advances in this field.

2.7 References

Allen C, Ball A and Protheroe B E (1981), 'The abrasive corrosive wear of stainless steels', *Wear*, **74**: 287–305.

Amstutz H C, Ma S M, Jinnah R H and Mai L L (1982), 'Revision of aseptic loose total hip arthroplasties', *Clinical Orthopedics*, **170**: 21–33.

Amstutz H C, Campbell P, Kossovsky N and Clarke I C (1992), 'Mechanism and clinical significance of wear debris-induced osteolysis', *Clinical Orthopedics*, **276**: 7–18.

Andrew T A, Flanagan J P, Gerundini M and Bombelli R (1996), 'The isoelastic, noncemented total hip arthroplasty', *Clinical Orthopedics*, **206**: 127–138.

Aspenberg P, Goodman S, Toksvig-Larsen S, Ryd L and Albrektsson T (1992), 'Intermittent micromotion inhibits bone ingrowth: titanium implants in rabbits', *Acta Orthopedica Scandinavia*, **63**: 141–145.

Barton J (1827),'On the treatment of ankylosis by the formation of artificial joints', *North American Medical Surgical Journal*, **3**: 279–400.

Boutin P (1972), 'Arthroplastie totale de la hanche par prothese en alumine frittee: etude experimentale et premieres applications cliniques', *Revue de Chirurgie Orthopedique*, **58**: 229–246.

Boutin P, Christel P, Dorlot J-M, Meunier A, deRoquancourt B D et al. (1988), 'The use of dense alumina–alumina ceramic combination in total hip replacement', *Journal of Biomedical Materials Research*, **22**: 1203–1232.

Boyle C and Kim I Y (2011), 'Comparison of different hip prosthesis shapes considering micro-level bone remodeling and stress-shielding criteria using three-dimensional design space topology optimization', *Journal of Biomechanics*, **44**: 1722–1728.

Bozic K J, Kurtz S M, Lau E, Ong K, Vail T P et al. (2009), 'The epidemiology of revision total hip arthroplasty in the United States', *Journal of Bone and Joint Surgery, American*, **91**: 128–133.

Brashear W (1852), 'First case of amputation at the hip-joint in the United States', *Transactions of the Kentucky State Medical Society*, **2**: 265.

Carrerot H, Rieu J, Bousquet G and Rambert A (1990), 'Alumina plasma spray coatings on stainless steels and titanium alloys for prosthesis anchorage', in: *Bioceramics:*

Published by Woodhead Publishing Limited, 2013

Proceedings of the 2nd International Symposium on Ceramics in Medicine. Cologne, vol. 2, pp. 211–218.

Celis J-P, Ponthiaux P, Wenger F (2006), 'Tribo-corrosion of materials: Interplay between chemical, electrochemical, and mechanical reactivity of surfaces', *Wear*, **261**: 939–946.

Charnley J (1979), *Low Friction Arthroplasty of the Hip – Theory and Practice*. Berlin: Springer.

Clarke I C, Green D D, Williams P A, Kubo K, Pezzotti G et al. (2009), 'Hip-simulator wear studies of an alumina-matrix composite (AMC) ceramic compared to retrieval studies of AMC balls with 1–7 years follow-up', *Wear*, **267**: 702–709.

Essner A, Sutton K and Wang A (2005), 'Hip simulator wear comparison of metal-on-metal, ceramic-on-ceramic and crosslinked UHMWPE bearings', *Wear*, **259**: 992–995.

Fischmeister H and Roll U (1984), 'Passive layers on stainless steels: a survey of surface analysis results', *Fresenius' Zeitschrift für Analytische Chemie*, **319**: 639–645.

Fouvry S, Kapsa P, Zahouani H and Vincent L (1997), 'Wear analysis in fretting of hard coatings through a dissipated energy', *Wear*, **203/204**: 476–484.

Geringer J, Forest B and Combrade P (2005), 'Fretting-corrosion of materials used as orthopaedic implants', *Wear*, **259**: 943–951.

Geringer J, Forest B and Combrade P (2006), 'Wear analysis of materials used as orthopaedic implants', *Wear*, **261**: 971–979.

Geringer J, Atmani F and Forest B (2009), 'Friction–corrosion of AISI 316L/bone cement and AISI 316L/PMMA contacts: ionic strength effect on tribological behavior', *Wear*, **267**: 763–769.

Geringer J, Normand B, Alemany-Dumont C and Diemiaszonek R (2010), 'Assessing the tribo-corrosion

Published by Woodhead Publishing Limited, 2013

behaviour of Cu and Al by electrochemical impedance spectroscopy', *Tribology International*, **43**: 1991–1999.

Geringer J, Kim K and Boyer B (2011), 'Tribo-corrosion of passive metals and coatings', in: Landolt D and Mischler S (eds), *Fretting Corrosion in Biomedical Implants*. Sawston: Woodhead.

Geringer J, Macdonald D D (2012), 'Modeling fretting corrosion wear of 316L SS against Poly(methyl methacrylate) with the point defect model: fundamental theory, assessment and outlook', *Electrochimica Acta*, **79**: 17–30.

Geringer J, Pellier J, Cleymand F and Forest B (2012), 'Atomic force microscopy investigations on pits and debris related to fretting-corrosion between 316L SS and PMMA', *Wear*, **292/293**: 207–217.

Gluck T (1890), 'Die invaginationsmethode der Osteo- und Arthroplastik', *Klinische Wochenschrift (Berlin)*, **28**: 732–736.

Gomez P T and Morcuende J A (2005), 'Early attempts at hip arthroplasty 1700s to 1950s', *Iowa Orthopedic Journal*, **25**: 25–29.

Greenwood J A and Williamson J B P (1966), 'Contact of nominally flat surfaces', *Proceedings of the Royal Society of London. Series A, Mathematical and Physical Sciences*, **295**: 300–319.

Hallab N J, Jacobs J J and Lawrence Katz J (2004), 'Orthopedic applications', in: Ratner B D, Hoffman D, Schoen F J and Lemons J E (eds), *Biomaterials Science: An Introduction to Materials in Medicine*, pp. 526–555. San Diego, CA: Elsevier.

Henrichsen E, Jansen K and Krough-Poulsen W (1952), 'Experimental investigation of the tissue reaction to acrylic plastics', *Acta Orthopedica Scandinavia*, **22**: 141–146.

Published by Woodhead Publishing Limited, 2013

Hertz H (1882), 'Über die berührung fester elastischer körper', *Journal für die reine und angewandte Mathematik*, **92**: 156–171.

Heuer A H, Kahn H, Natishan P M, Martin F J and Cross L E (2011), 'Electrostrictive stresses and breakdown of thin passive films on stainless steel', *Electrochimica Acta*, **35**: 157–160.

Hills D A, Nowell D and Sackfield A (1993), *Mechanics of Elastic Contact*. Oxford: Butterworth-Heinemann.

Holtzwarth U and Cotogno G (2012), *State of the Art, Challenges and Prospects*. European Commission, Joint Research Centre, Institute for Health and Consumer Protection, *http://publications.jrc.ec.europa.eu/repository/handle/111111111/25991*.

Jacobs J J, Hallab N J, Urban R M and Wimmer M (2006), 'Wear particles', *Journal of Bone and Joint Surgery, American*, **88**: 99–102.

Jakob R P, Jacobi M and Lobenhoffer P (2008), in: *Osteotomies Around the Knee*. Stuttgart: Theime, pp. XIII–XXII.

Jiang J and Stack M M (2006), 'Modelling sliding wear: from dry to wet environments', *Wear*, **261**: 954–965.

Jiang J, Stack M M and Neville A (2002), 'Modelling the tribo-corrosion interaction in aqueous sliding conditions', *Tribology International*, **35**: 669–679.

Johnson K L (1985), *Contact Mechanics*, pp. 84–106. Cambridge: Cambridge University Press.

Joshi G, Miller F and Santare M H (2000), 'Analysis of a femoral hip prosthesis designed to reduce stress shielding', *Journal of Biomechanics*, **33**: 1655–1662.

Judet R and Judet J (1949), 'Essais de reconstruction prothétique de la hanche après résection de la tête fémorale', *Journal de Chirurgie*, **65**: 17–24.

Kovacs P, Davidson J A and Daigle K (1997), 'Correlation between the metal ion concentration and the fretting wear

Published by Woodhead Publishing Limited, 2013

volume of orthopaedic implant metals', in: *Particulate Debris from Medical Implants: Mechanisms of Formation and Biological Consequences*, *ASTM STP 1144*. pp. 160–176. West Conshohocken, PA: ASTM International.

Langlais F (1993), 'Prothèses totales de hanche. Facteurs biologiques et mécanismes de tolérance', in Langlais F and Delagoutte J P (eds), *Cahiers d'enseignement de la SOFCOT 44*, pp. 3–22. Paris: Expansion Scientifique Française.

Lopez A and Rieu J (1990), 'Mechanical behaviour of ceramic–metal interface in the femoral head prosthesis conical fitting', in: *Bioceramics: Proceedings of the 2nd International Symposium on Ceramics in Medicine*, Cologne, vol. 2, pp. 166–171.

Macdonald D D (1999), 'Passivity – the key to our metals-based civilization', *Pure and Applied Chemistry*, **71**: 951–978.

Macdonald D D (2011), 'The history of the Point Defect Model for the passive state: a brief review of film growth aspects', *Electrochimica Acta*, **56**: 1761–1772.

Macdonald D D and McKubre M C H (1982), 'Impedance measurements in electrochemical systems', in: Bockris J O'M, Conway B E and White R E (eds), *Modern Aspects of Electrochemistry*, vol. 14, p. 61. New York: Plenum Press.

Macdonald D D, Real S and Urquidi-Macdonald M (1986), 'Application of Kramers–Kronig transforms in the analysis of electrochemical impedance data. II. Transformations in the complex plane', *Journal of the Electrochemical Society*, **133**: 2018–2024.

McKee G K (1982), 'Total hip replacement-past, present and future', *Biomaterials*, **3**: 130–135.

Mathew M T, Ariza E, Rocha L A, Fernandes A C and Vaz F (2008a), 'TiC*x*O*y* thin films for decorative applications: tribo-corrosion mechanisms and synergism', *Tribology International*, **41**: 603–615.

Published by Woodhead Publishing Limited, 2013

Mathew M T, Stack M M, Matijevic B, Rocha L A and Ariza E (2008b), 'Micro-abrasion resistance of thermochemically treated steels in aqueous solutions: mechanisms, maps, materials selection', *Tribology International*, **41**: 141–149.

Mathew M T, Srinivasa P, Pourzal R, Fisher A and Wimmer M A (2009), 'Significance of tribo-corrosion in biomedical applications: overview and current status', *Advances in Tribology*, **9**: 1–12.

Mathew M T, Ariza E, Rocha L A, Vaz F, Fernandes A C et al. (2010), 'Tribo-corrosion behaviour of TiC*x*O*y* thin films in bio-fluids', *Electrochimica Acta*, **56**: 929–937.

Mischler S (2008), 'Triboelectrochemical techniques and interpretation methods in tribo-corrosion: a comparative evaluation', *Tribology International*, **41**: 573–583.

Mischler S, Spiegel A and Landolt D (1999), 'The role of passive oxide films on the degradation of steel in tribo-corrosion systems', *Wear*, **225/229**: 1078–1087.

Murphy J B (1913), 'Original memoirs: arthroplasty,' *Annals of Surgery*, **57**: 593–647.

Nevelos J E, Ingham E, Doyle C, Streicher R, Nevelos A et al. (2000), 'Microseparation of the centers of alumina–alumina artificial hip joints during simulator testing produces clinically relevant wear rates and patterns', *Journal of Arthroplasty*, **15**: 793–795.

Nevelos J E, Ingham E, Doyle C, Nevelos A B and Fisher J (2001), 'Wear of HIPed and non-HIPed alumina–alumina hip joints under standard and severe simulator testing conditions', *Biomaterials*, **22**: 2191–2197.

Nicic I and Macdonald D D (2008), 'The passivity of Type 316L stainless steel in borate buffer solution', *Journal of Nuclear Materials*, **379**: 54–58.

Niinimaki T J, Puranen J P and Jalovaara P K A (1995), 'Revision arthroplasty with an isoelastic uncemented femoral stem', *International Orthopaedics*, **19**: 298–303.

Published by Woodhead Publishing Limited, 2013

Niinomi M and Nakai M (2011), 'Titanium-based biomaterials for preventing stress shielding between implant devices and bone', *International Journal of Biomaterials*, **11**: 1–10.

Oliveira A L, Lima R G, Cueva E G and Queiroz R D (2011), 'Comparative analysis of surface wear from total hip prostheses tested on a mechanical simulator according to standards ISO 14242-1 and ISO 14242-3', *Wear*, **271**: 2340–2345.

Pellier J, Geringer J and Forest B (2011), 'Fretting-corrosion between 316L SS and PMMA: influence of ionic strength, protein and electrochemical conditions on material wear. Application to orthopaedic implants', *Wear*, **271**: 1563–1571.

Ponthiaux P, Richard C and Wenger F (2007), 'Tribo-corrosion', *Techniques de l'ingénieur*, COR60.

Postel M, Kerboul M, Evrard J and Courpied J P (1985), *Arthroplastie totale de hanche*. Berlin: Springer.

Pramanik S, Agarwal A K and Rai K N (2005), 'Chronology of total hip joint replacement and materials development', *Trends in Biomaterials and Artificial Organs*, **19**: 15–26.

Rieu J (1993), 'Ceramic formation on metallic surfaces (ceramization) for medical applications', *Clinical Materials*, **12**: 227–235.

Rubin P J, Rakotomanana R L, Leyvraz P F, Zysset P K, Curnier A et al. (1993), 'Frictional interface micromotions and anisotropic stress distribution in a femoral total hip component', *Journal of Biomechanics*, **26**: 725–739.

Schmalzried T P, Fowble V A, Bitsch R G and Choi E S (2007), 'Total hip resurfacing', in: Callaghan J J, Rosenberg A G and Rubash H E (eds), *The Adult Hip*, vol. 2, pp. 969–979. Philadelphia, PA: Lippincott Williams & Wilkins.

Simon P (2005), 'Fractures de l'extremite superieure du femur', Faculty of Medicine Strasbourg DCEM 1 Module

Published by Woodhead Publishing Limited, 2013

12B Appareil locomoteur. Available from: *http://lmm.univ-lyon1.fr/internat/download/item239.pdf*.

Simpson J M and Villar R N (2010), 'Focus on hip resurfacing arthroplasty', *Journal of Bone and Joint Surgery, British*, **2010**: 1–3.

Spence W T (1954), 'Form-fitting plastic cranioplasty', *Journal of Neurosurgery*, **11**: 219–225.

Srinivasa P P, Mathew M T, Stack M M and Rocha L A (2008), 'Some thoughts on neural network modelling of microabrasion–corrosion processes', *Tribology International*, **41**: 672–681.

Stack M M (2002), 'Mapping tribo-corrosion processes in dry and in aqueous conditions: some new directions for the new millennium', *Tribology International*, **35**: 681–689.

Stack M M and Abd El Badia T M (2008), 'Some comments on mapping the combined effects of slurry concentration, impact velocity and electrochemical potential on the erosion–corrosion of WC/Co–Cr coatings', *Wear*, **264**: 826–837.

Stack M M and Abdelrahman G H (2010), 'Mapping erosion-corrosion of carbon steel in oil exploration conditions: some new approaches to characterizing mechanisms and synergies', *Tribology International*, **43**: 1268–1277.

Stack M M and Chi K (2003), 'Mapping sliding wear of steels in aqueous conditions', *Wear*, **255**: 456–465.

Stack M M and Pungwiwat N (2004), 'Erosion–corrosion mapping of Fe in aqueous slurries: some views on a new rationale for defining the erosion–corrosion interaction', *Wear*, **256**: 565–576.

Stack M M, Jawan H and Mathew M T (2005), 'On the construction of micro-abrasion maps for a steel/polymer couple in corrosive environments', *Tribology International*, **38**: 848–856.

Published by Woodhead Publishing Limited, 2013

Stack M M, Rodling J, Mathew M T, Jawan H, Huang W et al. (2010), 'Micro-abrasion–corrosion of a Co–Cr/UHMWPE couple in Ringer's solution: an approach to construction of mechanism and synergism maps for application to bio-implants', *Wear*, **269**: 376–382.

Stewart T D, Williams S, Tipper J L, Ingham E, Stone M H et al. (2003), 'Advances in simulator testing of orthopaedic joint prostheses', *Tribology Series*, **41**: 291–296.

Uribe J, Geringer J and Forest B (2012), 'Shock machine for the mechanical behaviour of hip prostheses: a description of performance capabilities', *Lubrication Science*, **24**: 45–60.

Wan Z, Dorr L D, Woodsome T, Ranawat A and Song M (1999), 'Effect of stem stiffness and bone stiffness on bone remodeling in cemented total hip replacement', *Journal of Arthroplasty*, **14**: 149–158.

Waterhouse R B (1982), 'Occurrence of fretting in practice and its simulation in the laboratory, Materials evaluation under fretting conditions', *ASTM STP 780*, pp. 3–16. West Conshohocken, PA: ASTM International.

Watson S W, Friedersdorf F J, Madsen B W and Cramer S D (1995a), 'Methods of measuring wear-corrosion synergism', *Wear*, **181/183**: 476–484.

Watson S W, Madsen B W and Cramer S D (1995b), 'Wear-corrosion study of white cast irons', *Wear*, **181/183**: 469–475.

Wegrelius L, Falkenberg F and Olefjord I (1999), 'Passivation of stainless steels in hydrochloric acid', *Journal of the Electrochemical Society*, **146**: 1397–1406.

Wiles P (1958), 'The surgery of the osteoarthritic hip', *British Journal of Surgery*, **45**: 488–497.

Wiltse L L (1957), 'Experimental studies regarding the possible use of self-curing acrylic in orthopaedic surgery', *Journal of Bone and Joint Surgery, American*, **39A**: 961–972.

Published by Woodhead Publishing Limited, 2013

Wimmer M A, Fischer A, Büscher R, Sprecher C M, Hauert R et al. (2010), 'Wear mechanisms in metal-on-metal bearings: the importance of tribochemical reaction layers', *Journal of Orthopedic Research*, **28**: 436–443.

Wood R J K (2010), 'Tribo-corrosion', *Shreir's Corrosion*, **2**: 1005–1050.

Yan Y, Neville A and Dawson D (2007), 'Biotribo-corrosion of CoCrMo orthopaedic implant materials', *Tribology International*, **40**: 1492–1499.

Yan Y, Neville A, Dowson D, Williams S and Fisher J (2009), 'Effect of metallic nanoparticles on the biotribo-corrosion behaviour of metal-on-metal hip prostheses', *Wear*, **267**: 683–688.

Zhang H, Brown L T, Blunt L A, Jiang X and Barrans S M (2009), 'Understanding initiation and propagation of fretting wear on the femoral stem in total hip replacement', *Wear*, **266**: 566–569.

Published by Woodhead Publishing Limited, 2013

3

Application of biomedical-grade titanium alloys in trabecular bone and artificial joints

Yong Luo, Li Yang and Maocai Tian, China University of Mining and Technology

DOI: 10.1533/9780857092205.181

Abstract: This chapter introduces the application of biomedical-grade titanium (Ti) alloys in trabecular bone and artificial joints. It is focused on the tribological properties of Ti alloys and treated or modified Ti alloys. In the application of Ti alloys in trabecular bone, the factors influencing the coefficient of friction, including sliding speed, lubrication and bone type, were researched. Additionally, in order to simulate artificial joints, the tribological performance of Ti alloy and carburized Ti alloy against ultra-high-molecular-weight polyethylene under dry friction and bovine serum lubrication was studied.

Key words: titanium alloy, artificial joint, biotribology, biomaterial.

Published by Woodhead Publishing Limited, 2013

3.1 Introduction to biomedical-grade titanium alloys

Titanium (Ti) alloys are metallic materials that contain a mixture of Ti and other chemical elements. Such alloys have very high tensile strength and toughness, light weight, extraordinary corrosion resistance, and the ability to withstand extreme temperatures.

The crystal structure of Ti at ambient temperature and pressure is hexagonal close-packed (h.c.p.) α-phase with a *c*/*a* ratio of 1.587. At about 882 °C, the Ti undergoes an allotropic transformation to a body-centered cubic (b.c.c.) β-phase that remains stable to the melting temperature. Some alloy elements raise the α-to-β transition temperature while others lower the transition temperature.

Aluminum (Al), gallium (Ga), germanium (Ge), carbon (C), oxygen (O) and nitrogen (N) are α stabilizers, whereas molybdenum (Mo), vanadium (V), tantalum (Ta), niobium (Nb), manganese (Mn), iron (Fe), chromium (Cr), cobalt (Co), nickel (Ni), copper (Cu) and silicon (Si) are β stabilizers.

Based on the two phases of Ti, Ti alloys are generally classified into three classes: α, β and α + β alloys (Li et al., 2011). Due to their low density, high specific strength, high melting temperature and superior corrosion resistance, Ti alloys are widely used in space technology and ship technology (Ren et al., 2007). However, their high friction coefficient, high sensitivity to adhesive wear and fretting wear, as well as their poor resistance to high temperature oxidation and low wear resistance, have restricted the application of Ti alloys (Wang et al., 2008). Therefore, many modification technologies, such as laser surface modification technology, anodic oxidation, ion implantation and deposition, are used to solve these problems.

Published by Woodhead Publishing Limited, 2013

3.1.1 Titanium alloys applied as biomaterials

The use of Ti has increased in importance since it was first applied in the aerospace industry in the 1950s. Nowadays, a large number of alloys with variable compositions and microstructures are available, and they can be employed in different fields, like in the manufacturing of aerospace components and orthopedic implant devices. Pure Ti and Ti alloys show very interesting characteristics, such as high strength-to-weight ratio, admirable corrosion resistance and excellent biocompatibility, which make such materials appropriate for use in orthopedic and dental implants. The use of pure Ti as a biomedical material began in the 1960s. Despite the fact that pure Ti shows superior corrosion resistance and tissue acceptance when compared with other biomedical materials, it has disadvantages in terms of strength and stiffness, and difficulty in polishing when applied as a medical metal (Iijima et al., 2003).

In order to overcome such restrictions, Ti6Al4V alloy, which has higher strength than pure Ti and sufficient corrosion resistance, is used to substitute the pure Ti in medical applications (Chen and Gao, 2009). Ti6Al4V alloy is a representative $\alpha + \beta$ alloy type, where the α-phase is stabilized by Al and the β-phase is stabilized by V. Ti6Al4V alloy contains enough stabilizing elements to modify the $\alpha + \beta$-phase field in such a way that both phases are present at room temperature. It is considered as a good surgical implant material; however, some studies found that this kind of alloy would release V ions in long-term implantation and V ions may react with the tissues in the human body. In addition, recent research has led to the conclusion that V is toxic to the human body. According to Ito et al. (1995) and Okazaki et al. (1996), V can accumulate in some body parts, such as

Published by Woodhead Publishing Limited, 2013

bone, kidneys and liver. Also, when compared with other metals like Ni and Cr, V may be more toxic. An interesting alternative to solve this problem is the replacement of V with Nb in the Ti α + β alloy type. Therefore, two new Ti alloys, Ti6AlNb and Ti5Al2.5Fe α + β-type alloys, were used to replace Ti6Al4V alloy. As compared with Ti6Al4V alloy, due to the lower Ti concentrations, the Ti–Al–Nb alloys are considered as one of the most attractive materials for biomedical implant applications. Finally, the castings of these alloys show slightly lower strength and about 40% higher elongation (Iijima et al., 2003; Boehlert et al., 2008).

3.1.2 Mechanical properties

Titanium alloys are applied as biomedical materials mainly in hard tissue replacement, which requires a modulus similar to human bone and high fatigue strength. The typical mechanical properties of biomedical Ti alloys are listed in Table 3.1 (Long and Rack, 1998; Mitsuo, 1998). As shown in Table 3.1, the elastic modulus of Ti alloys ranges from 55 to 114 GPa and it was noticed that Ti alloys exhibit a lower elastic modulus when compared with other metallic biomedical materials, such as 316L stainless steel and Co-based alloys (Mitsuo, 1998). The elastic modulus of bone is generally between 10 and 30 GPa; therefore the elastic modulus of the implants is required to be much more similar to that of bone. Among the three types of Ti alloys, the β-type alloys have a smaller elasticity than the others.

It can be also found that, compared with pure Ti, the alloys that contain Al have a higher elastic modulus, since Al can increase the Young's modulus. As Nb and Zr can decrease

Published by Woodhead Publishing Limited, 2013

Table 3.1 **Mechanical properties of Ti alloys for biomedical applications**

Alloy	Tensile strength (UTS) (MPa)	Yield strength	Elongation (%)	Elastic modulus (GPa)
α type				
Pure Ti grade1	240	170	24	102.7
Pure Ti grade2	345	275	20	102.7
Pure Ti grade3	450	380	18	103.4
Pure Ti grade4	550	485	15	104.1
α + β type				
Ti–6Al–4V ELI (mill annealed)	860–965	795–875	10–15	101–110
Ti–6Al–4V (annealed)	895–930	825–869	6–10	110–114
Ti–6Al–7Nb	900–1050	880–950	8.1–15	114
Ti–5Al–2.5Fe	1020	895	15	112
Ti–5Al–1.5B	925–1080	820–930	15–17.0	110
Ti–15Zr–4Nb–4Ta–0.2Pd				
Annealed	715	693	21	89
Aged	919	806	10	103
Ti–15Zr–4Nb–4Ta–0.2Pd				
Annealed	715	693	28	94
Aged	919	806	18	99
β type				
Ti–13Nb–13Zr (aged)	973–1037	836–908	10–16	79–84
Ti–12Mo–6Zr–2Fe	1060–1100	100–1060	18–22	74–85
Ti–15Mo (annealed)	874	544	21	78
Ti–15Mo–5Zr–3Al	852–1100	838–1060	18–25	80
Ti–15Mo–2.8Nb–0.2Si	979–999	945–987	16–18	83
Ti–35.3Nb–5.1Ta–7.1Zr	596.7	547.1	19.0	55.0
Ti–29Nb–13Ta–4.6Zr	911	864	13.2	80

Published by Woodhead Publishing Limited, 2013

the Young's modulus, Ti alloyed with Nb and Zr has a lower modulus (Raducanu et al., 2011). The tensile strength of pure Ti ranges from 240 to 550 MPa and up to 1100 MPa for alloys strengthened by alloy elements, since the alloy elements lead to solid-solution strengthening or second-phase strengthening. The ductility is measured by the elongation and ranges from 10% to 28%. The analysis of slip systems in different crystal structures reveals that it is easier for a highly close-packed crystal surface and orientation to promote plastic deformation; plastic deformation occurred in the b.c.c. crystal structure rather than the h.c.p. structure. The fatigue strengths at 10^7 cycles of biomedical Ti alloys are given in Figure 3.1. It is shown that the fatigue strength of α + β alloy can reach 810 MPa, and under different conditions or treatments the fatigue strength varies, since the α-phase has a h.c.p. crystal structure, which is anisotropic.

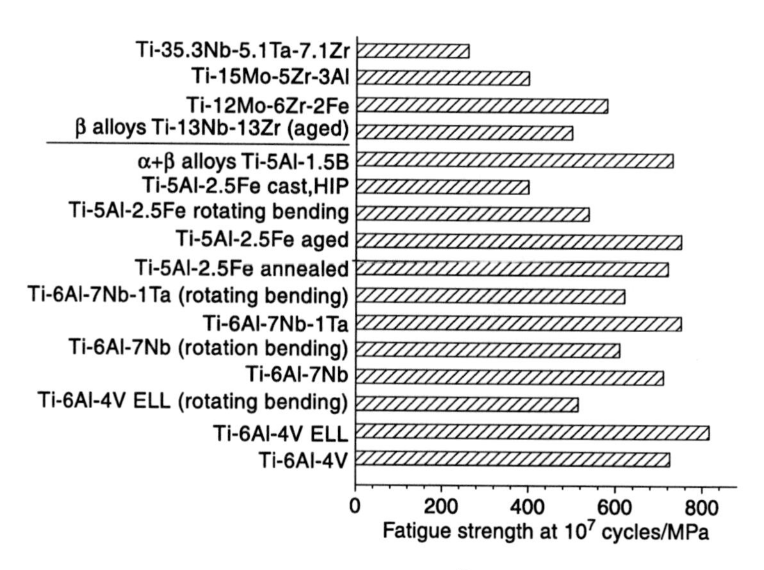

Figure 3.1 Fatigue strength at 10^7 cycles of biomedical Ti alloy.

Published by Woodhead Publishing Limited, 2013

3.1.3 Corrosion resistance

Corrosion resistance is one of the main properties of biomedical materials. Thus, it should be carefully examined before application in the human body. It has been documented in the literature that the pH value of the fluids in the human body, under normal conditions, is about 7.4 and may increase up to 7.8 or decrease to 5.5 after a surgical procedure, and the value will return back to normal a few days later. In such an environment, Ti and its alloys exhibit better corrosion resistance than Co-based alloys and 316L stainless steel.

Atapour and Pilchak (2011) investigated the corrosion resistance of β biomedical Ti alloys Ti13Mo7Zr3Fe (TMZF) and Ti35Nb7Zr5Ta (TiOsteum) in 0.9% NaCl and 5 mol/L HCl solutions. The average values of the corrosion potential, the corrosion current density and the high-potential passive current density for these alloys are given in Table 3.2. It was found that all of the alloys showed very low corrosion current density in the NaCl solution and TiOsteum exhibited a lower corrosion current density than the other two alloys. In 5 M HCl, all of the alloys exhibited dissolution of the surface oxide film. TMZF (metastable β) and TiOsteum showed significantly extreme low weight loss even though corrosion rates were similar to Ti6Al4V.

The good corrosion resistance of Ti alloys is attributed to a stable and protective layer that is obtained through the reactions between Ti alloys and body liquids, which consist of water molecules, dissolved ions and proteins. Recently, X-ray diffraction analysis of the layers indicated that orthorhombic TiO_2 films were formed on the surfaces of pure Ti, Ti6Al4V ELI ('Extra-Low Interstitial') and Ti–10% Ta alloys (Zhou et al., 2005).

Published by Woodhead Publishing Limited, 2013

Table 3.2 Experimental corrosion potentials, corrosion current densities and high-potential passive current densities of the Ti–6Al–4V ELI, TiOsteum, TMZF (as-received $\alpha + \beta$) and TMZF (metastable β) alloys in Ringer's solution at 37 °C after 1 h immersion

Material	Corrosion potential (mV(SCE))	Corrosion current density (nA/cm^2)	Passive current density ($\mu A/cm^2$)
TMZF ($\alpha + \beta$)	−421 ± 12	29 ± 15	2.2 ± 0.1
TMZF (β)	−343 ± 83	20 ± 10	2.1 ± 0.1
TiOsteum	−292 ± 6	12 ± 5	1.9 ± 0.4
Ti–6Al–4V ELI	−380 ± 65	31 ± 13	2.9 ± 0.4

3.1.4 Biocompatibility

Biocompatibility is the ability of a material to remain biologically innocuous when applied inside a living creature (Long and Rack, 1998). A variety of interactions and reactions between implants and the human body will lead to injury as follows. (i) The metallic implant will release ions that may interfere with physiological movement of ions in neural cells. (ii) The enrichment of metallic ions in the human body may cause local adverse tissue reactions and allergic reactions. This release of ions depends on the corrosion rate of the alloy and the solubility of the first-formed corrosion products. Once corrosion products are formed, their further behavior depends on the nature of the film substances, such as the electrical, chemical and mechanical properties (Zhou et al., 2005). Therefore, consideration of corrosion product stability in tissues becomes important. The alloy elements, Ta, Nb, V and Zr, produce essentially insoluble oxides and their corrosion products can have good stability in the human body.

Published by Woodhead Publishing Limited, 2013

3.1.5 Osseointegration

The ideal biomaterial should have excellent biocompatibility characteristics and osseointegration. Several studies on the osseointegration of Ti alloys have been performed both *in vitro* and *in vivo*. Nails made of Ti (Ti6Al4V) were implanted into healthy and osteopenic rats to evaluate the osseointegration of Ti alloys, and the *in vitro* study also used cells cultured from the same animals (Fini et al., 2011). After 2 months, it was found that the osseointegration of Ti6Al4V happened in normal and osteopenic bone, and the rate of osseointegration in normal bone was greater than that in osteopenic bone. Several studies have reported on the bone remodeling activity on Ti implants with different surface roughness values; a rough surface supplies a stable bone–implant interface and promotes the osseointegration of Ti implants (Suzuki et al., 1997; Huang et al., 2011). A special surface treatment method has been used to promote bone growth on the Ti surface by increasing the bone–implant interface. More recently, some elements, such as Nb, Ta, Zr and Mo, have been used as alloying elements to develop some new alloys, such as Ti22Nb6Zr. Those new alloys present a good electrochemical behavior in physiological fluids and can induce better osseointegration; as a result they are expected to become promising candidates for biomedical applications (Li et al., 2004; Satendra and Sankara, 2008; Daniel et al., 2009; Raducanu et al., 2011).

3.1.6 Medical applications

Titanium and Ti alloys are common in biomaterials. The applications of Ti and its alloys can be classified as cardiovascular applications, osteosynthesis and hard tissue replacements (Liu et al., 2004).

Published by Woodhead Publishing Limited, 2013

The idea to support a failing heart with extracorporeal circulation was first suggested in the early nineteenth century. In 1951, an artificial pump sustained a dog successfully. The pump consisted of two side-by-side membrane sacs attached to an external drive shaft. A new heart–lung machine was implanted in 2011; both the blood sacs and the valves were made of a novel polyether-based polyurethane plastic encased in a Ti shell (Gray et al., 2006). A Ti6Al4V artificial heart valve ring was coated with nanocrystalline diamond by Jozwik and Karczemska (2007), and the structure and thickness of the coating remained the same after long-term mechanical fatigue experiments. The coating showed high resistance to wear, which seems to be the result of loads acting on the heart valve placed in the aortic position. Recently, the use of shape memory Ni–Ti alloy in intravascular devices, such as stents and occlusion coils, has received considerable attention (Liu et al., 2004).

Titanium alloys are sometimes used in osteosynthesis, such as bone fracture fixation. Acero et al. (1999) analyzed the behavior of Ti when used in bone repair after facial fractures or osteotomies and good ultrastructural osseointegration of the Ti osteosynthesis material was shown in most cases. It was found that Ti and its alloys with rough surfaces or bioactive surfaces can improve osteointegration because they bond tightly to the bone, thereby reducing relative motions.

The hard tissue replacements of Ti and its alloys include artificial joints, and recently Ti and its alloys have been applied as trabecular bone. In addition, Ti and Ti alloys are common in dental implants. Researchers found a new Ti alloy had no irritation response to the oral mucous membrane (Xu et al., 2006). Recently, many surface modification technologies have been utilized to improve the osseointegration ability of Ti dental implants. The

Published by Woodhead Publishing Limited, 2013

applications of Ti alloys in trabecular bone and artificial joints will be discussed in Section 3.2 and 3.3.

3.2 Application of titanium alloys in trabecular bone

3.2.1 Introduction

Trabecular bone is situated at the end of the long bones and in the spinal column, where it fills all of the inner vertebral space and has a complex three-dimensional architecture (Thurner et al., 2007). As shown in Figure 3.2 (Thomsen et al., 2002), with increasing age, the trabecular structure changes and will lead to osteoporosis. More seriously, it will lead to osteonecrosis of the femoral head (ONFH). ONFH is a common disease in both the young and adults. The useful time of an artificial joint cannot reach the lifetime of the patient. Many efforts were undertaken to slow down ONFH by using artificial trabecular bone for the treatment of early-stage osteonecrosis. Tantalum is a widely used material for artificial trabecular bone and the elastic modulus of Ta is about 3GPa, which is much more similar to bone

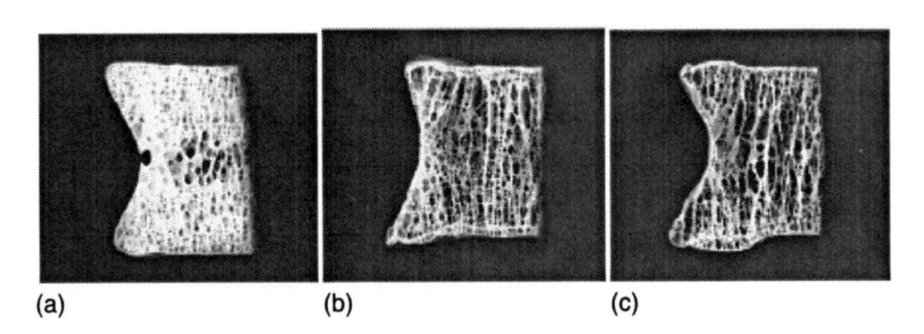

Figure 3.2 Regional changes in trabecular structure with age: (a) 37-year-old woman, (b) 72-year-old woman and (c) 81-year-old woman.

Published by Woodhead Publishing Limited, 2013

(Wang and Wang, 2010). The Ta implantation may not stop ONFH, but it can improve the function of bone during early-stage osteonecrosis. Titanium alloy can be recommended for the treatment of ONFH. Wang et al. (2007) used a Ti alloy cage implantation for the treatment of ONFH in dogs, and found that the Ti alloy cage could provide structural support to the subchondral bone and prevent collapse. Finally, it was found that the peripheral holes can have a good osteoconductivity (Wang et al., 2007).

One application of Ti alloy in trabecular bone is the trabecular structure-like Ti on the surface of the acetabular cup. Marin et al. (2010) obtained the structure on the acetabular cup by EBM (electron beam melting) technology (Figure 3.3) and found this structure can have good osseointegration. In order to understand the friction and contact between the Ti and bone, our group performed a large number of experiments using the trabecular structure Ti and porcine bones. Therefore, we will mainly discuss the coefficient of friction (COF) of this structure

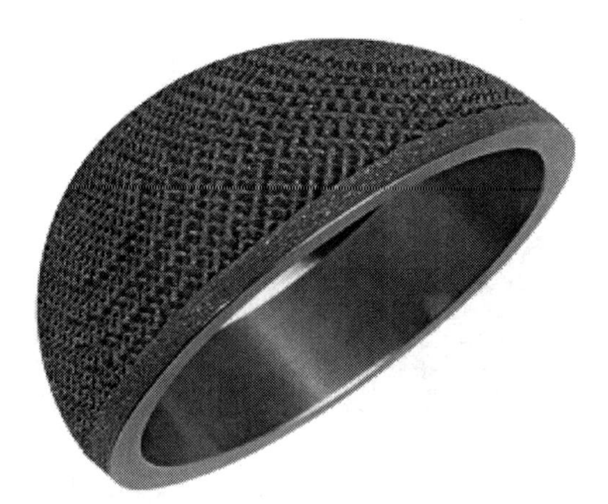

Figure 3.3 Acetabular cup in trabecular Ti for use in primary acetabular surgery.

Published by Woodhead Publishing Limited, 2013

wear against porcine bone under different lubricating conditions.

3.2.2 Materials

The artificial trabecular bone was made of Ti6Al4V in the form of a cellular solid structure by EBM, and the dimensions were 10 mm (diameter) × 30 mm. The three-dimensional structure of the Ti specimen is shown in Figure 3.4. The compact bone and cancellous bone used in this procedure were from the porcine femur. The lubricating fluids in this procedure include deionized water, saline water with 0.9 wt% NaCl and bovine serum at a concentration of 25%.

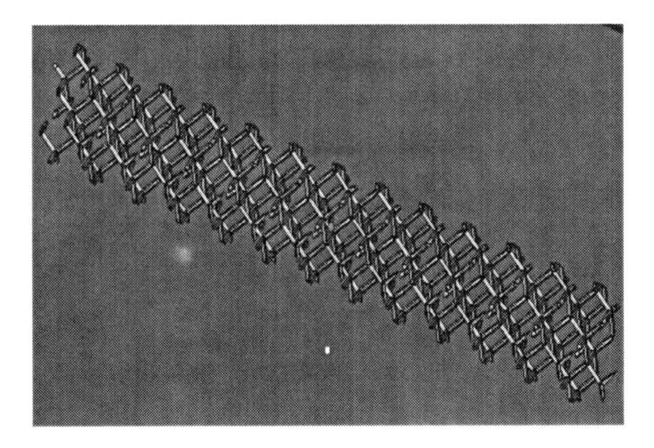

Figure 3.4 Three-dimensional structure of the Ti specimen.

3.2.3 Procedure

The compact bone used in this procedure was cut from the porcine femoral diaphysis and the cancellous bone from the porcine femoral head. First, we eliminated the soft tissue, fat and marrow of the femur, and then reserved the femoral

Published by Woodhead Publishing Limited, 2013

head and diaphysis. Then, the femoral head was cut into dimensions of 5 mm × 15 mm × 25 mm and the surface area was 15 × 25 mm^2. The thickness of the specimen from the porcine diaphysis was about 3 mm and then the diaphysis was machined to 15 × 25 mm^2 surface area. As shown in Figure 3.5, in order to get a large surface, the compact bone should be sanded with an average roughness of 0.5 μm. The left image is the cancellous bone specimen and the right image is the compact bone specimen.

The COF of Ti cellular solid structure wear against the two bones was measured on a universal multifunctional tester (UMT) developed at CETR (Campbell, CA). The wear tests were performed in a pin-on-flat model with reciprocating motion. The sliding velocities of the Ti alloy cellular solid structure pin against the bone plate were 0.01, 0.05 and 0.1 mm/s, respectively. Lubrication fluids (deionized water, saline water with 0.9 wt% NaCl and bovine serum at a concentration of 25 wt%) were used in the friction and wear test. The normal load applied in this procedure was

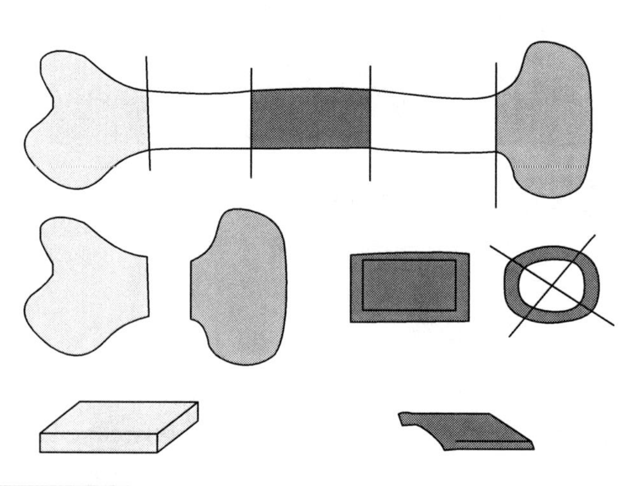

Figure 3.5 Schematic of bone specimen preparation.

Published by Woodhead Publishing Limited, 2013

10 N and the sliding displacement was 4 mm. Each process lasted for 3 min.

3.2.4 Results and discussion

The COFs of the bone sliding against Ti alloy with trabecular structure at low sliding speeds in the sliding process were obtained and discussed. It was found that some fluctuations appeared on the COF curves at speeds of 0.05 and 0.1 mm/s under different lubricating conditions.

Effect of sliding speed on COF

Figure 3.6–3.8 show the variation of the COF of a Ti pin with trabecular structure sliding against bone under different lubrications as a function of testing time (T) at different sliding speeds.

Figure 3.6 gives the COF of a Ti pin with trabecular structure sliding against bone under deionized water lubrication. For compact bone specimens, as shown in Figure 3.6(a), the COF kept stable at a sliding speed of 0.01 mm/s and it had an average value of 0.36. With the

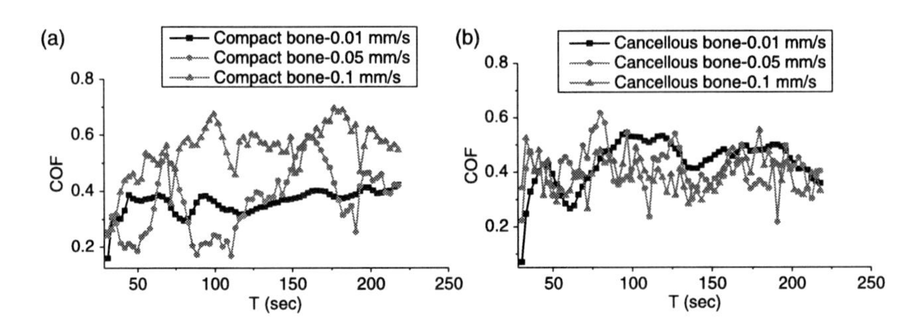

Figure 3.6 COF of Ti pins sliding against bone in deionized water at different sliding speeds.

Published by Woodhead Publishing Limited, 2013

increase of sliding speed, there was a large fluctuation of the COF at the sliding speed of 0.05 mm/s and some obvious peak values observed on the curve obtained at the speed of 0.05 mm/s. When the sliding speed increased to 0.1 mm/s, the curve became stable and gave the highest COF value.

For cancellous bone specimens in water, as shown in Figure 3.6(b), the variation of COF was undistinguishable at the three sliding speeds as time went by.

Figure 3.7 shows the COF of a Ti pin with trabecular structure sliding against bone under lubrication with saline water with 0.9 wt% NaCl. Figure 3.7(a) shows the COF of compact bone and the COF for the sliding speed at 0.01 mm/s remained stable. As the sliding speed increased, the COF value became larger. It should be noted that the COF at the sliding speed of 0.05 mm/s showed an increasing tendency as time went by. At the sliding speed of 0.1 mm/s, a peak appeared and the COF value decreased at first and then increased, and the value eventually remained stable at the value of 0.6.

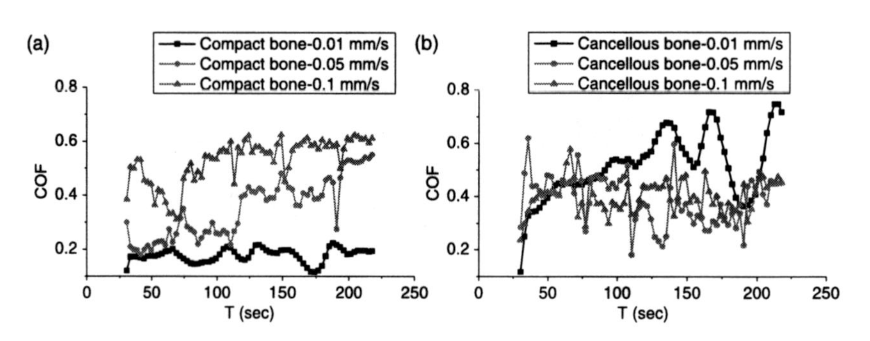

Figure 3.7 COF of Ti pins sliding against bone under lubrication with saline water at different sliding speeds.

Published by Woodhead Publishing Limited, 2013

The COF of cancellous bone at 0.01 mm/s gave the lowest value at first. Then the COF value increased and met the highest value under lubrication with saline water. With the increase of sliding speed, the COF at the sliding speed of 0.05 mm/s stayed the highest value at first and some large fluctuations appeared in the curve. When the sliding speed was 0.1 mm/s, the variation of the COF value reached 0.4.

Figure 3.8(a) presents the COF of compact bone under lubrication with bovine serum at various sliding speeds. For compact bone, the COF at the sliding speed of 0.01 mm/s had a stable value of 0.65 and then increased to a higher value. As time went by, the value decreased to the lowest. It was found that the COF remained stable around the value of 0.6 at the sliding speeds of 0.05 and 0.1 mm/s.

For cancellous bone under lubrication with bovine serum, as shown in Figure 3.9, the COF at the speed of 0.01 mm/s showed a decreasing tendency. With the increase of sliding speed, the COF changed irregularly at sliding speeds of 0.05 and 0.1 mm/s.

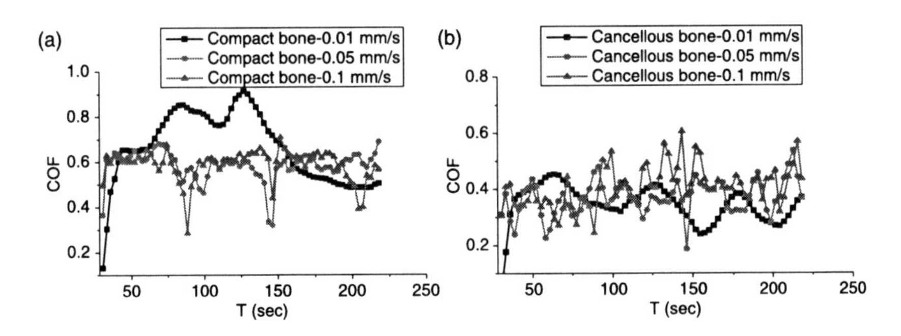

Figure 3.8 COF of Ti pins sliding against bone under lubrication with bovine serum at different sliding speeds.

Published by Woodhead Publishing Limited, 2013

Effect of lubricating fluids on COF

Figure 3.9–3.11 show the variation of COF of a Ti pin sliding against bone at different sliding speeds as a function of testing time (*T*) under different lubricating conditions.

Figure 3.9 shows the COF of a Ti pin sliding against bone specimens at a sliding speed of 0.01 mm/s under different lubricating conditions. The COF for compact bone kept a stable value of 0.4 under lubrication with deionized water, while the COF value decreased to a lower value, although it still remained stable, under lubrication with saline water. It was obvious that the COF reached the highest value under lubrication with bovine serum. For the cancellous bone under lubrication with deionized water, a continuous fluctuation appeared in the COF curve. Under lubrication with saline water, the COF of a Ti pin against cancellous bone reached a lower value at first and then showed an increasing tendency. It was also noticed that some fluctuations appeared in the COF curve under all three lubrication conditions as time went by. The COF value of a Ti pin against cancellous bone remained the lowest under lubrication with bovine serum.

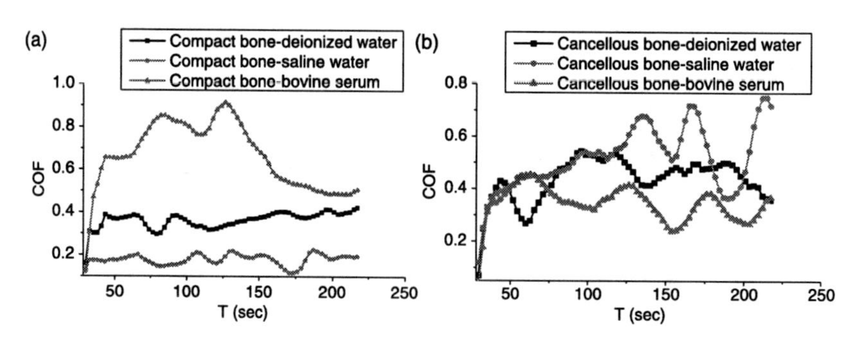

Figure 3.9 COF of Ti pins sliding against bone at a sliding speed of 0.01 mm/s under different lubricating conditions.

Published by Woodhead Publishing Limited, 2013

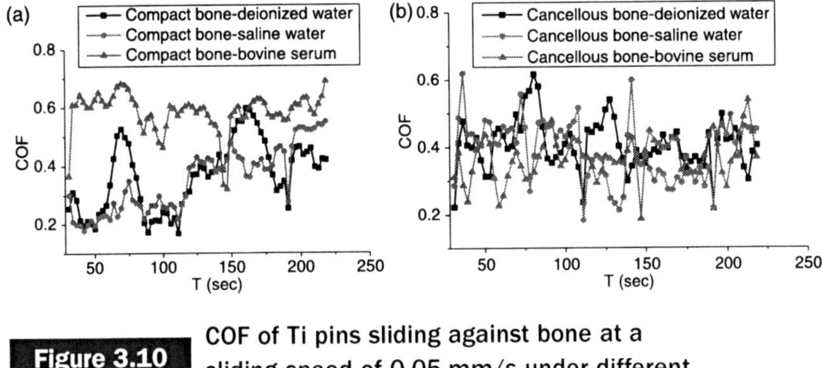

Figure 3.10 **COF of Ti pins sliding against bone at a sliding speed of 0.05 mm/s under different lubricating conditions.**

Figure 3.10 presents the COF of a Ti pin sliding against bone at a sliding speed of 0.05 mm/s under different lubricating conditions. For compact bone specimens, the COF of a Ti alloy pin showed an increasing tendency and similar values under lubrication with both saline water and deionized water. It was revealed that the COF of a Ti alloy pin against compact bone specimens remained at the highest value of 0.6 under lubrication with bovine serum. It should be noted the COF curve fluctuated under lubrication with deionized water. For cancellous bone specimens, the COF of a Ti alloy pin showed fluctuations and a similar value of 0.4 under all three lubrication conditions.

Figure 3.11 shows the COF of a Ti pin sliding against bone at a sliding speed of 0.1 mm/s under different lubricating conditions. The variation of the COF had a similar trend for compact bone specimens under all three lubrication conditions, as shown in Figure 3.11(a). Under all of the three lubrication conditions, the COF of a Ti pin sliding against compact bone showed a little fluctuation and had an average value around 0.6. For the cancellous bone specimens, a similar situation occurred. It was noticed that the variation of the COF had a similar trend for cancellous bone specimens

Published by Woodhead Publishing Limited, 2013

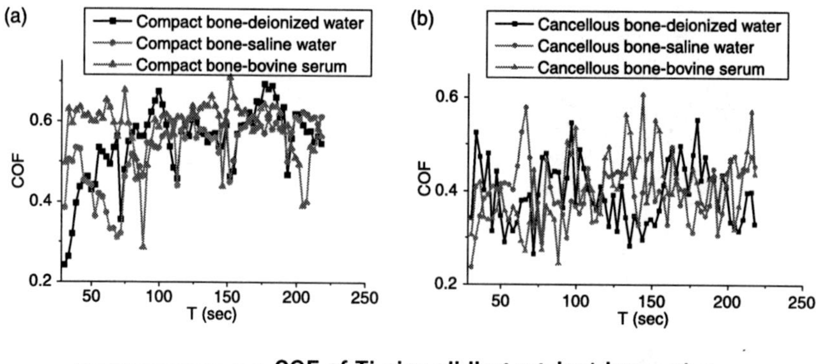

Figure 3.11 COF of Ti pins sliding against bone at a sliding speed of 0.1 mm/s under different lubricating conditions.

under all three lubrication conditions, as shown in Figure 3.11(b). Under all of the three lubrication conditions, the COF of a Ti pin sliding against cancellous bone showed a little fluctuation and had an average value around 0.4.

Effect of the bone type on COF

Figures 3.12–3.14 show the variation in COF of a Ti pin sliding against different types of bone at different sliding speeds as a function of testing time (*T*) under three lubricating conditions.

Figure 3.12 shows the COF of Ti alloy specimens against different bones at a sliding speed of 0.1 mm/s under different lubricating conditions. In deionized water, the fluctuation of the COF curve for compact bone was larger than that of cancellous bone and the COF value of cancellous bone was smaller than that of compact bone. As presented in Figure 3.12(b), both compact bone and cancellous bone showed some obvious fluctuations in the COF curve and the compact bone had a higher COF value than cancellous bone. Under lubrication with bovine serum, the COF value of compact bone was more stable than that of cancellous bone.

Published by Woodhead Publishing Limited, 2013

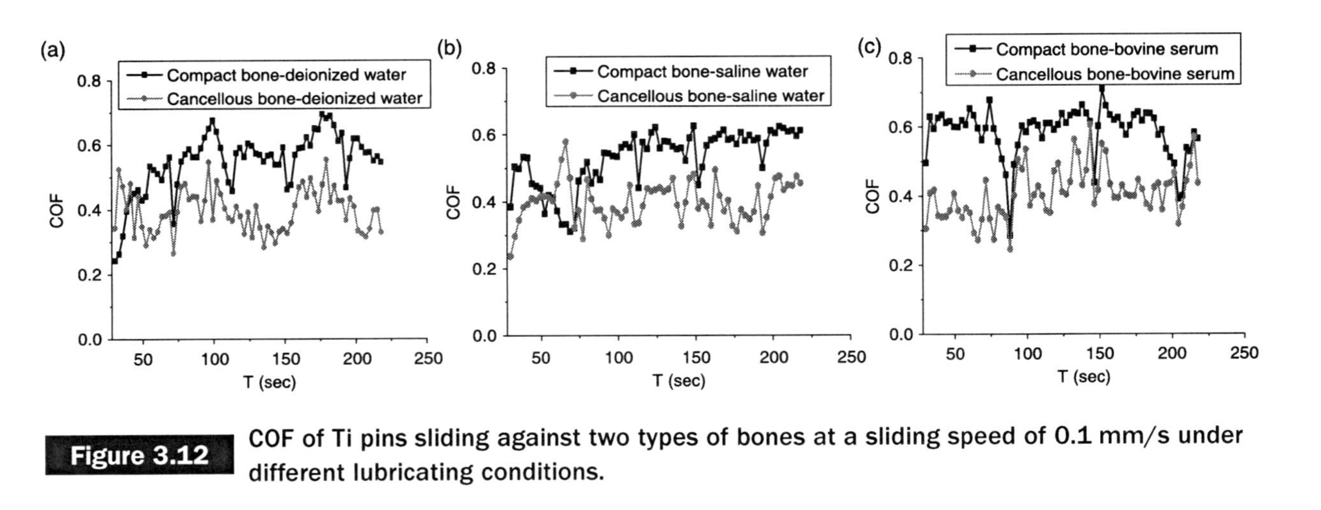

Figure 3.12 COF of Ti pins sliding against two types of bones at a sliding speed of 0.1 mm/s under different lubricating conditions.

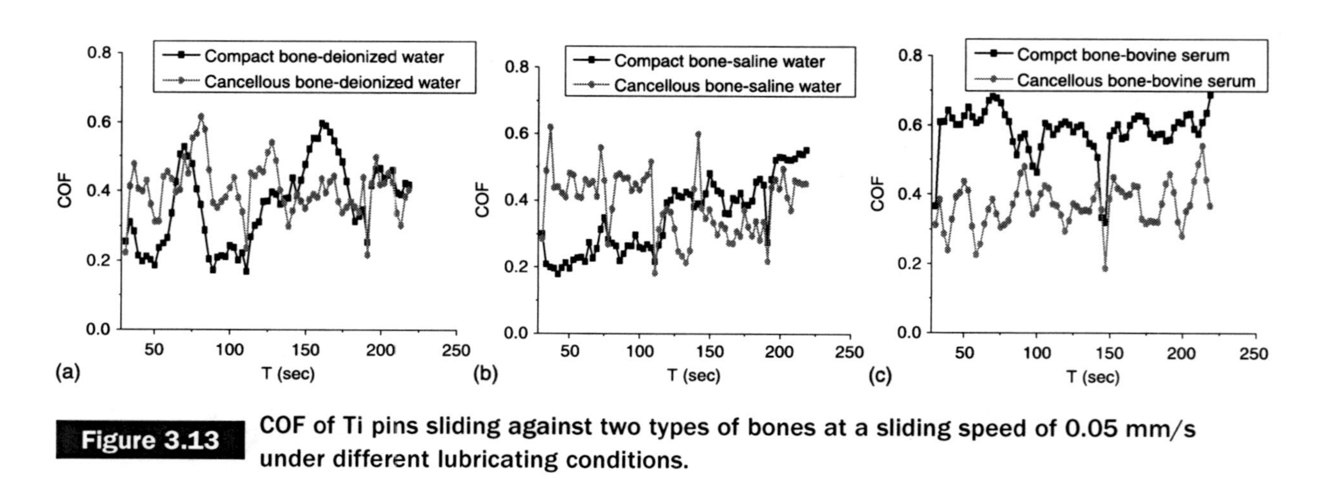

Figure 3.13 COF of Ti pins sliding against two types of bones at a sliding speed of 0.05 mm/s under different lubricating conditions.

Figure 3.13 shows the COF of a Ti pin sliding against two types of bones at a sliding speed of 0.05 mm/s under different lubricating conditions. Under lubrication with deionized water, there was no apparent difference between the two COF curves of compact and cancellous bone, respectively. Under lubrication with saline water, the COF value of compact bone showed an increasing tendency, but the COF value of cancellous bone indicated a decreasing tendency. Under lubrication with bovine serum, the compact bone had a higher COF value than cancellous bone.

Figure 3.14 presents the COF of a Ti pin sliding against two bones with a sliding speed of 0.01 mm/s under different lubricating conditions. The cancellous bone had a higher COF value than the compact bone under lubrication with deionized water and saline water. Under lubrication with bovine serum, the compact bone had a higher COF value than cancellous bone.

First peak COF value

The Ti alloy specimen with trabecular structure could keep the acetabular cup stable after implantation in the human body. Measurement of the static friction coefficient between the Ti specimen with trabecular structure and bone is needed. In this part, as shown in Table 3.3, the first peak COF value was defined as the static friction coefficient.

In order to express the first peak value intuitively, a histogram was taken to represent the variations of the first COF peak values. As shown in Figure 3.15, it was revealed that the first COF peak value increased with the sliding speed. For compact bone, the lubricating conditions played an important role on the first COF peak values. It was also found that the sliding speed could affect the first COF peak values under different lubricating conditions. For cancellous

Published by Woodhead Publishing Limited, 2013

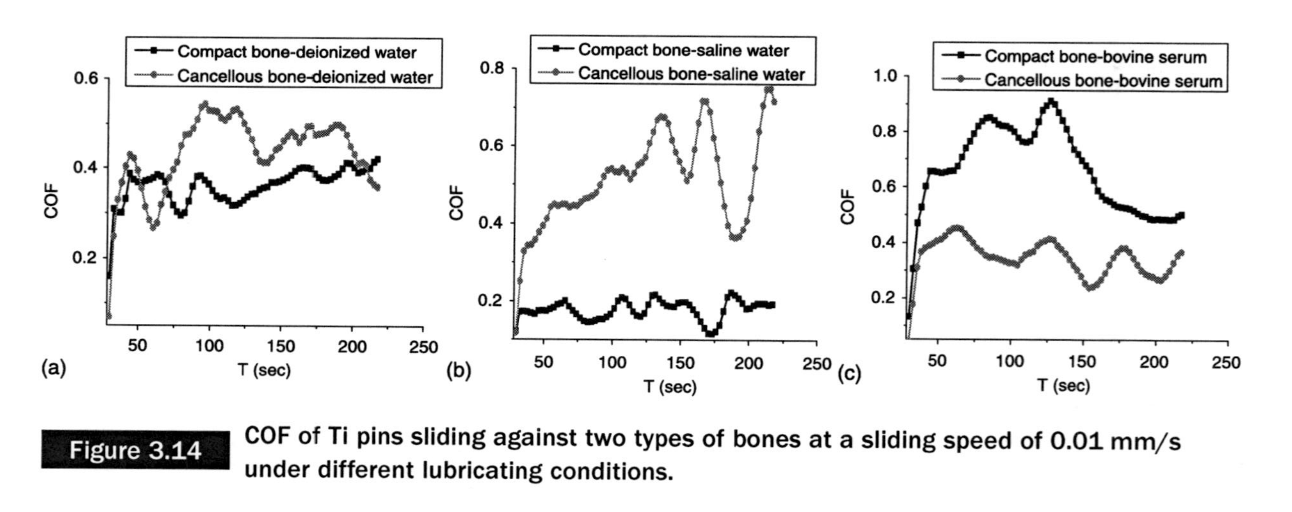

Figure 3.14 COF of Ti pins sliding against two types of bones at a sliding speed of 0.01 mm/s under different lubricating conditions.

Published by Woodhead Publishing Limited, 2013

Table 3.3 First COF peak value of Ti specimens with trabecular structure sliding against bone under different lubricating conditions

	Speed (mm/s)		
	0.01	0.05	0.1
Compact bone/deionized water	0.320	0.3295	0.4706
Compact bone/saline water	0.201	0.3688	0.4896
Compact bone/bovine serum	0.5438	0.6063	0.6116
Cancellous bone/deionized water	0.3057	0.4234	0.4036
Cancellous bone/saline water	0.3149	0.3365	0.3692
Cancellous bone/bovine serum	0.3117	0.4572	0.4722

bone, the sliding speeds played a greater role in the first COF peak value than the lubricating conditions, and obvious differences of the first COF peak values are observed with the increase of sliding speed, especially under lubrication with deionized water and bovine serum.

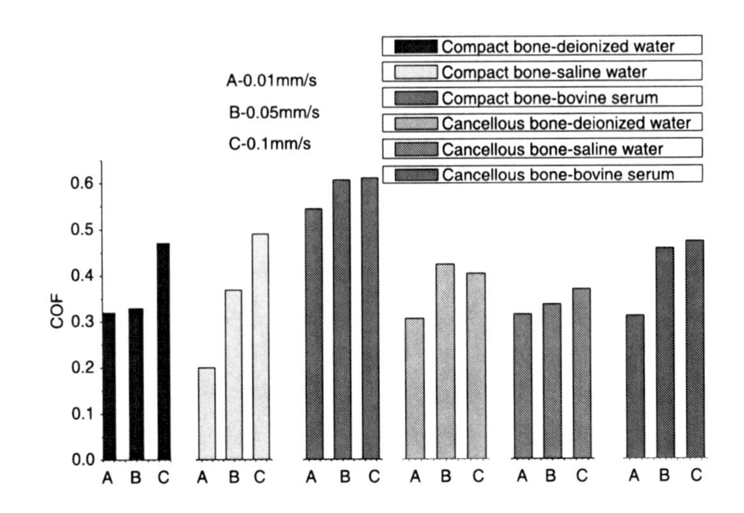

Figure 3.15 First peak COF values of Ti trabecular structure sliding against bone under different lubricating conditions.

Published by Woodhead Publishing Limited, 2013

3.3 Application of titanium alloys in artificial joints

3.3.1 Introduction

Artificial joints need to be strictly tested before implantation. As a joint prosthesis, the material must have high strength, good corrosion resistance, excellent wear resistance and outstanding biocompatibility (Santavirta et al., 1998). It is generally accepted that artificial joint materials include metal, polymer and bioceramics. Ultra-high-molecular-weight polyethylene (UHMWPE) is the main polymer used for joints, and it is widely used as acetabular cup material due to its superior biocompatibility, high impact strength and non-toxicity. Ceramics, such as alumina (Al_2O_3) and zirconia (ZrO_2) ceramics, have been used extensively in total joint bearings for their high oxidation levels, good chemical stability, excellent resistance to corrosion and reliable long-term behavior. Silicon carbide, classified as a non-oxide ceramic, has higher strength and hardness characteristics than those of Al_2O_3 (Sonny et al., 2006). In spite of this, metals are still alternative materials due to their good elasticity and wear resistance. Stainless steel, Co-based alloys and Ti-based alloys are the most widely used metallic materials in orthopedic implants (Luo et al., 2009b). Titanium and its alloys are known as the best potential candidates for artificial joints, due to their good corrosion resistance, low elastic modulus, high strength and superior biocompatibility (Jayanthi et al., 2010). However, their poor tribological performance limits their use in wear-related engineering applications, especially in artificial joints (Atar et al., 2008). Many early works were made to improve the tribological performance of Ti alloys by using different surface modifications, including physical vapor deposition

Published by Woodhead Publishing Limited, 2013

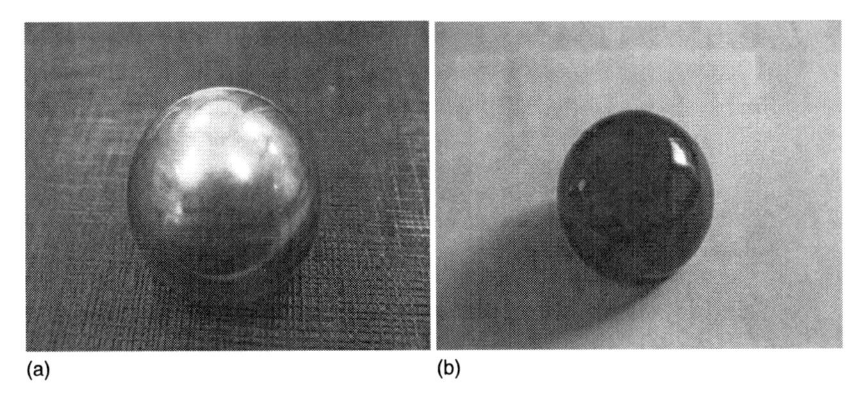

(a) (b)

Figure 3.16 **Photographs of Ti6Al4V femoral head before (a) and after (b) being carburized.**

(PVD), ion implantation, thermal plasma and laser nitriding, etc. Titanium carbide is a material of great commercial importance due to its superior hardness, high melting point, and excellent thermal and chemical stability. Many methods were attempted to synthesize Ti carbide, such as magnetron sputtering, pulsed ion beam assisted carburization and plasma immersed ion implantation (Ajikumar et al., 2012). As reported recently, Ti carbide was synthesized by our group at high-temperature exposure of Ti alloys to different concentrations of acetylene and for different exposure durations, as shown in Figure 3.16.

In this section, the tribological properties between UHMWPE and carburized Ti alloy are analyzed under different conditions. The wear mechanisms of UHMWPE against Ti alloy and carburized Ti alloy are also discussed.

3.3.2 Materials

The Ti alloys used in the procedure were Ti6Al4V alloy with dimensions of 15 mm × 15 mm × 5 mm. The carburized Ti

Published by Woodhead Publishing Limited, 2013

alloys and UHMWPE pins in this procedure were processed to meet the satisfactory criteria. The UHMWPE pins were made from UHMWPE powder with a molecular weight of 1 million.

3.3.3 Procedure

The Ti alloys were ultrasonically cleaned in acetone for 30 min and then placed in a high-temperature carburization furnace to carburize Ti alloys with C_2H_2. The surface of the carburized Ti alloys must be polished with an average roughness of 0.05 μm after carburizing. To transform the UHMWPE powder into pins, we placed the powder into a mould and heated at 200 °C under a pressure of 15 MPa for 2 h to get a UHMWPE block. Then, the UHMWPE block was machined to UHMWPE pins with dimensions 4 mm (diameter) × 30 mm. The circular cross-section of each UHMWPE pin should also be polished.

The tests were measured on a UMT developed at CETR. The tests were performed in a pin-on-disc model with reciprocating motion under conditions of dry friction and bovine serum lubrication. The normal load applied in this procedure was 10 N and the sliding speed was 2 mm/s for each process with a sliding displacement of 4 mm. The time for each process was 120 min.

Before or after the wear tests, the specimen should be ultrasonically cleaned in anhydrous alcohol for about 1 h. The specimens were then heated to 60 °C for 24 h for UHMWPE pins and 2 h for Ti specimens. The specimens were weighed after heat treatment to obtain the mass loss of each specimen; each specimen should be weighed three times and the average value taken. The wear rate and the mechanism of UHMWPE pins against Ti6Al4V and carburized Ti6Al4V will now be discussed.

Published by Woodhead Publishing Limited, 2013

3.3.4 *Results and discussion*

COF

Figure 3.17 presents the COF curves of Ti6Al4V alloy and the carburized Ti6Al4V alloy against the UHMWPE pin under dry sliding and bovine serum lubrication.

The average COF value was measured when the friction curve remained constant after certain testing periods. The common features of friction curves of carburized Ti6Al4V are slight fluctuation under both dry and bovine serum lubrication, and the value of them was around 0.085. In the case of Ti6Al4V alloy, bovine serum caused an abrupt reduction in COF values and fluctuations when compared with the dry sliding condition. It was observed that the value of COF decreased from 0.112 to 0.070 and the variance of COF decreased from 0.035 to 0.02. Wear debris covering the worn surface of Ti6Al4V led to fluctuation of the COF curve, while the carburized Ti6Al4V alloy had a stable COF due to its unique porous structure that could store wear debris. Table 3.4

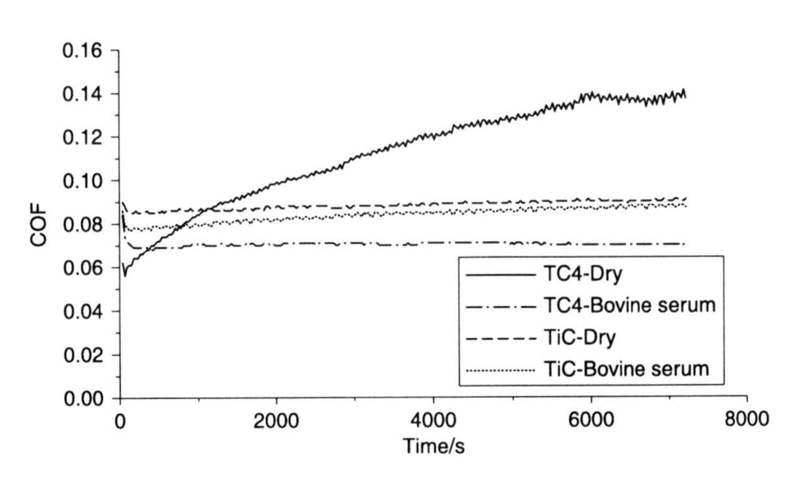

Figure 3.17 COF of Ti6Al4V and carburized Ti6Al4V under dry friction and serum lubricant conditions.

Published by Woodhead Publishing Limited, 2013

Table 3.4 COF and variance of Ti6Al4V (TC4) and carburized Ti6Al4V alloy (TiC)

Lubrication	Sample	Average COF	Variance
Dry friction	TC4	0.11180	0.03495
	TiC	0.08892	0.01315
Bovine serum lubrication	TC4	0.07026	0.02004
	TiC	0.08476	0.01919

gives the values of COF and variance of Ti6Al4V (TC4) and carburized Ti6Al4V alloy (TiC).

It should be noted that the COF of Ti6Al4V alloy under dry sliding increased continuously during the whole testing process and bovine serum lubrication could not provide a considerable beneficial effect on the wear resistance of the Ti6Al4V alloy for the higher fluctuations, even though the COF was reduced. All of the results provided a good explanation why the untreated Ti alloys were not suitable for artificial joints. The carburized Ti6Al4V alloy displayed excellent tribological properties for the stem material in artificial joints, especially its stability.

Wear performance

It was found that the mass loss of Ti alloy after the wear test became a minus value due to the formation of the transfer film on the Ti alloy surface. Some visible scratches were found on the surface of Ti alloys. However, for carburized Ti, no visible scratches were found on the surface after the wear process.

Due to the transfer film that appeared in the wear process, it is difficult to measure the wear rate of Ti alloy specimens. In order to account for the changes of wear properties of Ti alloy and carburized Ti alloy, the wear rates of UHMWPE pins against Ti6Al4V and carburized Ti6Al4V were

Published by Woodhead Publishing Limited, 2013

Table 3.5 **Mass loss of UHMWPE pins for different friction pairs**

Lubrication condition	Friction pairs	Mass loss (kg)	Wear rate (kgN^{-1} m^{-1})
Dry friction	UHMWPE pin on TC4	0.9×10^{-7}	6.38×10^{-10}
	UHMWPE pin on TiC	0.5×10^{-7}	3.54×10^{-10}
Bovine serum lubrication	UHMWPE pin on TC4	0.3×10^{-7}	2.12×10^{-10}
	UHMWPE pin on TiC	0.1×10^{-7}	0.71×10^{-10}

measured. Table 3.5 presents the mass loss of UHMWPE pins for different friction pairs. For the UHMWPE pin sliding on Ti alloy, the mass loss is the highest under dry friction and its wear rate was 6.38×10^{-10} kgN^{-1} m^{-1} under the condition of dry friction. It was found that the wear rate was reduced to 2.12×10^{-10} kgN^{-1} m^{-1} under lubrication with bovine serum, i.e. a decrease of 66.8%. Adhesive wear occurred under dry friction; the bovine serum reduced the adhesive wear and improved wear resistance effectively. For the UHMWPE pin sliding on carburized Ti alloy, the wear rate was 3.54×10^{-10} kgN^{-1} m^{-1} under dry friction, i.e. decreased by 44.5% compared with the UHMWPE pin sliding against Ti alloy under the same condition. Titanium carbide ceramics formed on the surface of carburized Ti alloy improved the hardness of the surface and the free state carbon atoms improved the friction environment effectively, therefore reducing the COF and wear (Luo et al., 2009a). The wear rate of the UHMWPE pin sliding against carburized Ti alloy was 0.71×10^{-10} kgN^{-1} m^{-1} under lubrication with bovine serum. The wear rate of the UHMWPE pin sliding against carburized Ti alloy under bovine serum lubrication decreased by 80% compared with that under dry friction.

The COF of carburized Ti6Al4V was steady under both dry and bovine serum lubrication, while the COF of Ti6Al4V

Published by Woodhead Publishing Limited, 2013

fluctuated heavily, especially under dry friction. The carburized Ti alloy has higher wear resistance than Ti alloys and it causes less harm to the UHMWPE due to lubrication with the free state carbon atoms.

3.4 Conclusions

Titanium alloys have been extensively applied in the aerospace, chemical and biomedical industries due to the excellent combination of their mechanical properties. The tribological behaviors of Ti alloys are dissatisfactory, but treated or modified Ti alloys could exhibit the required properties, including mechanical properties and tribology properties, when used as trabecular bone and artificial joints.

3.5 Acknowledgements

The authors wish to thank the National Natural Science Foundation of China under grant 51005234, the Fundamental Research Funds for the Central Universities under grant 2012QNA06 and the Vital Foundational 973 Program of China under grant 2011CB707603.

3.6 References

Acero J, Calderon J, Salmeron I, Verdaguer J and Somacarrera L (1999), 'The behaviour of titanium as a biomaterial microscopy study of plates and surrounding tissues in facial osteosynthesis', *Journal of Cranio-Maxillofacial Surgery*, 27: 117–123.

Published by Woodhead Publishing Limited, 2013

Ajikumar P, Vijayakumar M, Kamruddin M, Kalavathi S and Kumar N (2012), 'Effect of reactive gas composition on the microstructure, growth mechanism and friction coefficient of TiC overlayers', *International Journal of Refractory Metals and Hard Materials*, **31**: 62–70.

Atapour M and Pilchak A L (2011), 'Corrosion behavior of β titanium alloys for biomedical applications', *Materials Science and Engineering C*, **31**: 885–891.

Atar E, Kayali E S and Cimenoglu H (2008), 'Characteristics and wear performance of borided Ti6Al4V alloy', *Surface and Coatings Technology*, **202**: 4583–4590.

Boehlert C J, Cowen C J, Quast J P, Akahori T and Niinomi M (2008), 'Fatigue and wear evaluation of Ti–Al–Nb alloys for biomedical applications', *Materials Science and Engineering C*, **28**: 323–330.

Chen H and Gao W (2009), 'An overview on biomedical porous titanium and its alloys', *Southern Metals*, 8 (4): 26–28.

Daniel M, Romeu C and Gordin D (2009), 'Comparative corrosion study of Ti–Ta alloys for dental applications', *Acta Biomaterialia*, 5: 3625–3639.

Fini M, Giavaresi G, Torricelli P, Krajewski A, Ravaglioli A et al. (2011), 'Biocompatibility and osseointegration in osteoporotic bone', *Journal of Bone and Joint Surgery*, **83**: 139–143.

Gray N, Selzman C and Hill M (2006), 'Current status of the total artificial heart', *American Heart Journal*, **152**: 4–10.

Huang C, Zhao C, Han P, Ji W, Guo S et al. (2011), 'Histological and biomechanical evaluation in the interface between nano-surface titanium alloy implants and bone', *Journal of Clinical Rehabilitative Tissue Engineering Research*, 5: 3867–3870.

Iijima D, Yoneyama T, Doi H, Hamanaka H and Kurosaki N (2003), 'Wear properties of Ti and

Published by Woodhead Publishing Limited, 2013

Ti–6Al–7Nb castings for dental prostheses', *Biomaterials*, **24**: 1519–1524.

Ito A, Okazaki Y, Tateishi T and Ito Y (1995), '*In vitro* biocompatibility, mechanical properties, and corrosion resistance of Ti–Zr–Nb–Ta–Pd and Ti–Sn–Nb–Ta–Pd alloys', *Journal of Biomedical Materials Research*, **29**: 893–899.

Jayanthi P, Binil S, Shivakumar R and Christensen A (2010), 'Mechanical evaluation of porous titanium (Ti6Al4V) structures with electron beam melting (EBM)', *Journal of the Mechanical Behavior of Biomedical Materials*, **3**: 249–259.

Jozwik K and Karczemska A (2007), 'The new generation Ti6Al4V artificial heart valve with nanocrystalline diamond coating on the ring and with Derlin disc after long-term mechanical fatigue examination', *Diamond and Related Materials*, **16**: 1004–1009.

Li H, Lei T, Fan S and Huang G (2011), 'Research progress of biomedical titanium alloys', *Metallic Functional Materials*, **18**: 70–73.

Li S J, Yang R and Li S (2004), 'Wear characteristics of Ti–Nb–Ta–Zr and Ti–6Al–4V alloys for biomedical applications', *Wear*, **257**: 869–876.

Liu X, Chu P and Ding C (2004), 'Surface modification of titanium, titanium alloys and related materials for biomedical applications', *Materials Science and Engineering R*, **47**: 49–121.

Long M and Rack H J (1998), 'Titanium alloys in total joint replacement – a materials science perspective', *Biomaterials*, **19**: 1621–1639.

Luo Y, Ge S and Jin Z (2009a), 'Wettability modification for biosurface of titanium alloy by means of sequential carburization', *Journal of Bionic Engineering*, **6**: 219–223.

Luo Y, Ge S, Liu H and Jin Z (2009b), 'Microstructure analysis and wear behavior of titanium cermet femoral head with hard TiC layer', *Journal of Biomechanics*, **42**: 2708–2711.

Marin E, Fusi S, Pressacco M, Paussa L and Fedrizzi L (2010), 'Characterization of cellular solids in Ti6Al4V for orthopaedic implant applications: trabecular titanium', *Journal of the Mechanical Behavior of Biomedical Materials*, **3**: 373–381.

Mitsuo N (1998), 'Mechanical properties of biomedical titanium alloys', *Materials Science and Engineering A*, **243**: 231–236.

Okazaki Y, Ito Y, Kyo K and Tateishi T (1996), 'Corrosion resistance and corrosion fatigue strength of new titanium alloys for medical implants without V and Al', *Materials Science and Engineering A*, **213**:138–147.

Raducanu D, Vasilescu E, Cojocaru V D and Drob S I (2011), 'Mechanical and corrosion resistance of a new nanostructured Ti–Zr–Ta–Nb alloy', *Journal of the Mechanical Behavior of Biomedical Materials*, **4**: 1421–1430.

Ren X, Zhang Y, Zhou J and Ma Z (2007), 'Study of the effect of laser shock processing on titanium alloy', *Journal of Huazhong University of Science and Technology (Nature Science Edition)*, **35** (Supp1.): 150–152.

Santavirta Y, Konttinen R, Lappalainen A, Anttila S, Goodman SB et al. (1998), 'Materials in total joint replacement', *Current Orthopaedics*, **12**: 51–57.

Satendra K and Sankara T (2008), 'Corrosion behaviour of Ti–15Mo alloy for dental implant applications', *Journal of Dentistry*, **36**: 500–507.

Sonny B, Jonathan G, Michael R and Mohamed R (2006), 'Ceramic materials in total joint arthroplasty', *Seminars in Arthroplasty*, **17**: 94–101.

Published by Woodhead Publishing Limited, 2013

Suzuki K, Aoki K and Ohya K (1997), 'Effects of surface roughness of titanium implants on bone', *Bone*, **21**: 507–514.

Thomsen J S, Ebbesen E N and Mosekilde L (2002), 'Zone-dependent changes in human vertebral trabecular bone: clinical implications', *Bone*, **30**: 664–669.

Thurner P J, Erickson B, Jungmann R, Schriock Z and Hansma P K (2007), 'High-speed photography of compressed human trabecular bone correlates whitening to microscopic damage', *Engineering Fracture Mechanics*, **74**: 1928–1941.

Wang D, Tian Z, Shen L, Liu Z and Huang Y (2008), 'Research states of laser surface modification technology on titanium alloys', *Laser and Optoelectronics Progress*, **45**: 24–32.

Wang H and Wang J (2010), 'Progress of a porous tantalum implant for the treatment of early-stage osteonecrosis', *Journal of Clinical Orthopaedics*, **13**: 563–565.

Wang R, Zhang Q and Fu D (2007), 'Titanium alloy cage implantation for the treatment of the ischemic necrosis of femoral head in dogs', *Orthopedic Journal of China*, **15**: 538–540.

Xu Z, Zhang Y, Wang Z, Yu Z and Zhou L (2006), 'Oral mucous membrane irritation test on new medical titanium alloys', *Rare Metal Materials and Engineering*, **35**: 110–113.

Zhou Y, Mitsuo N, Toshikazu A, Hisao F and Hiroyuki T (2005), 'Corrosion resistance and biocompatibility of Ti-Ta alloys for biomedical applications', *Materials Science and Engineering A*, **398**: 28–36.

Published by Woodhead Publishing Limited, 2013

4

Fatigue strengthening of an orthopedic Ti6Al4V alloy: what is the potential of a final shot peening process?

Robert Sonntag and Joern Reinders, Heidelberg University Hospital, Germany, Jens Gibmeier, Karlsruhe Institute of Technology, Germany and J. Philippe Kretzer, Heidelberg University Hospital, Germany

DOI: 10.1533/9780857092205.217

Abstract: Mechanical surface treatments locally deform a metal substrate, introducing high compressive stresses at their surface. This has been shown to positively influence the fatigue endurance strength of cyclically loaded parts, e.g. in the aerospace industry. Hour-glass shaped specimens made of an orthopedic standard titanium alloy (Ti6Al4V) were shot peened and subjected to a simusoidal bending load condition up to a total of 10^7 cycles or until fracture occurred. Residual stress profiles were determined with high compressive stresses of over 800 MPa and a maximum penetration depth of 130 μm. Surface roughness was increased by 840% compared to the untreated condition. In conclusion, shot peening shows the potential

Published by Woodhead Publishing Limited, 2013

to increase fatigue strength by 12.3% and represents a great option for Ti6Al4V parts that are susceptible to high stresses, e.g. modular total joint replacements or implants for trauma surgery.

Key words: arthroplasty, Ti6Al4V, surface treatment, shot peening, fatigue failure

4.1 Titanium and its alloys

Materials that are used in load-bearing implants have to display a wide range of properties in order to work well in the human body. They need to maintain an appropriate mechanical (e.g. fatigue strength) and chemical performance (e.g. corrosion resistance) *in vivo* over time, and must have excellent biocompatibility, in other words insignificant local tissue reactions and systemic changes. In addition, manufacturing needs to be possible at an appropriate quality and at reasonable costs.

Standard metallic materials used in orthopedic and trauma surgery include stainless steels, cobalt–chromium alloys, pure titanium (Ti content: 98.9–99.6%) as well as titanium-based alloys. Today, an increasing number of devices are made of various titanium alloys (Table 4.1). They are used for osteosynthesis applications as well as load-carrying components for cementless total joint replacements (TJRs) among others.

Titanium and its alloys show several advantages that make them the most widely used metals in the field of medical implants: high biocompatibility, corrosion resistance and fatigue strength. Generally, Ti6Al4V, the most popular titanium alloy, has mechanical properties that exceed those of stainless steel, and an elasticity (Young's modulus) less than that of stainless steel and cobalt–chromium alloys. As a consequence, *stress* shielding is reduced which means that

Published by Woodhead Publishing Limited, 2013

Table 4.1 **Titanium and its standard alloys used in orthopedic applications**

Designation	Standards
Commercially pure titanium (CP-Ti, four grades)	ASTM F-67/ISO 5832-2
Titanium aluminum vanadium ELI ('Extra-Low Interstitial') alloy, wrought (Ti6Al4V)	ASTM F-136/ISO 5832-3
Titanium aluminum vanadium alloy, wrought (Ti6Al4V)	ASTM F-1472/ISO 5832-3
Titanium aluminum vanadium ELI ('Extra-Low Interstitial') alloy, forged (Ti6Al4V)	ASTM F-620/ISO 5832-3
Titanium aluminum vanadium alloy, cast (Ti6Al4V)	ASTM F-1108/ISO 5832-3
Titanium aluminum niobium (Ti6Al7Nb)	ASTM 1295/ISO 5832-11

the mechanical reaction to an external load after implantation is more similar to the physiological situation, enhancing the bone-to-implant load transfer. On the other hand, low shear strength and wear resistance are limiting factors for the use of titanium-based materials, such as in articulating components seen in TJRs. In addition, titanium is known for its high notch sensitivity, which increases the material's susceptibility to crack propagation and reduces its strength dramatically as can be the case in an inappropriate design. Table 4.2 summarizes the most important material properties of commercially pure titanium and Ti6Al4V standard alloy.

In vivo, titanium spontaneously forms a highly protective oxide layer (TiO_2) on the substate's surface of both the commercially pure form and its Ti6Al4V alloy. Although there is no dispute about the corrosion resistance that is provided by the oxide layer, there is still some disagreement in the literature about the exact oxide chemistry and biological performance at a molecular and tissue level (Brunski, 2004).

Table 4.2 **Mechanical properties of commercially pure titanium (CP-Ti) and Ti6Al4V**

	CP-Ti (Grade 4)	Ti6Al4V
Young's modulus (GPa)	105	110
Tensile strength (MPa)	692	850–900
Ultimate strength (MPa)	785	960–970
Fatigue strength at 107 cycles; *R* = –1 (MPa)	300	620–689
Hardness (HVN)	120–200	310
Elongation to fracture (%)	14–18	8
Titanium (Ti) content (wt%)	Balanced	88.3–90.8
Aluminum (Al) content (wt%)	–	5.5–6.5
Vanadium (V) content (wt%)	–	3.5–4.5
Iron (Fe) content (wt%)	Max. 0.5	Max. 0.25
Oxygen (O) content (wt%)	Max. 0.4	Max. 0.13
Carbon (C) content (wt%)	Max. 0.1	Max. 0.08
Nitrogen (N) content (wt%)	Max. 0.05	Max. 0.05
Hydrogen (H) content (wt%)	Max. 0.015	Max. 0.013

Source: Hallab et al., 2004; Navarro et al., 2008.

Newer titanium alloys seek to improve biocompatibility and lower the Young's modulus to one that is even closer to bone (thereby reducing 'stress shielding'), while maintaining other mechanical properties of the Ti6Al4V alloy. This can be done by substituting the relatively toxic vanadium with a less toxic metal, e.g. niobium (Ti6Al7Nb, ASTM 1295).

4.2 Fatigue failure after orthopedic surgical intervention

In the course of an implant's existence life span, ductile materials such as metals may fail due to breakage just like brittle materials

Published by Woodhead Publishing Limited, 2013

like ceramics can. National joint arthroplasty registers provide a good insight into the clinical failure mechanisms of hip and knee replacements. According to the data on total hip replacements, implant failure due to fracture of either the acetabular shell or the femoral stem component is seen in 1.5–2.0% of all revisions (Garellick et al., 2010; AOA, 2011). Although fracture is rare, complications are serious and painful for the patient (Figure 4.1). Revision needs to be performed carefully as implant fracture is often accompanied by damage to the surrounding bone and soft tissue.

Not only the choice of an appropriate material, but also the design has a substantial influence on the fatigue behavior and thus the long-term success of the implant. Critical geometric factors, such as small radii or notches that favor the crack initiation, may be one reason for early implant failure. Additionally, in the case of a recall of an inadequate

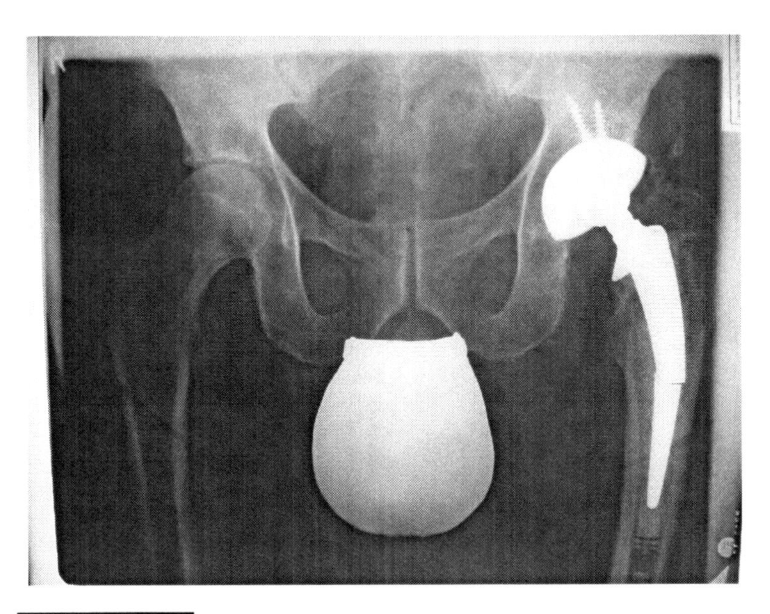

Figure 4.1 Failure of a hip stem four years after implantation.

system, patients who had been treated with such an implant are at increased risk of requiring revision surgery even if their implant is working well at that time.

In order to minimize soft tissue damage and the risk of infection during an operative intervention, minimally invasive approaches in both orthopedic and trauma surgery are becoming more frequent. To allow for these newer approaches, new implant designs have been introduced which tend to be more sophisticated. Additionally, today's patients are generally younger and more active, causing larger loads onto the implants. These trends are putting implants under larger duress, challenging today's material science. Another trend that contributes to the risk of early failure is the use of modular systems. Such systems are mainly used in revision arthroplasty and consist of multiple components. They are applied in order to restore the normal physiological situation of the patient intraoperatively, in other words to adjust the neck extension length, retro-version–anteversion discrepancy, or to restore a

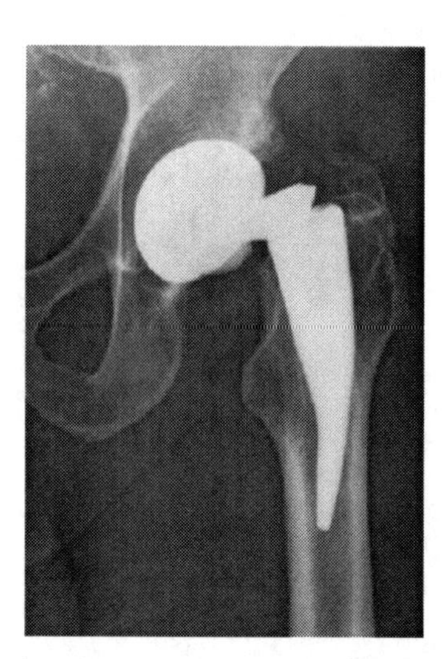

Figure 4.2 Failure of a modular titanium neck adapter.

(***Source***: Grupp et al. (2010))

joint presenting large bony defects. Therefore, adapters with mechanical tapered connections are used, which also increase the risk for implant fracture due to excessive fretting (Figure 4.2). There is an ongoing discussion on whether or not micro-motions within the taper junction induce *in vivo* crevice corrosion (Gilbert et al., 1993; Chu et al., 2000), Corrosive wear not only weakens the implant, but might also have a direct biological impact on the periprosthetic environment (Cook et al., 1994; Kretzer et al., 2009). In addition to orthopedic applications, periostal reactions and osteolysis around a modular conjunction have been reported for intramedullary femoral nails in trauma surgery (Jones et al., 2001).

4.3 Mechanical surface treatments

Mechanical surface treatments are widely applied for cyclically loaded titanium parts in the fields of mechanical and aerospace engineering in order to increase the resistance to the initiation and the early growth of fatigue cracks, such as in turbine blades in aircraft.

4.3.1 Shot peening

The most widely applied mechanical surface treatment for improvement of a material's fatigue strength is shot peening, which shows great flexibility regarding the geometry of the component to be treated. Shot peening is a cold-working process that is based on the random elastic/plastic impact of a shot material on the component's surface at high velocities (Figure 4.3). These shots introduce small rounded shallow indentations or dimples. Shot peening induces local stochastic deformation at the surface and an increase in dislocation

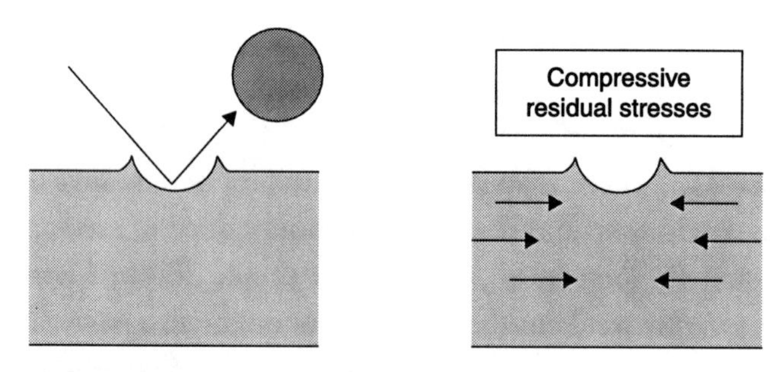

Figure 4.3 Shot peening process.

density that results in work-hardening of the surface layers and compressive residual stresses. These stresses are opposed to the tensile stresses that appear during physiologic loading.

In practice, small beads mostly made of spherically cast steel, rounded cut wire, ceramics or glass with diameters around 0.5–1 mm are accelerated (using air blast systems or centrifugal blast wheels) and bombarded onto the metal surface. The most important process parameters are listed in Table 4.3. The intensity of the peening process is measured using Almen strips (A, N or C type). It is a function of the substrate's hardness and the residual stresses distributions in the near surface layer.

Table 4.3 Shot peening process parameters

Parameter	
Peening system	Air blast system or centrifugal blast wheel
Shot distance	Distance from the workpiece: approx. 15 cm
Shot material and size	Cast steel, cut wire, ceramics or glass; typical diameter: 0.2–1.5 mm
Impact velocity and angle	–
Coverage ratio	Typically: 98% of the total surface (time dependent)

Published by Woodhead Publishing Limited, 2013

It is important to remember that the peening parameters need to be adopted to the size of the part to be treated. In the case of thin components, such as bone plates in trauma surgery the compressive stresses at the surface may tend to curve the component and the peened side will become convex. This effect is used for the so-called 'peen forming' process in the aerospace industry (Miao et al., 2010).

4.3.2 Residual stress measurements

Depth profiles of the residual stresses can be recorded using destructive X-ray diffraction (XRD) techniques. To do this, XRD stress analyses are repeatedly measured after an incremental layer removal by electrochemical polishing. The sum of all of the measurements at the different levels gives a depth profile of the residual stresses. For XRD analyses on metals, a monochromatic X-ray beam interacts with the crystallites of the near surface region. Constructive diffraction occurs when the Bragg equation

$$2d_{\{hkl\}}\sin\theta = n\lambda \qquad [4.1]$$

is fulfilled. Using a monochromatic X-ray beam with a known wavelength λ, the interplanar distances of a family of lattice planes of type $\{hkl\}$ $d_{\{hkl\}}$ can be determined when the diffraction angle θ of the diffracted beam is measured by means of an X-ray diffractometer (Bragg's law; see Figure 4.4). Crystal lattice strain can be determined according to the total differential of Bragg's law with:

$$\varepsilon_{\{hkl\}}^{\text{lattice}} = \frac{d_{\{hkl\}} - d_{0,\{hkl\}}}{d_{0,\{hkl\}}} = -\frac{1}{2}\cot\theta_0 \Delta 2\theta \qquad [4.2]$$

where d_0 and θ_0 are the interplanar lattice spacing and the corresponding Bragg angle of the unstressed crystal lattice.

Published by Woodhead Publishing Limited, 2013

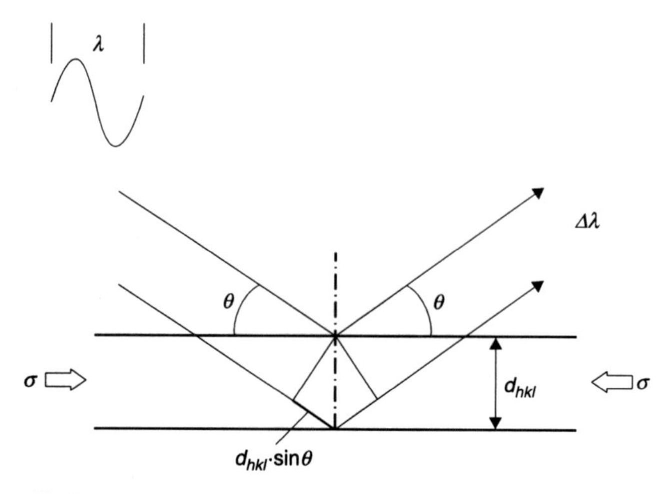

Figure 4.4 Bragg's law.

Stresses can be calculated from the lattice strains by using the generalized Hooke's law and the diffraction elastic constants. The most frequently applied technique for XRD analysis is the $\sin^2\psi$ method (Macherauch and Mueller, 1961).

The residual stress depth distribution in the near-surface region is affected by the mechanical surface treatment parameters and the material state. Typically, the maximum compressive residual stress is located at or slightly below (<100 µm) the component's surface (McClung, 2007). An example of the qualitative residual stress depth profile is shown in Figure 4.5 with a total depth of compressive penetration after shot peening of typically less than 1 mm.

4.3.3 Influences of residual stresses on the fatigue strength

Fatigue endurance strength is mainly influenced by how fast cracks are built within a component and how fast they can

Published by Woodhead Publishing Limited, 2013

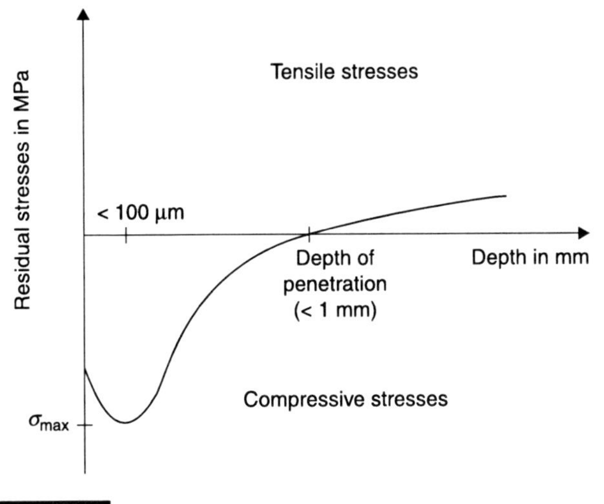

Figure 4.5 Qualitative residual stress profile.

propagate. Generally, cracks are built in the superficial area around (micro-) notches which cause very high local stresses. Thus, fatigue strength can be significantly increased when the crack initiation and propagation near the surface is delayed which is meant to be achieved by a mechanical surface treatment.

Orthopedic implants and those used in trauma surgery are subjected to a cyclic bending loading that induces both tensile and compressive stresses. These stresses show a linear distribution within the component with a maximum stress at the surface (Figure 4.6a). Here, the line of no stress at the center of the beam's cross-section separates the region of compressive from that of tensile stresses and is called the 'neutral fiber'. As metals are more susceptible to tensile than to compressive stresses, crack initiation is likely to take place in the superficial regions subjected to maximum tensile stresses. This may not only be the case under a pure bending or tensile load, but also under a multi-axial load situation and a combined corrosive environment or micro-motions.

Published by Woodhead Publishing Limited, 2013

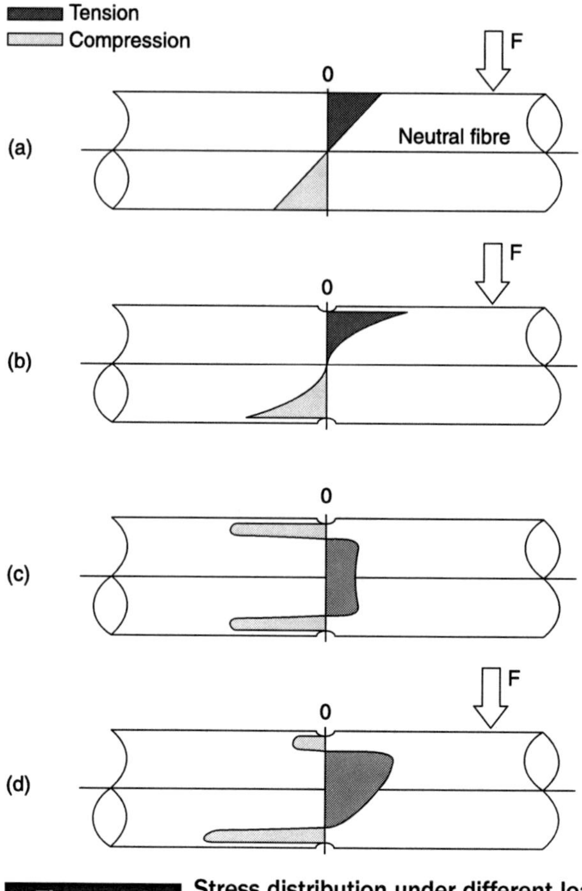

Figure 4.6 Stress distribution under different loading conditions: (a) untreated rod under bending load, (b) notched rod under bending load, (c) residual stresses after mechanical surface treatment (no external load) and (d) notched rod after mechanical surface treatment under bending load.

Mechanical surface treatments aim at work hardening the component's near-surface region and introducing compressive residual stresses, where the first can inhibit crack initiation and the latter serve accessorily as a buffer against crack propagation under tensile loading conditions (Song and Wen, 1999). Figure 4.6(b) shows the stress distribution within a

Published by Woodhead Publishing Limited, 2013

superficially notched and loaded beam under bending conditions. Here, tensile as well as compressive stresses are maximal in the ground of the notch (multi-axial stress state). A typical residual stress distribution after a shot peening treatment is shown in Figure 4.6(c) (unloaded conditions). In order to maintain the beam in a mechanical stress equilibrium, tensile stresses are built up inside the component as compressive stresses are introduced at the surface. Loading of a mechanically treated and notched component leads to a superposition of the latter two scenarios under consideration of their stress distributions (Figure 4.6d). The compressive residual stresses at the surface regions are reduced before tensile stresses are experienced in this region. Thus, higher bent loading conditions can be applied to the component before reaching the material's critical tensile strength.

Due to the superposition of tensile stresses inside the part subsequent to bend loading, the risk of crack initiation in the core is increased (over-peening effect), in particular in the case of a small component. Therefore, even if the volume subjected to compressive load is small in relation to the total volume and tensile residual stresses are negligible, the introduction of compressive stresses at the surface is limited to a certain extent.

As shot peening is mainly applied in the field of mechanical engineering, studies on orthopedic titanium and its alloys are quite rare. However, previous investigations report possible positive effects on the fatigue strength, with improvements up to 10–25% for different titanium alloys and load conditions (Franz and Olbricht, 1987; Sridhar et al., 1996; Jiang et al., 2007).

4.4 Materials and methods

In this study, standard hour-glass-shaped Ti6Al4V specimens with a minimum diameter of 10 mm were machined

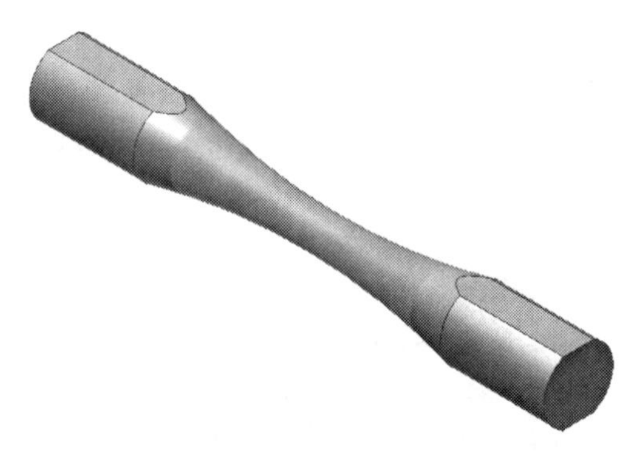

Figure 4.7 Hour-glass-shaped Ti6Al4V specimens (relieved part: surface treated region).

(Figure 4.7). In order to produce a standardized reference, any residual stresses introduced during manufacturing were eliminated by a subsequent annealing treatment at 620 °C for 10 h in an inert nitrogen environment followed by an acid cleaning process overnight.

A high-intensity shot peening treatment using rounded cut wire was applied on the relieved part of eight Ti6Al4V specimens. In order to avoid possible steel contamination from the peening medium, the component was subsequently subjected to a cleaning process using glass beeds (two-step peening).

Arithmetic mean roughness (R_a) measurements were taken on the annealed surfaces and after shot peening (Mahr Perthometer M2; Germany). In addition, residual stress depth profiles prior to and after shot peening were determined in the treated region of the specimen by electrochemical layer removal in combination with XRD stress analysis. The residual stress was analyzed by means of an X-ray diffractometer (XRD3000 PTS; Rich. Seifert Ltd, Germany) configuration using Fe-filtered Co-Kα radiation. The stress analyses were carried out for the {114} lattice planes of the α-Ti phase according to the $\sin^2\psi$ method. For

Published by Woodhead Publishing Limited, 2013

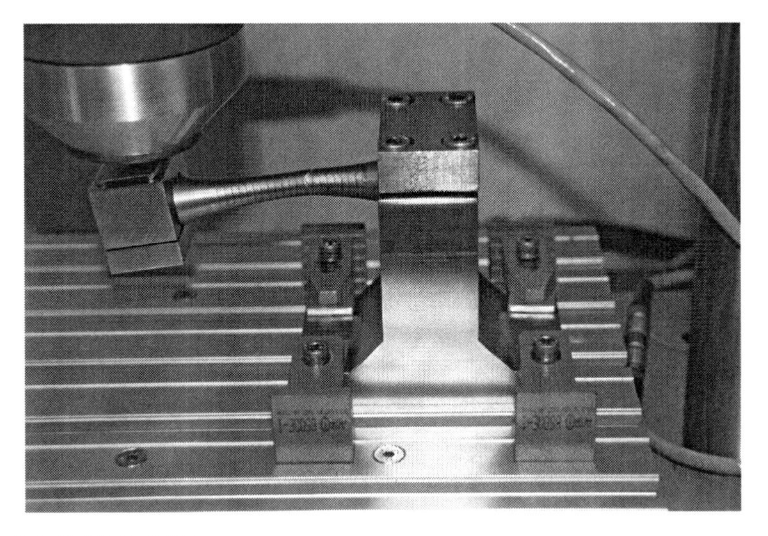

Figure 4.8 Fatigue testing set-up.

stress calculation, the following material constants were used: $E_{\{114\}}$ = 129 GPa and $\nu_{\{114\}}$ = 0.31.

Cyclic tests were performed on a servo-hydraulic uniaxial test device (Bosch Rexroth, Germany) at 10 Hz and a load ratio (F_{max}/F_{min}) of R = 0.1 under dry conditions (Figure 4.8). All tests were performed up to a total number of 10^7 cycles (high-cycle fatigue testing) or until fracture occurred. Subsequent to mechanical testing, the fracture surfaces were optically inspected using a microscope and field emission gun scanning electron microscopy (FEG-SEM, Zeiss, Germany).

4.5 Results and discussion

The surface roughness (Figure 4.9) drastically increases by 840% after the combined cut wire and glass peening treatment (R_a = 2.02 ± 0.16 μm) when compared to the annealed reference (R_a = 0.24 ± 0.09 μm) ($p < 0.01$).

Published by Woodhead Publishing Limited, 2013

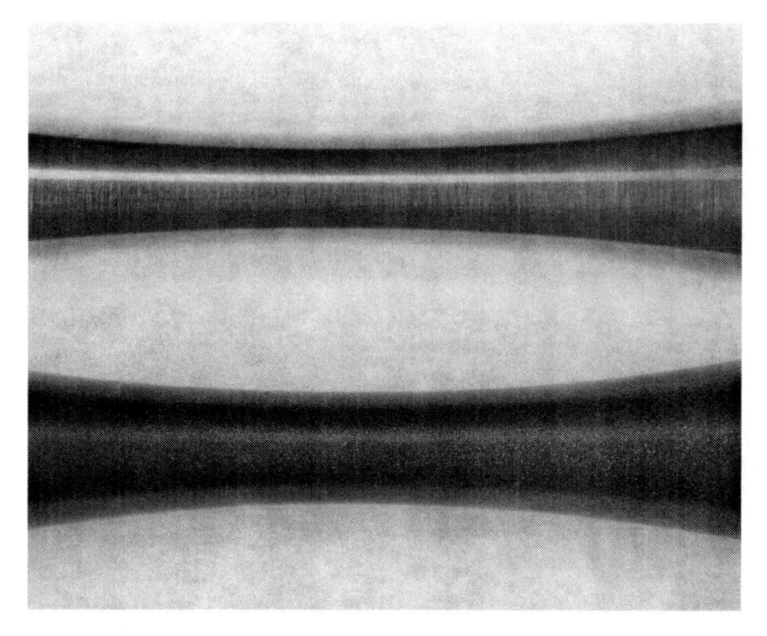

Figure 4.9 Surfaces: top, annealed; bottom, after shot peening.

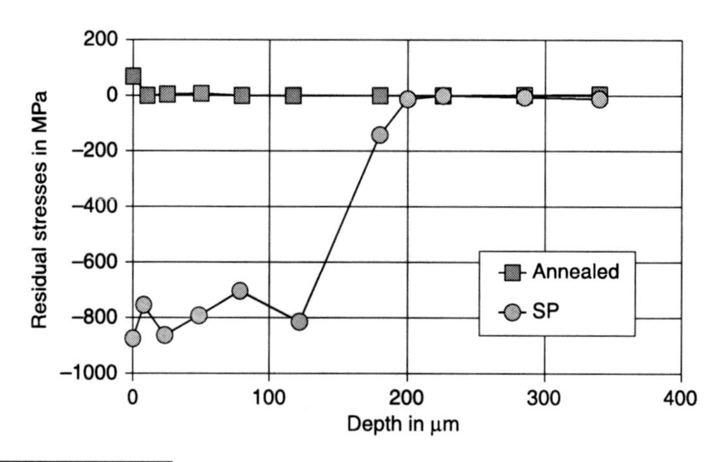

Figure 4.10 Residual stress depth profiles (longitudinal).

Published by Woodhead Publishing Limited, 2013

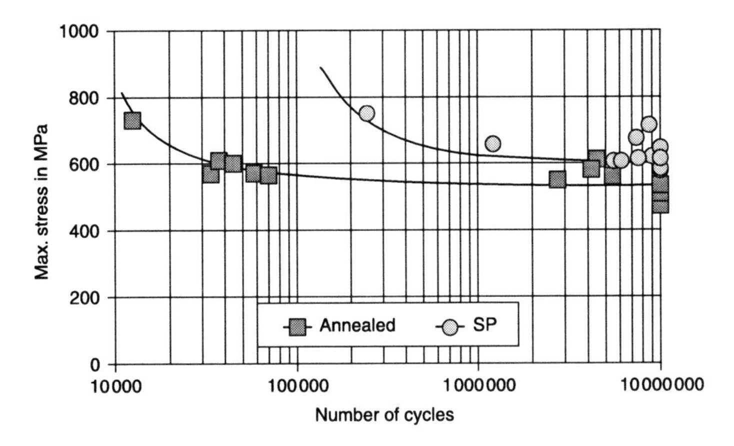

Figure 4.11 Woehler diagram.

Residual stresses are introduced during the peening process as a superposition of plastic deformation and Hertzian stresses. They were measured up to a depth of 200 μm (Figure 4.10). Maximum compressive stresses of around 800 MPa are observed near the surface (depth below 130 μm).

Fatigue endurance strength was determined by destructive testing of single fatigue tests. In the Woehler diagram (Figure 4.11), the maximum stress at the surface is given on the y-axis and the number of cycles on the x-axis. Every dot (shot-peened) or square (asannealed) represents a failed specimen, except at the total of 10^7 cycles representing fatigue-tested specimens without any rupture. The (high-cycle) fatigue is then identified as the asymptotic stress at 10^7 cycles. Thus, an increase in fatigue strength after shot peening of 12.3% relative to the annealed and cleaned condition is reported.

Figure 4.12 exemplarily shows the fatigue fracture pattern of a shot-peened specimen that fractured after a total of 8 840 279 cycles. The fracture origin is located near the

Published by Woodhead Publishing Limited, 2013

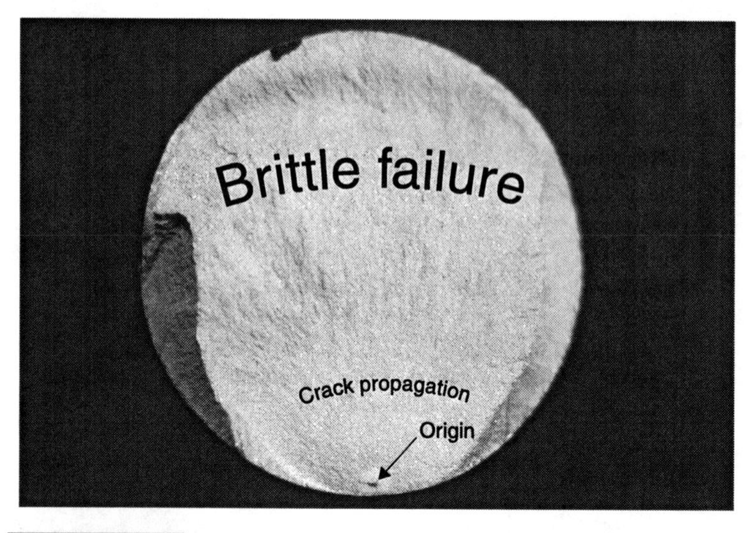

Figure 4.12 Fracture pattern of a failed shot-peened specimen.

surface where the highest tensile stresses occur. Microscopic analyses serve to identify the direction of crack propagation until brittle fracture occurs.

4.6 Conclusion

Surface treatments represent a widely used standard process in mechanical and aerospace engineering for cyclically highly loaded titanium parts. However, they are rarely applied in the orthopedic or trauma surgical field. The potential of a final shot peening process on high-cycle fatigue of a standard Ti6Al4V alloy was investigated. Fatigue strength was significantly improved and mechanical surface treatments seem to be a good option for implants that have a critical design and, thus, suffer high tensile stresses under service load. Main changes in surface layer properties, e.g. roughness, residual stresses and dislocation density, are introduced

Published by Woodhead Publishing Limited, 2013

during treatment. However, roughness did not seem to affect the fatigue strength performance in this study. It is likely that the influence after introduction of micro-notches is superposed by other effects such as higher hardness or residual stresses. Additionally, it will be interesting to study the effect of osseointegration on surfaces that have been strengthened by a final shot peening treatment on either a blank titanium alloy or even bioactive coatings, e.g. hydroxyapatite.

Preliminary studies using a roller-burnished Ti6Al7Nb alloy have shown the potential to increase fatigue strength and lower the degree of contamination introduced by shot peening (Schuh et al., 2006). Other surface treatments, such as roller burnishing, may be an alternative and need to be further considered with respect to their strengthening potential as well as applicability to orthopedic implants. In concusion, using a combined shot peening process with cut wire and glass beads increases fatigue strength of 12.3% compared to as annealed specimens.

4.7 References

AOA (2009), *National Joint Replacement Registry. Annual Report*. Adelaide: Australian Orthopaedic Association.

Brunski J B (2004), 'Metals', in: Ratner B D, Hoffman A S, Schoen F J and Lemons J E (eds), *Biomaterials Science: An Introduction to Materials in Medicine*, pp. 137–153. London: Elsevier.

Chu Y H, Elias J J, Duda G N, Frassica F J and Chao E Y S (2000), 'Stress and micromotion in the taper lock joint of a modular segmental bone replacement prosthesis', *Journal of Biomechanics*, **33**: 1175–1179.

Cook S D, Barrack R L and Clemow A J (1994), 'Corrosion and wear at the modular interface of uncemented femoral

Published by Woodhead Publishing Limited, 2013

stems', *Journal of Bone and Joint Surgery, British*, **76B**: 68–72.

Franz H E and Olbricht A (1987), 'Optimization of shot peening to improve the fatigue strength', in: Wohlfahrt H, Kopp R and Vöhringer O (eds), *Shot Peening*, pp. 439–446. Kassel, DGM.

Garellick G, Kärrholm J, Rogmark C and Herberts P (2010), *Swedish Hip Arthroplasty Register. Annual Report*. Göteborg: Swedish Hip Arthroplasty Register.

Gilbert J L, Buckley C A and Jacobs J J (1993), '*In vivo* corrosion of modular hip prosthesis components in mixed and similar metal combinations. The effect of crevice, stress, motion and alloy coupling', *Journal of Biomedical Materials Research*, **27**: 1533–1544.

Grupp T, Weik T, Bloemer W and Knaebel H P (2010), 'Modular titanium alloy neck adapter failures in hip replacement – failure mode analysis and influence of implant material', *BMC Musculoskeletal Disorders*, **11**: 1–12.

Hallab N J, Jacobs J J and Katz J L (2004), 'Orthopedic application', in: Ratner B D, Hoffman A S, Schoen F J and Lemons J E (eds), *Biomaterials Science: An Introduction to Materials in Medicine*, pp. 526–555. London: Elsevier.

Jiang X P, Man C S, Shepard M J and Zhai T (2007), 'Effects of shot-peening and re-shot-peening on four-point bend fatigue behavior of Ti–6Al–4V', *Materials Science and Engineering A*, **468–470**, 137–143.

Jones D M, Marsh J L, Nepola J V, Jacobs J J, Skipor A K et al. (2001), 'Focal osteolysis at the junctions of a modular stainless-steel femoral intramedullary nail', *Journal of Bone and Joint Surgery, American*, **83**: 537–548.

Kretzer J P, Jakubowitz E, Krachler M, Thomsen M and Heisel C (2009), 'Metal release and corrosion effects of

Published by Woodhead Publishing Limited, 2013

modular neck total hip arthroplasty', *International Orthopaedics*, **33**: 1531–1536.

Macherauch E and Mueller P (1961), 'Das sin^{2}psi-Verfahren der röntgenographischen Spannungsmessung', *Zeitschrift für angewandte Physik*, **13**: 305–312.

McClung R C (2007), 'A literature survey on the stability and significance of residual stresses during fatigue', *Fatigue and Fracture of Engineering Materials and Structures*, **30**: 173–205.

Miao H Y, Demers D, Larose S, Perron C and Levesque M (2010), 'Experimental study of shot peening and stress peen forming', *Journal of Materials Processing Technology*, **210**: 2089–2102.

Navarro M, Michiardi A, Castano O and Planell J A (2008), 'Biomaterials in orthopaedics', *Journal of the Royal Society Interface*, **5**: 1137–1158.

Schuh A, Zeller C, Holzwarth U, Kachler W, Wilcke G et al. (2006), 'Deep rolling of titanium rods for application in modular total hip arthroplasty', *Journal of Biomedical Materials Research B*, **81**: 330–335.

Song P S and Wen C C (1999), 'Crack closure and crack growth behaviour in shot peened fatigued specimen', *Engineering Fracture Mechanics*, **63**: 295–304.

Sridhar B R, Ramachandra K and Padmanabhan K A (1996), 'Effect of shot peening on the fatigue and fracture behaviour of two titanium alloys', *Journal of Materials Science*, **31**: 5953–5960.

Published by Woodhead Publishing Limited, 2013

5

Wear determination on retrieved metal-on-metal hip arthroplasty: an example of extreme wear

Sebastian Jaeger, Joern Reinders, Johannes S. Rieger and J. Philippe Kretzer, Heidelberg University Hospital, Germany

DOI: 10.1533/9780857092205.239

Abstract: We present a method to determine wear of metal-on-metal hip replacement and a case of extreme wear. The high wear rates resulted in adverse reactions to metal debris and dramatically increased the blood serum metal ion concentration.

Key words: hip replacement, metal-on-metal bearing, ion concentration, wear measurement, cup inclination, pseudotumor, arthroplasty.

5.1 Introduction

The history of metal-on-metal (MoM) articulating surfaces in total hip arthroplasty started over 70 years ago (Amstutz

Published by Woodhead Publishing Limited, 2013

and Grigoris, 1996). High failure rates of historical designs occurred because of metallurgy and imprecise manufacturing technology (Schmalzried et al., 1996; Heisel et al., 2004). Friction between the two metallic bearing surfaces leads to the release of metal particles and ions into the body. The biological interactions caused by the released metal ions and particles are still a cause for concern, and much research is being performed in this area (Kwon et al., 2009; Watters et al., 2010). Even modern MoM designs may have high failure rates due to osteolysis or adverse reactions to metal debris (ARMD) (e.g. pseudotumors), and the failure rates are currently rising (Smith et al., 2012). Retrieved MoM hip implants often showed high wear rates and a prevalence of edge loading (Glyn-Jones et al., 2011; Hart et al., 2012; Matthies et al., 2012). However, if the bearing is well implanted, and appropriate patient and implant selection performed, MoM bearings showed lower wear rates compared with conventional metal-on-polyethylene bearings. Even so, as metal particles are much smaller than polyethylene particles, the number of particles produced by MoM bearings can be much higher (Doorn et al., 1998). The surface-to-volume ratio and therefore the total surface area of the metal particles are higher than those of polyethylene particles. As a consequence, increased systematic (e.g. serum, blood, urine) ion levels of chromium and cobalt are reported (Jacobs et al., 1996; Brodner et al., 1997). The ions and particles may have both local and systemic effects. Thus, documentation and analysis of retrieved MoM bearings are important to understand the failure mechanism of these implants. We therefore present the following case.

Published by Woodhead Publishing Limited, 2012

5.2 Case

A 63-year-old woman (height 1.50 m, weight 75.5 kg, body mass index 33.6 kg/m^2) underwent a right hip resurfacing for coxarthrosis using an articular surface replacement (ASR) with a femoral head size of 41 mm and an acetabular cup size of 46 mm (DePuy/Johnson & Johnson, Leeds, UK). The postoperative course was without incident. Four years later, after a history of squeaking and necrosis of the femoral head with loosening of the femoral component, the patient underwent revision surgery. The ASR cup remained *in situ* and a cementless total hip arthroplasty consisting of a Corail stem size 8 and an ASR Femoral Modular XL Head size 41 mm with a 5-mm Sleeve Adapter (DePuy/Johnson & Johnson) was implanted (Figure 5.1).

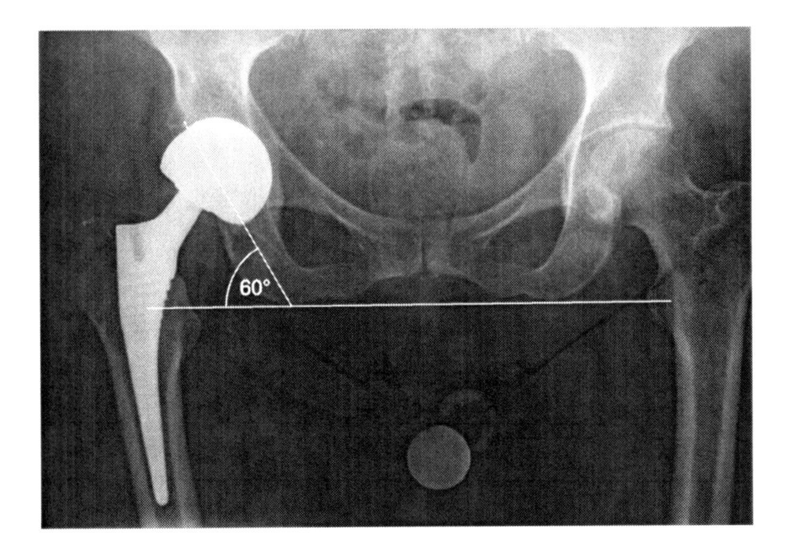

Figure 5.1 Four years after primary surgery the first revision was performed without replacing the ASR cup. A cementless total hip arthroplasty and a MoM bearing (ASR-XL) were implanted.

Published by Woodhead Publishing Limited, 2012

Another 2 years later she presented at our institution with distinctive noises like squeaking and grinding during normal walking and symptoms of subluxation. X-rays showed a high cup inclination of more than 60° (Figure 5.1). Magnetic resonance imaging (MRI) was performed that showed pronounced metalosis caused by the metal debris. Also, whole-blood metal ion concentrations (cobalt and chromium) were dramatically increased.

During the second revision (6 years after initial hip resurfacing) pronounced black coloring of the soft tissue with localization of fluid collection and metallic wear debris were found. A pseudotumor with a solid mass of 4 cm × 3 cm × 2 cm was excised at the trochanteric ridge. All MoM components were revised (Figure 5.2). A pronounced metalosis was detected behind the cup after extraction. After extensive debridement a 50-mm cementless cup with a polyethylene

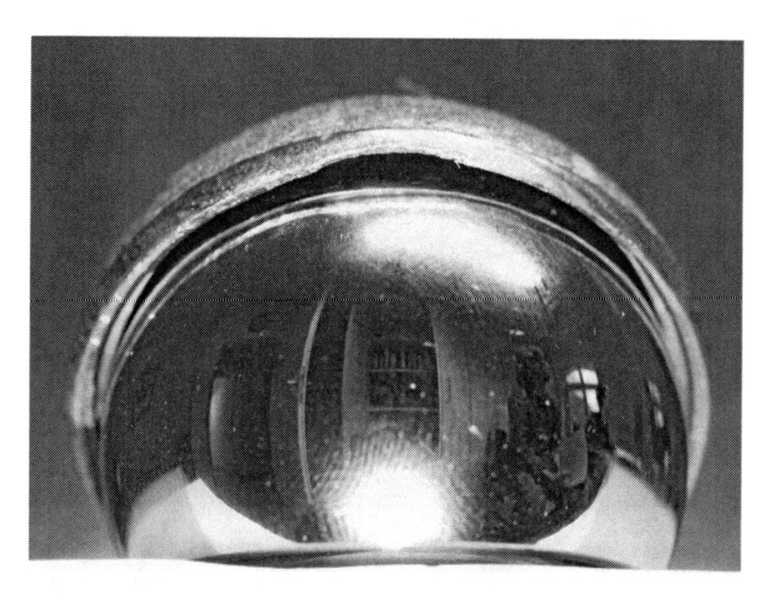

Figure 5.2 Revised cup and head. The material is visibly worn at the edge of the cup.

Published by Woodhead Publishing Limited, 2012

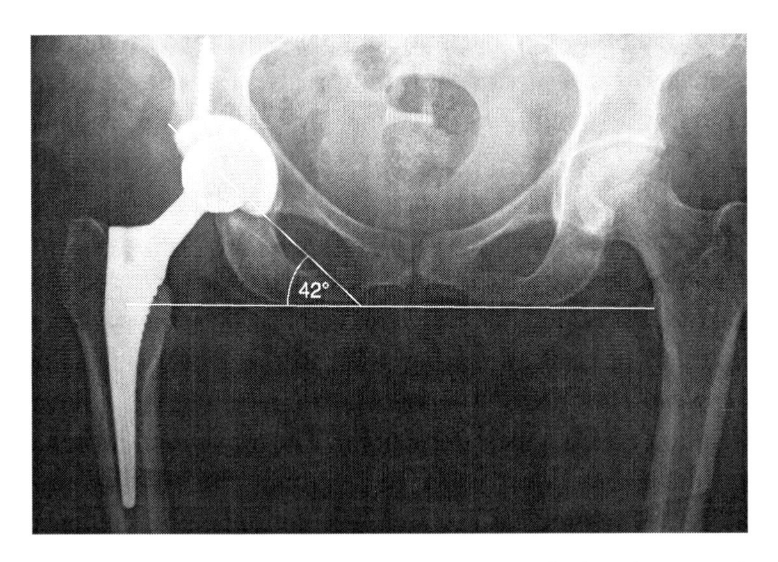

Figure 5.3 Six years after initial hip resurfacing the second revision was performed. The ASR cup and the ASR-XL head were revised to a cementless cup with a polyethylene insert and a metallic head (32 mm).

insert and a 32/+8 mm CoCr-head size XL was implanted. A cup inclination of 42° could be achieved (Figure 5.3). The convalescence was uneventful and the hip was stable.

5.3 Wear measurement

The volumetric and linear wear of the retrieved cup and head were measured using a coordinate measuring machine (CMM) (Mahr Multisensor MS 222; Göttingen, Germany). First, the accuracy and precision of the CMM were determined using a certificated calibration sphere, and were found to be 4 μm or less in all cases. Then, the surface of the head and cup were measured in steps of 2° in the longitudinal and latitudinal directions. This resulted in a point cloud of

Published by Woodhead Publishing Limited, 2012

8100 points for the head and 6300 points for the cup. All geometrical measurements were repeated three times under standardized conditions in a temperature-controlled room at 22.0 °C. The following process was used to determine the volumetric and linear wear.

If the wear scars were visually present, the wear scar areas were excluded for a following best-fit algorithm to fit a sphere into the point cloud (least-squares best fit). Then the deviation (residual) of each measuring point to the sphere (including the wear scar area) was calculated, resulting in a linear deviation for each measuring point. The maximum deviation was defined as linear wear. To determine the wear volume, the corresponding surface area was multiplied by the linear deviation of each measuring point. In general, linear deviations below the determined accuracy of the CMM were not considered in this calculation. If the wear scars were not visibly present on the articulating surface a sphere was fitted with the entire point cloud. Following this, measuring points showing the maximum deviations to the sphere were excluded and the process was repeated. This interactive process was repeated multiple times, aiming to identify the unworn areas. However, using this approach, two aspects need to be considered. On the one hand, excluding too many points will reduce the precision of the fitted sphere. We therefore aimed to keep at least 30–50% of the initial point cloud to calculate the best-fit sphere. On the other hand, deviations in roundness (as a result of the initial manufacturing) of the components have to be considered. Typically, deviations on roundness are below 10 μm (Heisel et al., 2009). Therefore, the point-excluding process (to identify the unworn areas) needs to balance these two aspects and remains a subjective process.

The systematic metal ion concentration was measured according to a well-established protocol (Krachler et al., 2009) using high-resolution inductively coupled plasma-mass spectrometry (HR-ICP-MS) (Element2; Thermo Fisher Scientific, Bremen, Germany) with a detection limit of 0.03 μg/l for cobalt and 0.05 g/l for chromium.

Additionally, the wear pattern on the retrieved cup was investigated using field emission gun scanning electron microscopy (FEG-SEM) (Leo 1530; Oberkochen, Germany).

5.4 Results

The results of linear and volumetric wear measurements are shown in Figures 5.4 and 5.5. The femoral head showed a mean linear wear of 116.93 ± 0.44 μm and a mean volumetric wear of 29.27 ± 0.14 mm^3. The cup showed a mean linear wear of 1169.25 ± 43.31 μm and a mean volumetric wear of 44.63 ± 6.11 mm^3. This results in an annual overall linear

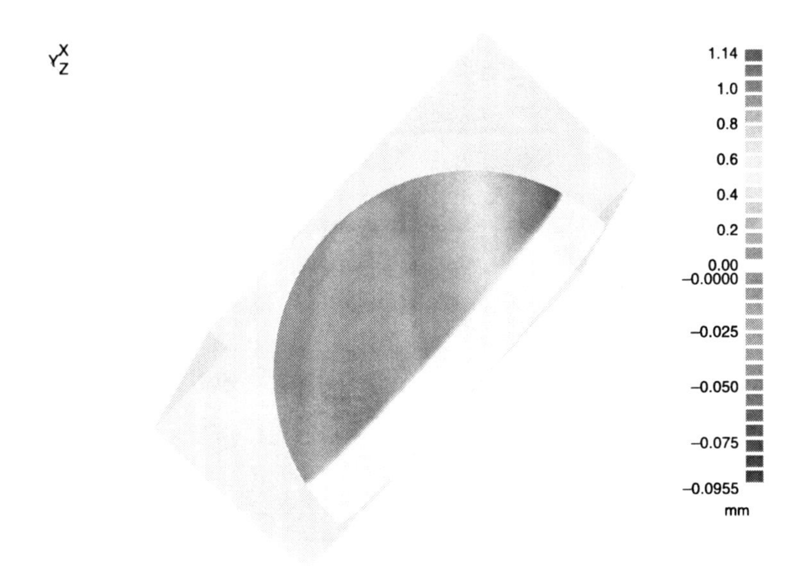

Figure 5.4 Deviation of the worn geometry relative to the unworn geometry: cup.

Published by Woodhead Publishing Limited, 2012

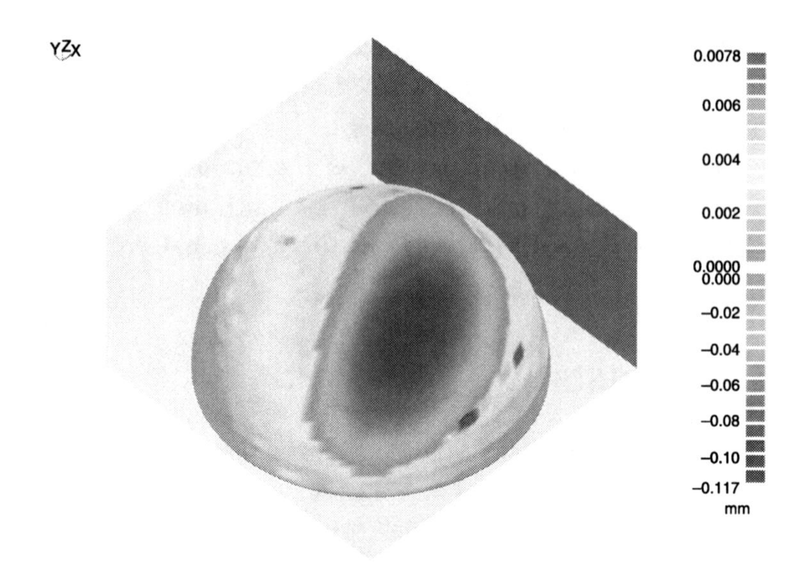

Figure 5.5 Deviation of the worn geometry relative to the unworn geometry: head.

wear rate of 253.33 μm/year and an annual overall volumetric wear rate of 22.08 mm^3/year.

5.4.1 Metal ion concentration analysis

The systemic metal ion concentration measured prior to the second revision showed a cobalt concentration of 158.7 μg/l and a chromium concentration of 64.0 μg/l. Ten months after this revision (revising to a metal-on-polyethylene bearing), cobalt decreased to 2.1 μg/l and chromium decreased to 24.0 μg/l.

5.4.2 SEM

The retrieved cup showed carbides that were fully or partially pulled out of the matrix material within the wear zone (Figure 5.6).

Published by Woodhead Publishing Limited, 2012

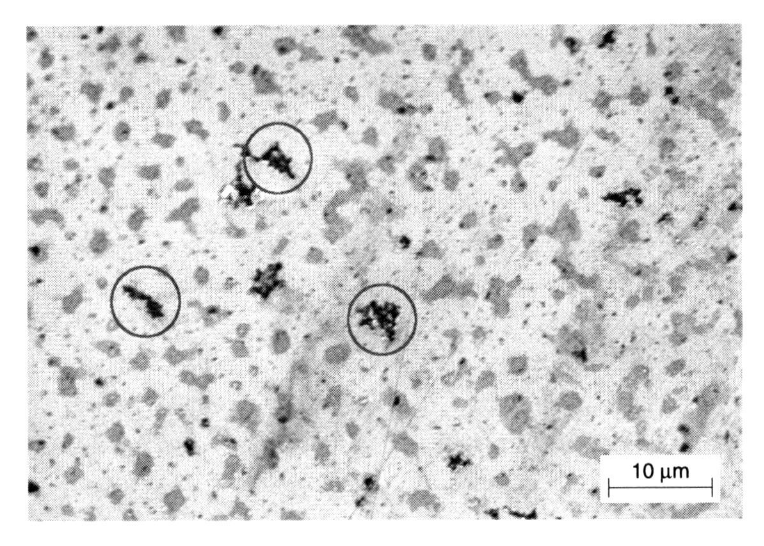

Figure 5.6 Wear pattern (FEG-SEM): carbide pulled out of the matrix of the cup (circled).

5.5 Discussion

MoM hip resurfacing arthroplasty shows good clinical results with appropriate patient selection and in experienced surgical hands (Jameson et al., 2012). However, the revision rates for MoM bearings have increased over recent years (Smith et al., 2012). The reasons for revisions of conventional total hip arthroplasty are osteolysis, aseptic loosening, infection, fracture and dislocation (Department of Orthopedics, 2010). Beside these, ARMD (like pseudotumors) are frequently reported (Morlock et al., 2008; Hart et al., 2009; Matthies et al., 2012) for MoM bearings. It has been shown that the cup position is an essential parameter regarding the wear behavior of resurfacing implants. A steep cup orientation leads to higher wear rates, as also seen in this case (Haan et al., 2008; Morlock et al., 2008). The metallurgy and carbide structure seem to affect the wear properties, as

Published by Woodhead Publishing Limited, 2012

seen in the FEG-SEM analysis (Heisel et al., 2008). Furthermore, implant design parameters like the head size, clearance, arc of coverage and manufacturing are important parameters (Haan et al., 2008; Shimmin et al., 2010; Desy et al., 2011). Well-functioning second-generation MoM bearings have been shown to generate mean linear wear rates of approximately 5 μm/year and mean volumetric wear rates of approximately 1 mm^3/year (Rieker et al., 2004). The determined volumetric and linear wear rates in this case were multiple times higher. Consequently, increased metal ion levels were found. Normally, patients with well-functional MoM hip replacements show cobalt and chromium levels in the range of approximately 2 μg/l (Heisel et al., 2008). The results of this case confirm that MoM hip replacements are at higher risk for reduced implant survival and increased wear and ion release compared with other bearing surfaces (Smith et al., 2012).

5.6 Conclusion

The current example demonstrates that MoM bearings are highly sensitive to patient selection, implantation techniques and design parameters regarding their wear behavior and clinical outcome.

5.7 References

Amstutz H C and Grigoris P (1996), 'Metal on metal bearings in hip arthroplasty', *Clin. Orthop. Relat. Res.*, **329** (Suppl.): S11–S34.

Brodner W, Bitzan P, Meisinger V, Kaider A, Gottsauner-Wolf F et al. (1997), 'Elevated serum cobalt with

Published by Woodhead Publishing Limited, 2012

metal-on-metal articulating surfaces', *J. Bone Joint Surg. Br.*, **79**: 316–321.

Department of Orthopedics (2010), *Swedish Hip Arthroplasty Register. Annual Report*. Göteborg: Swedish Hip Arthroplasty Register.

Desy N M, Bergeron S G, Petit A, Huk O L and Antoniou J (2011), 'Surgical variables influence metal ion levels after hip resurfacing', *Clin. Orthop. Relat. Res.*, **469**: 1635–1641.

Doorn P F, Campbell P A, Worrall J, Benya P D, Mckellop H A et al. (1998), 'Metal wear particle characterization from metal on metal total hip replacements: transmission electron microscopy study of periprosthetic tissues and isolated particles', *J. Biomed. Mater. Res.*, **42**: 103–111.

Glyn-Jones S N, Roques A, Taylor A, Kwon Y-M, Mclardy-Smith P et al. (2011), 'The *in vivo* linear and volumetric wear of hip resurfacing implants revised for pseudotumor', *J. Bone Joint Surg. Am.*, **93**: 2180–2188.

Haan R D, Pattyn C, Gill H S, Murray D W, Campbell P A et al. (2008), 'Correlation between inclination of the acetabular component and metal ion levels in metal-on-metal hip resurfacing replacement', *J. Bone Joint Surg. Br.*, **90**: 1291–1297.

Hart A J, Sabah S, Henckel J, Lewis A, Cobb J et al. (2009), 'The painful metal-on-metal hip resurfacing', *J. Bone Joint Surg. Br.*, **91**: 738–744.

Hart A J, Satchithananda K, Liddle A D, Sabah S A, McRobbie D et al. (2012), 'Pseudotumors in association with well-functioning metal-on-metal hip prostheses: a case-control study using three-dimensional computed tomography and magnetic resonance imaging', *J. Bone Joint Surg. Am.*, **94**: 317–325.

Heisel C, Kleinhans J A, Menge M and Kretzer J P (2009), 'Ten different hip resurfacing systems: biomechanical

Published by Woodhead Publishing Limited, 2012

analysis of design and material properties', *Int. Orthop.*, **33**: 939–943.

Heisel C, Silva M and Schmalzried T P (2004), 'Bearing surface options for total hip replacement in young patients', *Instr. Course Lect.*, **53**: 49–65.

Heisel C, Streich N, Krachler M, Jakubowitz E and Kretzer J P (2008), 'Characterization of the running-in period in total hip resurfacing arthroplasty: an *in vivo* and *in vitro* metal ion analysis', *J. Bone Joint Surg. Am.*, **90** (Suppl. 3): 125–133.

Jacobs J J, Skipor A K, Doorn P F, Campbell P, Schmalzried T P et al. (1996), 'Cobalt and chromium concentrations in patients with metal on metal total hip replacements', *Clin. Orthop. Relat. Res.*, (329 Suppl.): S256–S263.

Jameson S S, Baker P N, Mason J, Porter M L, Deehan D J et al. (2012), 'Independent predictors of revision following metal-on-metal hip resurfacing: a retrospective cohort study using National Joint Registry data', *J. Bone Joint Surg. Br.*, **94**: 746–754.

Krachler M, Heisel C and Kretzer J P (2009), 'Validation of ultratrace analysis of Co, Cr, Mo and Ni in whole blood, serum and urine using ICP-SMS', *J. Anal. Atom. Spectrom.*, **24**: 605–610.

Kwon Y-M., Xia Z, Glyn-Jones S, Beard D, Gill H S et al. (2009), 'Dose-dependent cytotoxicity of clinically relevant cobalt nanoparticles and ions on macrophages *in vitro*', *Biomed. Mater.*, **4**: 025018.

Matthies A K, Skinner J A, Osmani H, Henckel J and Hart A J (2012), 'Pseudotumors are common in well-positioned low-wearing metal-on-metal hips', *Clin. Orthop. Relat. Res.*, **470**: 1895–1906.

Morlock M M, Bishop N, Zustin J, Hahn M, Rüther W et al. (2008), 'Modes of implant failure after hip resurfacing:

Published by Woodhead Publishing Limited, 2012

morphological and wear analysis of 267 retrieval specimens', *J. Bone Joint Surg. Am.*, **90** (Suppl. 3): 89–95.

Rieker C B, Schöön R and Köttig P (2004), 'Development and validation of a second-generation metal-on-metal bearing: laboratory studies and analysis of retrievals', *J. Arthroplasty*, **19**: 5–11.

Schmalzried T P, Szuszczewicz E S, Akizuki K H, Petersen T D and Amstutz H C (1996), 'Factors correlating with long term survival of McKee–Farrar total hip prostheses', *Clin. Orthop. Relat. Res.*, **329** (Suppl.): S48–S59.

Shimmin A J, Walter W L and Esposito C (2010), 'The influence of the size of the component on the outcome of resurfacing arthroplasty of the hip: a review of the literature', *J. Bone Joint Surg. Br.*, **92**: 469–476.

Smith A J, Dieppe P, Vernon K, Porter M, Blom A W et al. (2012), 'Failure rates of stemmed metal-on-metal hip replacements: analysis of data from the National Joint Registry of England and Wales', *Lancet*, **379**: 1199–1204.

Watters T S, Cardona D M, Menon K S, Vinson E N, Bolognesi M P et al. (2010), 'Aseptic lymphocyte-dominated vasculitis-associated lesion: a clinicopathologic review of an underrecognized cause of prosthetic failure', *Am. J. Clin. Pathol.*, **134**: 886–893.

Published by Woodhead Publishing Limited, 2012

6

Natural articular joints: model of lamellar-roller-bearing lubrication and the nature of the cartilage surface

Zenon Pawlak, Tribochemistry Consulting, USA and University of Economy, Poland, Wieslaw Urbaniak, University of Economy and Kazimierz Wielki University, Poland and Adekunle Oloyede, Queensland University of Technology, Australia

DOI: 10.1533/9780857092205.253

Abstract: The influence of pH on interfacial energy and wettability distributed over the phospholipid bilayer surface were studied, and the importance of cartilage hydrophobicity (wettability) on the coefficient of friction (*f*) was established. It is argued that the wettability of cartilage significantly depends on the number of phospholipid bilayers acting as solid lubricant; the hypothesis was proven by conducting friction tests with normal and lipid-depleted cartilage samples. A lamellar-roller-bearing lubrication model was devised involving two mechanisms: (i) lamellar frictionless movement of bilayers, and (ii) roller-bearing lubrication mode through structured synovial fluid, which operates when lamellar

Published by Woodhead Publishing Limited, 2013

spheres, liposomes and macromolecules act like a roller-bearing situated between two cartilage surfaces in effective biological lubrication.

Key words: joint lubrication, surface amorphous layer, cartilage, hydrophobicity, hydrophilicity, phospholipid, bilayer, wettability, coefficient of friction, lamellar-roller-bearing

6.1 Introduction

Articular cartilage is the unique connective tissue of the diarthrodial joints that functions in harsh biomechanical environments. Its principal function is to provide frictionless lubrication for articulation. Articular cartilage is hyaline cartilage, 2–4 mm thick, and has a limited capacity for intrinsic healing and repair; it has no blood vessels, no lymphatic systems or nerves; its nutrition is solely by diffusion. In this regard, the preservation and health of articular cartilage are of paramount importance to a joint's health. It is composed of a dense extracellular matrix (ECM) with a sparse distribution of highly specialized cells called chondrocytes. The ECM is principally composed of collagen, proteoglycans and water, with other non-collagenous proteins, glycoproteins and phospholipids occurring in lesser amounts.

These components facilitate the retention of water within the ECM, which is critical to maintain its unique mechanical properties. Due to its location, articular cartilage interacts with the synovial fluid, which is known to contain a phospholipid multibilayer (solid lubricant), biomacromolecules of hyaluronic acid, albumin and lubricin, and other polyelectrolytes that can attach to the surface of cartilage. It has been proposed that the roles of these constituents of the

Published by Woodhead Publishing Limited, 2013

synovial fluid are to modify viscosity, protect the membrane surface against wear and ensure minimal friction (Maroudas et al., 1968; Afara et al., 2011; Horvai, 2011).

Along with collagen's fibrillar ultrastructure and ECM, chondrocytes contribute to various zones of the articular cartilage, i.e. the phospholipidic zone, the superficial zone, the middle zone, the radial zone and the calcified zone (Figure 6.1a). The sketch in Figure 6.1(b) demonstrates an

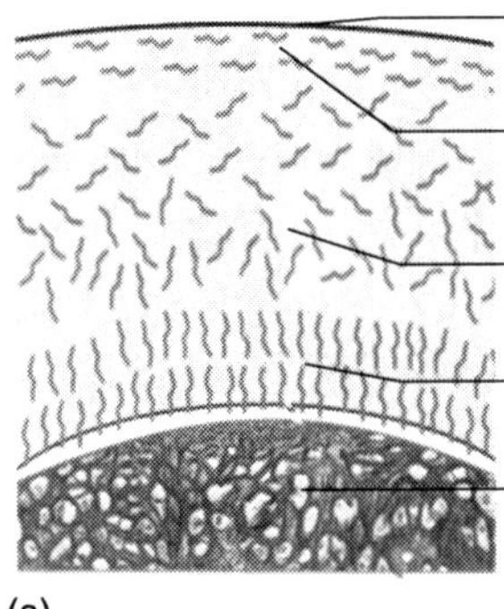

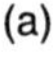

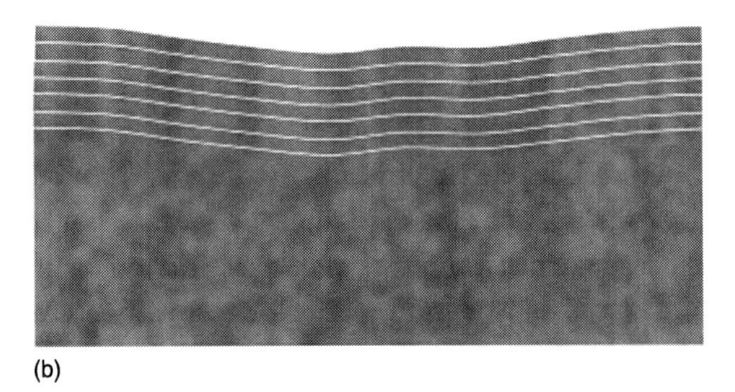
(b)

Figure 6.1 (a) Diagram of articular cartilage showing normal zones (traditionally four zones are identified) with the phospholipid solid lubricant at the surface illustrated. (b) Sketch showing the oligolamellar lining of six phospholipid bilayers on the articular cartilage surface.

Published by Woodhead Publishing Limited, 2013

oligolamellar (graphite-like) structure of surface-active phospholipids lining the articular surface of a human knee (Hills, 2002). The typical interlamellar spacing is about 45 Å. The hydrophobicity of the phospholipidic multibilayer depends on the degree of adsorption and cohesion. Cohesion of phospholipid molecules is due to the presence of the Ca^{2+} ions between phosphate ions (Hills, 2000; Richter et al., 2006). In normal joints the cartilage surface is perfectly smooth macroscopically, enabling joints to slide across one another without friction. Once the cartilage of the superficial zone starts to deteriorate, osteoarthritis could set in, triggering an irreversible process that eventually leads to the loss of the underlying layers of the cartilage until bone begins to grind painfully against bone. Osteoarthritis most commonly affects the spine, temporomandibular joints, shoulders, hands, hips and knees.

The focus of this chapter is on the tribological behavior of natural and so-called 'normal' synovial joints. In considering a model of lamellar-roller-bearing lubrication, three factors must be considered: (i) characteristics of the surface of articular cartilage, (ii) relation between surface energy, wettability and friction, and (iii) accuracy of the lamellar-roller-bearing lubrication model. The role played by phospholipid bilayers in frictionless lubrication between biological surfaces can be explained by surface parameters such as charge density, interfacial energy, friction coefficient, wettability and adsorption (or electrostatic interaction) processes.

6.2 Experimental

The articular cartilage specimens were collected from bovine knees (aged 15–20 months). Osteochondral plugs of two sizes, 5 and 10 mm in diameter, were harvested from the lateral and medial femoral condyles using a circular stainless steel cutter. Then, 3-mm diameter cartilage-on-bone discs were prepared from these osteochondral blocks. Two types of samples were tested: untreated bovine cartilage and bovine cartilage rinsed in a fat solvent (chloroform/methanol, v/v, 2:1) to remove the lipids from the surface of the cartilage. After preparation, the specimens were stored at –20 °C in saline of 0.15 M NaCl (or 0.9%) (pH 6.3) and fully defrosted prior to testing. The cartilage-on-bone samples were then glued to the disc and pin stainless surfaces to perform the lubrication test.

The contact angle between saline and the cartilage surface was measured using a KSV CAM100 tensiometer with multiple contact angles measured by placing a droplet of saline on the cartilage surface at five different locations on each sample. The measurements of the contact angle as a function of time were carried out over 110 min for both the normal and delipidized cartilage samples. The test was carried out at ambient laboratory temperature of around 22 °C and a relative humidity of around 45%. A total of five tests were performed using fresh samples for each experimental specimen and set-up.

The coefficient of friction was measured at room temperature using a sliding friction tester – a pin-on-disc tribotester manufactured by ITeR (Poland). The friction between two discs of cartilage soaked in saline (as the lubricating fluid) and subjected to a load, sliding velocities and time were measured. The tests were performed at a very low speed of 1 mm/s during 10 min and a load of 15 N (1.2 MPa), which corresponds to lubrication under physiological conditions. The cartilage samples were left for 1 h in saline before the test. Friction tests on delipidized samples were performed under the same conditions as

Published by Woodhead Publishing Limited, 2013

described above. A total of five tests were performed using fresh samples of each experimental specimen and set-up.

The delipidization of the cartilage surface was geared to gradual removal of the lipid bilayer structure covering the cartilage surface. The delipidization procedure was carried out as described elsewhere (Hills, 1989). Briefly, the cartilage samples were immersed in a fat-removing solvent (2:1 chloroform/methanol, v/v) for 4, 9 and 19 min, taking care to maintain the same meniscus. Immersion for 15 min was sufficient to remove phospholipid from the superficial phospholipid layer (SPL) (Little et al., 1969; Oloyede et al., 2004b). After each extraction, the sample was placed in saline solution for 60 min for rehydration and to remove organic solvent left on the surface of the cartilage. These samples were used in our experiments for determining surface wettability and lubrication characteristics (coefficient of friction). Both the normal intact and delipidized surfaces of articular cartilage were characterized by atomic force microscopy (AFM) (Pawlak et al., 2012b). Measurements were conducted with the samples immersed in saline in accordance with the protocol used previously (Jurvelin et al., 1996; Kumar et al., 2001). Osteochondral (3 mm × 3 mm) plugs with articular cartilage of full thickness that were still attached to their underlying bones (10 samples per patella) were imaged. The bone sublayer was dried with a paper towel and glued onto a Petri dish (1.5 cm in diameter) using two-sided adhesive tape and fast-drying Loctite® 454 glue. The normal and delipidized surface characterization was conducted on the same samples; lipid removal was done subsequent to the imaging of the normal intact specimen.

The apparatus used in the microelectrophoretic measurements and methods were described in a previous paper (Pawlak et al., 2010a).

Published by Woodhead Publishing Limited, 2013

6.3 Surface of articular cartilage – wettability, charge density, interfacial energy and friction

6.3.1 *Wettability of articular cartilage*

The surface properties of articular cartilage, such as hydrophobicity (wettability) and interfacial energy, affect the adsorption and chemical affinity of biomolecules that, in turn, influence the friction of this natural system. These properties underlie the mechanism that has been referred to as articular cartilage biofriction (Adamson, 1976; Chappuis et al., 1983; Hills, 1988). The tissue is a deformable, porous material with an average stiffness between 12 and 50 MPa, and surface roughness varying from 1 μm for infants, 2.25 μm for adults to 5.25 μm for osteoarthritis-affected cartilage (Wright and Dowson, 1976).

In a recent study, the conceptualization of articular cartilage as a giant reverse micelle with a mechanism of joint biocushioning and lubrication was proposed (Pawlak and Oloyede, 2008). It has also been hypothesized that a hydrophobic surface of articular cartilage that is composed of a highly hydrated three-dimensional network of phospholipids, namely the surface amorphous layer (SAL), on which phospholipid vesicles are formed, facilitates joint lubrication while sustaining the long-term efficacy of the articular surface in joint function (Hills, 2000; Gadomski, 2008; Pawlak and Oloyede, 2008). Synovial fluid is non-Newtonian in that its viscosity decreases non-linearly with an increase in the shear rate. In rheumatoid arthritis, the viscosity of synovial fluid depreciates, becoming more Newtonian in its rheological characteristics. Also, the fluid and protein content of synovial fluid is increased, while the content of hyaluronate and its length decrease in this

Published by Woodhead Publishing Limited, 2013

condition. The differences in the properties of synovial fluids of normal and arthritic joints are manifested in the dissimilarity in the values of their shear rate ($10\ s^{-1}$) and viscosity for normal ($1.1\ Ns/m^2$), arthritic ($0.3\ Ns/m^2$) and rheumatologic ($0.03\ Ns/m^2$) samples (Wright and Dowson, 1976). The bio-surface of cartilage in a normal joint is hydrophilic (with a wettability of around 0°) when undisturbed with its multibilayer membrane and hydrophobic (with a wettability of 105°) when air-dried (Chappuis et al., 1983; Hills, 1988; Pawlak et al., 2012b).

The presence of phospholipid bilayers on the surface of articular cartilage provides characteristics that are well adapted to wet and relatively dry conditions. This smart surface characteristic creates a hydrophobic/hydrophilic balance resulting in a functional hydrophilic surface in the intact joint. One of the quantitative indicators of surface tribochemical properties is hydrophobicity. This is measured as wettability or the contact angle between a drop of water and the reference surface (Pawlak et al., 2008b).

Wettability characterizes the surface of various substrates, which are defined as wettable (highly hydrophilic, $\theta \sim 0$–45°) or non-wettable (highly hydrophobic, $\theta \sim 90$–180°) (Figure 6.2). It is well known that polymers with hydrophobic groups ($-CH_2-$ and CH_3-) can be modified by oxygen plasma treatment to those carrying a hydrophilic group (–OH). This modification makes the surface hydrophilic with a small contact angle, which is effective in full aqueous lubrication (Lee and Spencer, 2005; Bongaerts et al., 2007).

Poor lubrication in animal joints, particularly on the articular surface of cartilage, can be attributed to deterioration of surface hydrophobicity, where the wettability or contact angle (θ) changes from 100° to less than 70° (Hills, 2000).

Published by Woodhead Publishing Limited, 2013

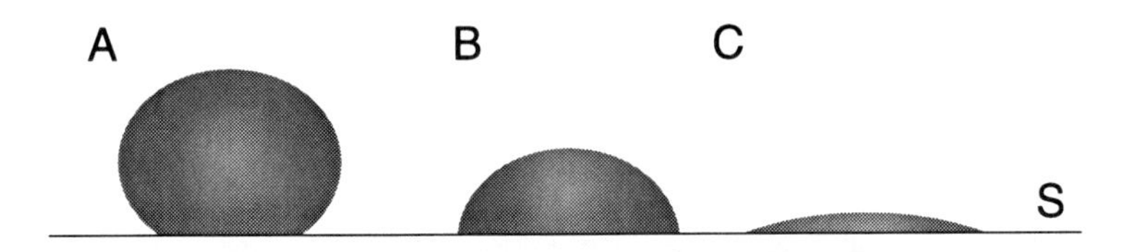

Figure 6.2 Wetting of different surfaces (S) with a drop of saline: (a) when placed on surface with contact angles (θ) greater than 150°, (b) when placed on normal (an intact, air-dried) bovine articular cartilage ($\theta \sim 100°$) and (c) when placed on articular surface of a human hip diagnosed with osteoarthritis ($\theta \sim 40°$).

Source: Hills (1988) (picture taken from Wikipedia).

Phospholipids form part of the porous solid matrix and any loss in their quantity through either abrasion or disease has been reported to change the wettability, which in turn results in a change of the frictional properties of the surface (Little et al., 1969; Hills and Monds, 1998a; Hills, 2000; Ballantine and Stachowiak, 2002). These phospholipids are also present in the synovial fluid, which has a pH of around 7.4 (Ropes and Bauer, 1953). The wetted surfaces of the phospholipid membranes are negatively ($-PO_4^-$) charged (Pawlak et al., 2008a).

In this study, we have assumed the Hills description of the articular surface of cartilage, which describes phospholipids as the major 'solid' component of the lubricant in articulating joints (Marti et al., 1995; Hills, 2000; Pawlak and Oloyede, 2008), the fluid being pressurized water (Oloyede and Broom, 1994). Following this model, it can be further argued that the phospholipids, in association with pressurized fluid, act as a hydrated semi-solid surfactant facilitating the almost frictionless lubrication of the mammalian joint (Oloyede et al., 2004a,b; Gudimetla et al., 2007). Biosurface wettability

Published by Woodhead Publishing Limited, 2013

can be measured relative to differences in the charge density of the functional amino ($-NH_3^+$) and phosphate ($-PO_4^-$) groups. In this regard, we note that Hills (1988) reported that the interfacial energy and wettability of a surface that is characterized by charged anionic phosphate ($-PO_4^-$) groups are lower than those of dry bilayer phospholipids surface by activating hydrophobic groups (see Figure 6.3) (Chen et al., 1989; Burke and Barrett, 2003a; Pawlak et al., 2010a,b).

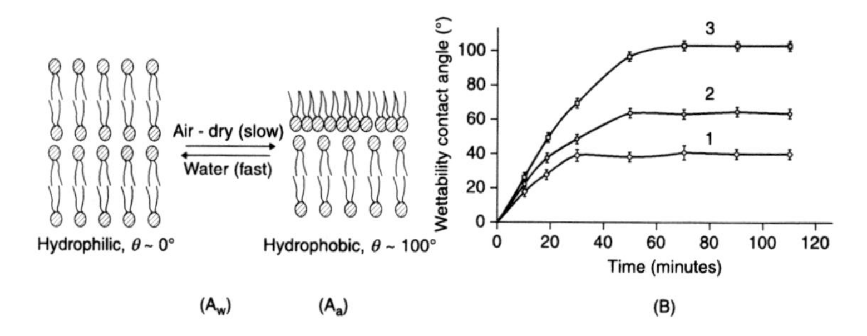

Figure 6.3 The smart-surface constitution of superficial phospholipid bilayers of articular cartilage in water (A_w) and air-dry (A_a) conditions. A change in surface energy leads to conformational changes in the surface of bovine patella from bilayer (super hydrophilic around 0° contact angle) to monolayer (hydrophobic). (B) Changes of the wettability contact angle as a function of air-drying time. Curve: (1) After 19-min delipidization in chloroform/methanol, v/v (2:1), contact angle of 40°, (2) after 9-min delipidization, contact angle of 63° and (3) normal articular surface, contact angle of 103°. Cartilage samples were immersed in saline for 30 min and then air-dried (n = 5, error bars = 95% confidence limit).

Published by Woodhead Publishing Limited, 2013

6.3.2 Surface charge density v. pH

Artificially prepared vesicles are known as liposomes. Liposomes have been used to mimic biological phospholipid membranes on articular cartilage surface where proteins are bound, ions are transported, energy is transduced and cellular processes take place. The charge density of the membrane was determined as a function of pH and electrolyte concentration from the interfacial energy method. Liposome membranes were prepared as an aqueous NaCl solution under various pH conditions. This procedure was used to examine the local acid/base equilibrium of the electrolytes at the membrane surface, which can be considered to mimic the phospholipid interface in articular cartilage.

The adsorbed ions (H^+, OH^-, Na^+, Cl^-) that are present in the electrically charged solutions of liposome membranes comprising phosphatidylcholine were found to exhibit pH-responsive quasi-periodic behavior. A novel model of the phospholipid bilayers of joints has been developed based on the liposome membrane. This model can be applied to the investigation of polyelectrolyte ions such as lubricin in articular cartilage. We have demonstrated that the acid/base processes occurring on charged surfaces provide a key mechanism facilitating lubrication in human joints. The hydrophilicity of the surface molecular groups, e.g. lipid head-groups, is affected by the electrolyte ions in solutions in such a way that, between negatively charged surfaces, short-range hydration repulsion increases with an increase in the number of adsorbed cations (Gale et al., 2007; Schmidt et al., 2007). A few molecular layers or a 1- to 2-nm layer of water in a 0.01 M KCl solution acts as a protective layer against adhesion-induced damage during sliding and a low friction coefficient of 0.02 is maintained under loads of up to 20 MPa (Israelachvili, 1986; Gale et al., 2007). The pH dependence of the surface charge of

Published by Woodhead Publishing Limited, 2013

the liposomal membrane in a 0.155 M NaCl solution and deionized water (control curve) is plotted in Figure 6.4.

It can be seen that, upon a decrease in the negative charge in the saline environment, the $-N^+$ and CH_3 groups of the phosphatidylcholine molecules are covered by OH^- ions, whereas the $-PO_4^-$ groups become uncovered. This fact indicates adsorption of the Na^+ ions. A similar tendency can be observed in acidic solution in the presence of sodium chloride: upon a decrease in positive charge, the $-PO_4^-$ groups are covered by H^+ ions, whereas the $-N^+$ and CH_3 groups become uncovered. This result indicates adsorption of the Cl^- ions (Pawlak et al., 2008a). If acid/base quasi-equilibria are

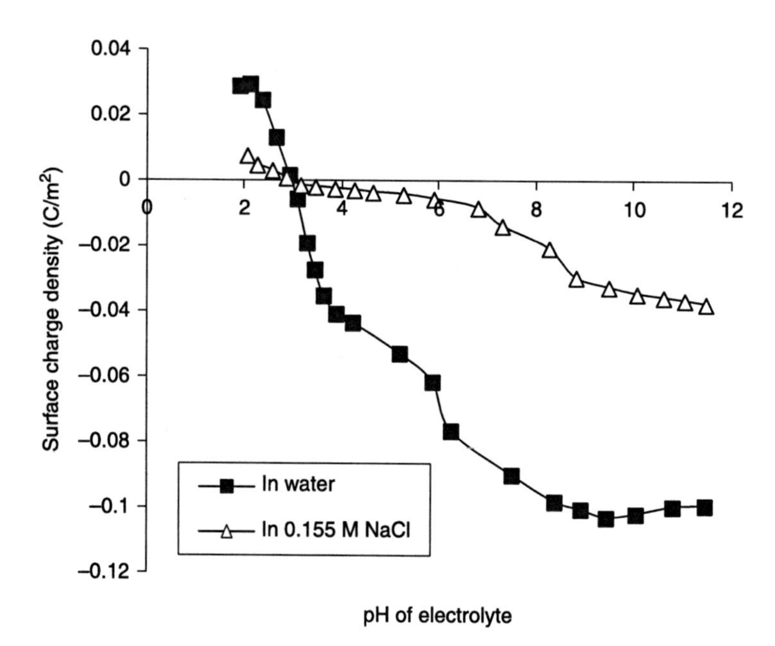

Figure 6.4 **pH dependence of the surface charge density of liposomal membranes formed from phosphatidylcholine in deionized water (squares) and a 0.155 M NaCl solution (triangles).**

Source: Pawlak et al. (2008a).

Published by Woodhead Publishing Limited, 2013

kept/recovered by the system, it is more resistive to wear (when static-friction treated); hydration of phospholipids assures that coagulation becomes ineffective – the layers involving hydrated phospholipids, and being electrostatically adsorbed at the surface(s) of articular cartilage, are also more mechanically robust. The latter gives rise to a weak friction promoting sliding effect, due to electrostatic repulsion, and opposes a (possible) peptization occurring; however, it depends upon maintaining a balance of salts within the system.

In our experiment, the pH range of 6.4–8.4 (7.4 is the physiological condition in synovial fluid) is of the utmost importance. Under this regime, we can conclude that interaction of the sodium and hydrogen ions with the $-PO_4^-$ group (or the degree of coverage of the phospholipid membrane surface) is high. Also, under physiological pH, the degree of coverage of the membrane by the OH^- ions is close to unity. Adsorption of the chloride ion, which is a very weak base, is not observed over the pH range of 6.4–8.4. Our results do indeed indicate that the surface charge strongly influences the acid/base equilibrium of the adsorbing species. Similarly to other experiments (Hills, 1990; Sader et al., 1999; Grant et al., 2006), we chose to alter the surface charge by changing the pH of the solution used to assemble the bilayer, since the pH affects the degree of dissociation of both polyelectrolytes (if present) and the charge density on the phospholipidic bilayer. This liposome bilayer is a model for phospholipidic bilayers and will be applied for investigation of the lubrication of contacting articular cartilage in general.

6.3.3 Wettability v. pH of phospholipid of amino and phosphate groups

With regard to wettability (contact angle θ), measurements of an amphoteric weak polyelectrolyte bilayer with phosphate and amino functional groups in the pH range 1–10 indicate that solution pH and salt concentration change the contact angle (Figure 6.5) (Burke and Barrett, 2003b). The amino group at low solution pH is in the $-NH_3^+$ form and as the pH increases the amino groups would lose their charge, resulting in an increased surface wettability. In the case of the phosphate functional group, the contact angle decreases with an increase in solution pH, screening the surface charges. Furthermore, the pH-dependent degree of dissociation of amino and phosphate surface bilayer compounds could increase or decrease the wettability, *f*, and swelling of weak polyelectrolyte (Burke and Barrett, 2003b; Pawlak at al., 2010a,b).

The often prevailing opinion in the literature is that phospholipids play a role in articular joint function, and that

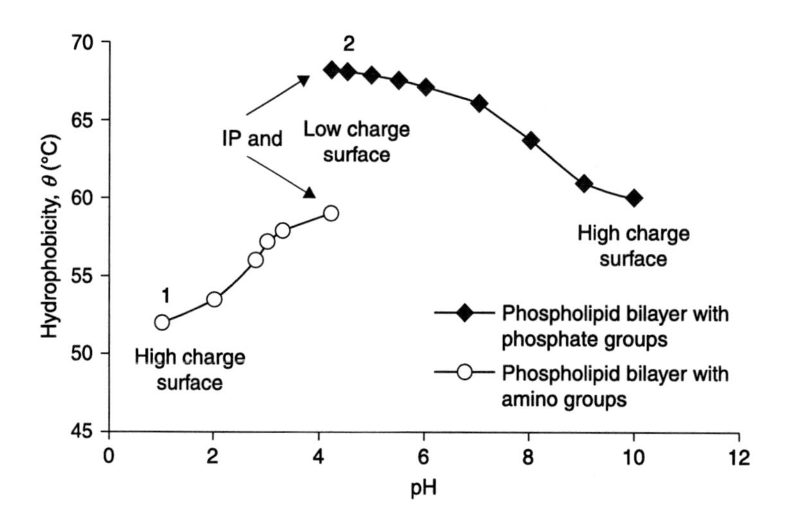

Figure 6.5 **Influence of solution pH on the wettability (θ) of the phosphatidylcholine bilayer surface of an amphoteric weak polyelectrolyte with both amino ($-NH_3^+/-NH_2$) and phosphate ($-PO_4H/-PO_4^-$) functional groups.**

Source: Pawlak et al. (2010b).

they depreciate in quality and quantity as the cartilage transforms from health to disease (Hills, 1996a). The degeneration is also often combined with changes in the pH of the synovial fluid with concomitant effects on the state of the cartilage surface wettability (Figure 6.5).

The relationships between solution pH and wettability (contact angle θ), interfacial energy (γ) and friction coefficient of a weak polyelectrolyte phospholipid bilayer membrane are presented in graphical form in Figure 6.5. Curve 1: the polyelectrolyte (phosphatidylcholine) with an amino group at pH 1.0 begins to pick up the charge from $-NH_3^+$, leaving the biomembrane with a more wettable character ($-NH_2$) as the solution pH is raised to 4.2, p*I*. Curve 2: the polyelectrolyte with a phosphate group ($-PO_4H$) at pH 4.2, p*I*, loses its proton, leaving the biomembrane with a less hydrophobic character ($-PO_4^-$) at pH 10. The phosphatidylcholine over the pH range 1.5–10 shows that wettability can be changed by charging both functional groups. The curves show that the phospholipid bilayer surface has an isoelectric point (p*I*) at a pH around 4.2. The wettability values of $-NH_3^+/-NH_2$ and $-PO_4H/-PO_4^-$ functional groups are adapted from Burke and Barrett (2003a). pH 7.4 ± 1 is a physiological condition of synovial fluid and we can conclude that the degree of coverage of the phospholipid membrane by negative $-PO_4^-$ groups is related to wettability, surface charge and biofriction processes (Pawlak et al., 2010a,b).

The lubrication system proposed by Hills is one in which phospholipid molecules are arranged in strongly cohesive sheets resembling natural membranes. The stacking of three to seven lipid bilayers separated by aqueous layers has been demonstrated for most biological rubbing surfaces (Hills, 1989). It is now a well-developed opinion that the gradual removal of or damage to this SPL or SAL is a key component of osteoarthritis (Hills, 2000; Ballantine and Stachowiak,

Published by Woodhead Publishing Limited, 2013

2002). Specifically, the SPL or SAL comprises lamellar bodies, charged macromolecules (lubricin, hyaluronate) and negatively charged vesicles (Hills, 1989; Kobayashi et al., 1995; Jurvelin et al., 1996; Graindorge et al., 2005) that create the hydrophilic condition that, in the presence of aqueous electrolyte, provides a most astonishing low sliding friction (see Figure 6.1) (Hills, 2000; Pawlak and Oloyede, 2008).

We hypothesize that the fundamental mechanism underlying the frictionless lubrication of articulating mammalian joints is the capacity of the SPL to transform itself through wetting or creation of a surface film from the hydrophobic to the hydrophilic condition. In other words, the function of the phospholipids (SPL) is to create surface hydrophobicity, which is the primary requirement for generating the basic surface 'wetness' to provide a water-facilitated and essentially frictionless surface (SAL). It can be argued that this characteristic is what is lost or reduced when articular cartilage degrades.

Based on experiments on engineering tribopairs, it has become increasingly apparent that the synovial fluid alone cannot facilitate effective lubrication (Gale et al., 2007; Pawlak et al., 2011). Cartilage literature has established that the synovial fluid in the joint is more than a vehicle for transporting phospholipid molecules to the cartilage–cartilage contact site. The major macromolecules of the synovial fluid are lubricin and hyaluronate. These constituents act as carriers for phospholipids and have been argued as contributory to good lubrication in the presence of vesicles (Hills, 1989; Schmidt et al., 2007).

Electron microscopy studies of the SAL structure revealed the presence of lamellated phospholipids (bilayers) on the articular surface (Hills, 1989). Lubricating systems, such as cartilage surfaces, show that phospholipids chemically

Published by Woodhead Publishing Limited, 2013

attached to the surfaces rubbing across an aqueous medium result in superior lubrication, which involves low sliding velocities under significant pressure. It has also been proposed that the articular friction system functions well with hydrophilic surfaces where the surface charge provides electrostatic 'double-layer' repulsion in addition to the 'steric' repulsion of the hydration layer of tightly bound water molecules (Israelachvili, 1986; Hills, 1988). The question as to what surface characteristics and mechanisms are responsible for the functional adhesion of the phospholipid liposomes and lamellar spheres that support the smooth lubrication of joints still remains largely unanswered.

When the standard procedure is used to measure wettability (contact angle θ) on a well-rinsed articular surface, values of between 100° and 105° are observed, indicating a very hydrophobic condition (Chappuis et al., 1983; Hills, 2000) that is similar to that measured in dry air. On the other hand, measurement of the contact angle on a wet cartilage surface returns a value of approximately 0°, indicating a highly hydrophilic condition. Drying of this surface in air results in (i) $\theta \sim 30°$ after 9 min, (ii) $\theta \sim 50°$ after 15 min, and (iii) $\theta \sim 100°$ after 50 min (Pawlak et al., 2012a).

6.3.4 Surface characterization of normal intact and delipidized articular cartilage by AFM

The results obtained from AFM imaging and characterization of the surface of normal intact and delipidized articular cartilage specimens are presented in this section. Figure 6.6 shows the plot of the height of the SAL of normal intact cartilage and cartilage whose surface has been subjected to different delipidization times in (chloroform/

Published by Woodhead Publishing Limited, 2013

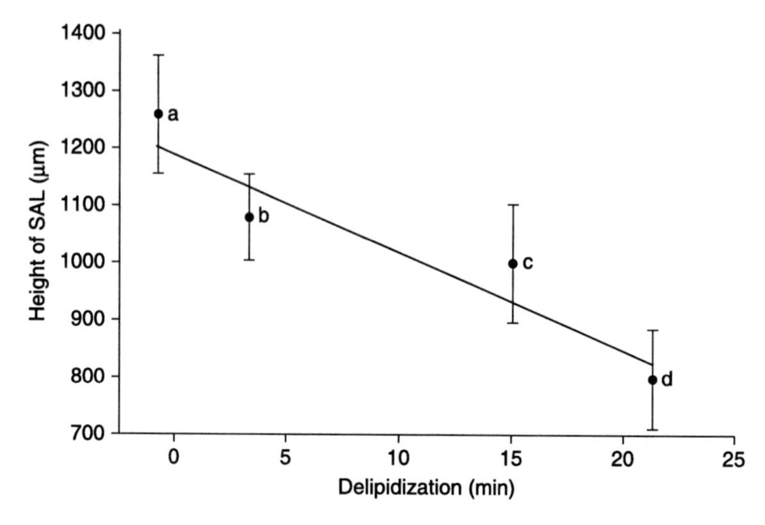

Figure 6.6 Variation of lipid lost (height of SAL, nm) with time following delipidization with chloroform:methanol, v/v, (2:1). (a) Normal/ intact 0-min delipidization; (b) 3-min delipidization; (c) 15-min delipidization; and (d) 21-min delipidization;

methanol, v/v, 2:1). In each of the delipidization groups, we observed a decrease in the heights of the SAL with time of exposure in lipid rinsing solvent (Yusuf et al., 2012).

Figure 6.7 shows the two-dimensional topographical (a) and deflection (b) images acquired simultaneously for normal intact articular cartilage. Figure 6.7 reveals that the normal cartilage is covered by a non-fibrous layer of organized surface structure. Hills (1989, 1990) described this structure as an oligolamella layer formed by the surface-active phospholipids (SAPLs). Figure 6.7 also shows the two-dimensional topographical (c, e) and deflection (d, f) images of the surface of articular cartilage

Published by Woodhead Publishing Limited, 2013

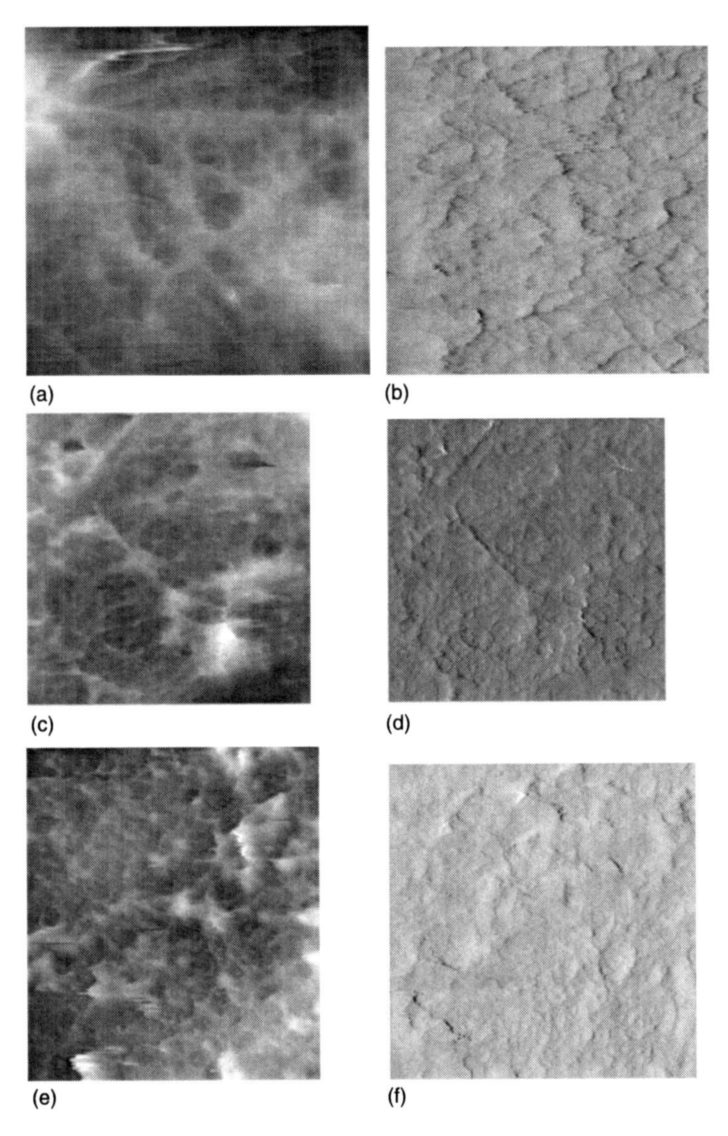

Figure 6.7 Topographical (a, c and e) and deflection (b, d and f) two-dimensional images of articular cartilage surface (frame size: 8 μm × 8 μm). Normal articular surface (a and b), after 3-min delipidization in chloroform/methanol (c and d) and after 21-min delipidization in chloroform/methanol (e and f).

Published by Woodhead Publishing Limited, 2013

exposed to chloroform/methanol (2:1) for 3 min (c, d) and 21 min (e, f) Rinsing the surface of normal cartilage with a lipid rinsing agent almost completely removed the organized SAL, but no fiber structure was noticed on the subsurface layer.

6.3.5 Interfacial energy forces v. pH of phospholipid membrane

Phospholipids, amphoteric molecules containing both positive and negative charges depending on the functional groups, are affected by the solution's pH. At low solution pH, the phospholipid amino group is in the protonated ($-NH_3^+$) form and $-PO_4H$ is in the molecular form – a situation that is characterized by low interfacial energy. As the pH of the solution is increased, the amino groups begin to lose partially their charge ($-NH_3^+ \rightarrow -NH_2$) and $-PO_4H$ groups begin to lose partially their proton ($-PO_4H \rightarrow -PO_4^-$), which causes an increase in the surface energy with the value approaching a maximum. This maximum would occur, as in Figure 6.8, at the *pI* that corresponds to the pH at which phospholipids or surface carriers have no net electrical charge, or where the negative and positive charges are equal (Adamson, 1976).

As the pH of the solution is increased, the amino groups begin to lose their charge ($-NH_3^+ \rightarrow -NH_2$) and more $-PO_4H$ groups begin to lose their proton ($-PO_4H \rightarrow -PO_4^-$), leaving the surface charged and leading to a decrease in the interfacial energy (See Figure 6.8). In this situation, the resulting surface would become less hydrophobic (See Figure 6.5) with a lower f (Burke and Barrett, 2003a). The maximum interfacial energy (γ_{max}) values of phosphatidylcholine and phosphatidylserine membranes were found to be 3.53 and 2.93 mN/m at pH values of 4.2 and 3.80, respectively. The pH of the solution influences changes in the electric charge of the membrane due

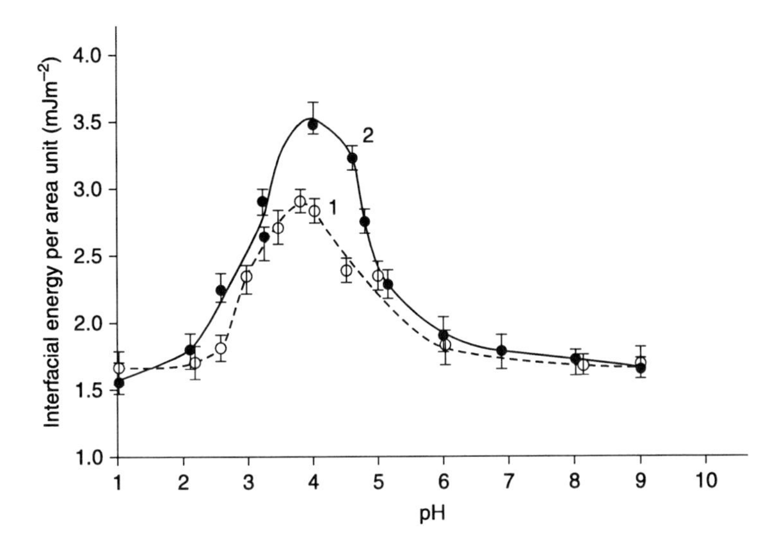

Figure 6.8 **Dependence of interfacial energy of phosphatidylserine (1) and phosphatidylcholine (2) membrane v. pH of the electrolyte solution with a maximum surface energy of 2.93 and 3.53 mN/m at pH equal to 3.8 and 4.1, respectively.**

to the variations in the acid/base equilibrium of the functional groups present in the membrane. The pH-dependent degree of dissociation of the surface functional $-NH_2$ and $-PO_4H$ groups can be used to vary and control the interfacial energy about the isoelectric point (p*I*) with a consequential change in coefficient of friction. This result strongly suggests a mechanism whereby the phospholipid bilayer surface can have a low charge around the p*I* and then transform into a highly charged surface through a change in pH. A noteworthy aspect of the result shown in Figure 6.8 is the closeness of the responses for the two different membranes used in this study. This is probably due to the similarity in the values of the acidity ($-PO_4H$) and basicity ($-NH_2$) of their functional groups, i.e. phosphatidylcholine: $pK_a = 2.58$, $pK_b = 5.68$;

Published by Woodhead Publishing Limited, 2013

phosphatidylserine: pK_a = 2.42, pK_b = 5.98 (Petelska et al., 2006; Pawlak et al., 2010a).

The density of packed phospholipid molecules on a biological surface can be expressed by the wettability contact angle (θ). The normal articular surface rinsed free of synovial fluid (washed with a detergent) has high hydrophobicity with contact angles between 100° and 105° (in dry-air condition) (Chappuis et al., 1983; Hills, 1989). After rigorous rinsing with lipid solvent, the wettability of the articular surface changes to a hydrophilic one with a contact angle of 37.4° (Table 6.1) (Gvozdanovic et al., 1975; Hills, 1989). The presence of phospholipids as surfactant in synovial fluid reduces surface tension and can transform a hydrophobic surface into a hydrophilic one. This can be argued to be an aggregation process in which phospholipid molecules arrange themselves into energetically favorable vesicles and lamellar spheres, forming reservoirs for the surfactants in the lubrication

Table 6.1 Wettability characteristics (hydrophobicity/hydrophilicity) of biological tissue surfaces

Biological tissue surface	Contact angle, θ (°)	Wettability characteristics
Normal articular cartilage, human	103–105	Hydrophobic
Normal bovine patella	100.1	Hydrophobic
Human knee	79.7	Hydrophobic
Hip (arthritic tissue)	56.3	Hydrophobic
Unworn knee (worn knee)	67.8 (62.9)	Hydrophobic
Articular cartilage degenerative	70	Hydrophobic
Articular cartilage rinsed with solvent (surface extracted with $CHCl_3$/MeOH, v/v, 2:1)	37.4	Hydrophilic
Articular cartilage with bilayer	<40	Hydrophilic

Note: Contact angle was determined under air-dry surface conditions.
Source: Chappuis et al., 1983; Hills and Monds, 1998a; Hills, 1989.

process (Gale et al., 2007; Gadomski et al., 2008a; Pawlak and Oloyede, 2008). It has also been shown that the combination of a low interfacial energy and large contact angle provides effective lubrication (Hills, 1988; Pawlak et al., 2012a).

6.4 Relation between surface energy, wettability and friction of a cartilage–cartilage tribopair

6.4.1 Influence of interfacial energy on coefficient of friction in joints

The characteristics of biosurfaces, i.e. surface smoothness/roughness, charge density and hydrophobic/hydrophilic balance, play a crucial role in certain processes such as adhesion, electrostatic flow and friction (Adamson, 1976). The interfacial energy between solid and air (γ_S) and the decrease in the interfacial energy between solid and liquid (γ_{SL}), together with the decrease of surface energy (in terms of the corresponding interfacial energy) of the lubricant containing surfactant (γ_L), lead to an increase in wettability in accordance with the Young–Dupree equation (Young, 1805):

$$\cos\theta = (\gamma_S - \gamma_{SL})/\gamma_L \qquad [6.1]$$

One of the ways in which proteins or surfactants lower their free energy is the removal of hydrophobic groups from contact with the aqueous environment. In this respect, the work of adhesion (W_{adh}) for proteins can be estimated from:

$$W_{adh} = \gamma_L(1 + \cos\theta) \qquad [6.2]$$

It should be noted that the value of $\cos\theta$ in Eq. [6.2] is estimated using an equilibrium value of the contact angle θ. The work of adhesion is an accurate reflection of the

Published by Woodhead Publishing Limited, 2013

wettability of a surface, which in turn correlates with the frictional properties of such a surface (Dela Volpe et al., 2002; Dhathathreyan and Meheshwari, 2002). When looking at Eq. [6.2] one sees that the work of adhesion can change periodically due to corresponding gradual changes in wettability characteristics from normal to degenerative articular cartilage (Table 6.1).

The relationship between wettability (contact angle θ) and interfacial energy (γ_L) of an aqueous solution of surfactants on, for example, polytetrafluoroethylene (PTFE; a hydrophobic solid, $\theta = 120°$) has been shown to be linear, while the same relationship for a hydrophilic glass surface with a contact angle of 37° and some aqueous solutions of non-ionic surfactants is non-linear (Szymczak and Janczuk, 2008). The wettability of soft tribopair-based lubricants is related to the characteristics of the frictional forces in the boundary area between the contacting surfaces, which decreases with decreasing contact angle (Lee and Spencer, 2005; Choo et al., 2007). Consequently, it can be inferred that the hydrophilization of a surface reduces the frictional forces in the associated water – a process that can be attributed to the elimination of unfavorable hydrophobic interaction. The coefficient of friction of the articular surface can be determined from the Coulomb-Amontons formula:

$$f = F/W \quad [6.3]$$

where force $F = (\gamma_L)L\cos\theta$ and γ_L is the corresponding interfacial energy, which is evaluated as force per wetted perimeter L, and θ is the contact angle (Hills, 1996b). It can be inferred that formula [6.3] is not readily applicable in situations where the loads are applied at the nanoscale level (Scherge and Gorb, 2001; Gadomski, 2008). It therefore appears that the pH dependence of the surface friction on the bilayer's phospholipid is of immense importance. The results

Published by Woodhead Publishing Limited, 2013

in this paper demonstrate that considerations of the charge density effect on cartilage–cartilage surfaces and the solution pH (lubricant) condition are required if we are to properly understand how the condition of articular cartilage, dealt with as a prone-to-restructuring solid/liquid interfacial system, may influence joint lubrication. For example, at solution pH 7.4, which is above the isoelectric point (p*I* ~ 4.2), the cartilage–cartilage surfaces and lubricant are both negatively charged (Gadomski et al., 2008a), with the charge density (repulsive interaction) of both increasing with increasing pH. This would lead to weak adhesion forces and very low coefficient of friction (Figure 6.9); in addition, the smallest

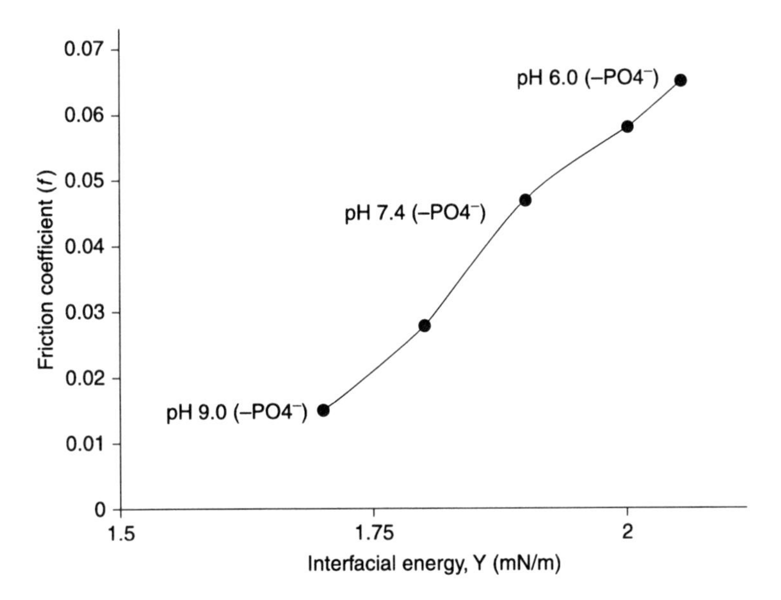

Figure 6.9 **Influence of interfacial energy on the coefficient of friction for phosphatidylcholine bilayer surface phosphate ($-PO_4H/-PO_4^-$) groups. Over the pH range 6–9, the phosphate group is charged ($-PO_4^-$), while the amino group ($-NH_2$) is neutral. The pH 7.4 is a working value when friction processes are taking place in joints.**

Published by Woodhead Publishing Limited, 2013

ions in the system, i.e. protons, being the most energetic ones, may also exhibit their biofriction-lowering role under a sufficient amount of permanent loading (Gadomski, 2008; Gadomski et al., 2008a; Pawlak et al., 2012a).

The isoelectric point (p*I*) for phosphate and amino functional groups for phosphatidylcholine and phosphatidylcholine is at solution pH 4.2 and interfacial energy γ_{max} = 3.53, as shown in Figure 6.8. The phosphate group ($-PO_4H/-PO_4^-$) is most charged over the pH range (see Figure 6.8) with low interfacial energy change (γ = 1.7–2.0), pH 6–9, shown in Figure 6.9. The friction coefficient values for the phosphate ($-PO_4H/-PO_4^-$) functional group were adapted from Burke and Barrett (2003a).

The biolubricant in the synovial joint contains hyaluronate, proteoglycan 4 (PRG4) which is also known as lubricin, and phospholipids as vesicles (Table 6.2); this mixture is mostly responsible for the ultra-low-friction mechanism in the joint (Schmidt and Sah, 2007). On the other hand, the phospholipid

Table 6.2 **Concentration of hyaluronate, PRG4 and phospholipids in synovial fluid**

Parameters	Healthy synovial fluid	Rheumatoid arthritis synovial fluid	Osteoarthritis synovial fluid
Hyaluronate (mg/ml)	1–4	0.8–1.5	0.7–1.1
PRG4 (μg/ml)	52–450	276–762	–
Phospholipids (mg/ml)	0.1–0.2	1.5–3.7	0.2–0.3
Protein (mg/ml)	15–25	36–54	29–39
Articular cartilage surface, θ (°)	100–105	<70	<70
pH of synovial fluid	7.30–7.43	7.4–8.1	7.4–7.6

Source: Bole and Peltier, 1962; Rabinowitz et al., 1983; Mazzucco et al., 2004; Jeleniewicz et al., 2005; Schmidt et al., 2007.

Published by Woodhead Publishing Limited, 2013

molecules that are not involved in the development/maintenance of the SAL gather to form a particular lamellar structure comprising both unilamellar and bilamellar folded spheres (Siegiel, 1984). We argue/hypothesize (Pawlak and Oloyede, 2008; Gadomski et al., 2008a,b) that this structure acts in the manner of vesicles (supplied by free phospholipids in synovial fluid), which dissipate energy and thus protect the cartilage from mechanical degradation. A stiff and flexible form of hyaluronate, which is known to possess unique water retention and proper viscoelasticity-promoting properties and hydrophobic interaction with vesicles, is a component of this lubricant, and is believed to control the pH of synovial fluid and its protein content. As has been shown in several publications (Higaki et al., 1998; Hills and Monds, 1998b; Murakami et al., 1998; Schwarz and Hills, 1998; Ozturk et al., 2004; Mazzucco et al., 2004), we support the notion in this work that lubricin is the carrier of phospholipids and the other macromolecules supporting and maintaining the structure responsible for the lubrication we have described (Figure 6.10).

Despite our present arguments, the form in which phospholipids exist in normal articular cartilage and synovial fluid as vesicles and lamellae spheres is poorly understood (Singer, 1971; Fox et al., 1991; Forsey et al., 2006). This is due to the limitation imposed on experiments, i.e. while the undisturbed surface of articular cartilage *in vivo* has the ability to build lamellar bodies, surfaces *in vitro* are incapable of doing this. This is also the case with the role of water in its pressurized and unpressurized conditions. Regardless, the experimental fact that normal synovial fluid diluted to a third of its concentration yielded similar results in friction tests as the unmodified one (Swann et al., 1981; Siegiel, 1984; Higaki et al., 1998; Murakami et al., 1998; Ozturk et al., 2004; Trunfio-Sfarghiu et al., 2007; Yarimitsu et al., 2009) provides a strong indication that the synovial fluid

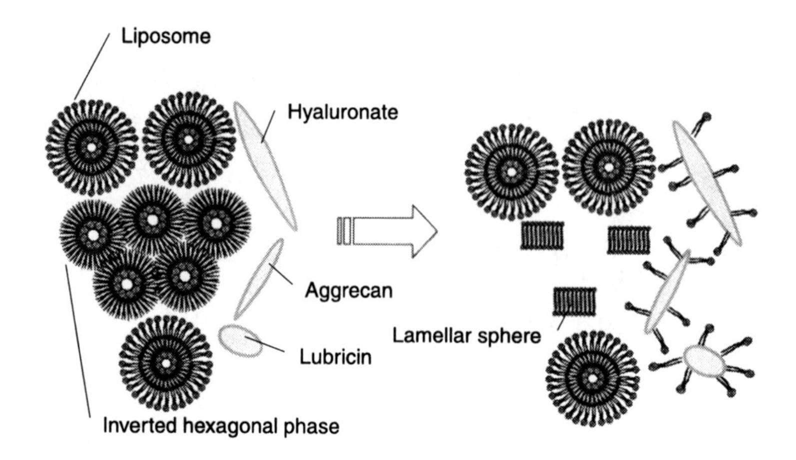

Figure 6.10 Equilibrium in synovial fluid between phospholipids and macromolecules (hyaluronate, aggrecan and lubricin) and liposomes, inverted hexagonal phase and lamellar spheres in the process of distribution on the surfaces in articular cartilage.

does not play a direct role in lubrication, but instead, and in accordance with our hypothesis, is a principal supplier of material for building and maintaining the near frictionless surface of articular cartilage.

The acid/base dissociation behavior of multilayer films of hyaluronic acid/poly(L-lysine), poly(acrylic acid)/poly(allylamine) or amphoteric bilayers of phospholipids is key in controlling factors such as wettability and surface friction, pH and ionic strength dependence, and some properties of the film, such as its swelling, wettability and surface friction. Increasing the salt concentration implies an increased screening of the surface charges, making the surface more hydrophobic in character, which causes an increase in contact angle. The strong evidence of differences between charged (NH_2^+, $-COO^-$) and uncharged ($-NH_2$, $-COOH$) phospholipid functional groups ($-NH_2$, $-PO_4H$) of interfacial

Published by Woodhead Publishing Limited, 2013

energy and hydrophobicity, as seen in Figures 6.5 and Figure 6.9, offers quantitative support for wettability and coefficient of friction (Burke and Barrett, 2003a; Pawlak et al., 2010a,b).

6.4.2 Wettability and friction of normal and delipidized cartilage–cartilage tribopairs

The present study is concerned with the wettability of the cartilage surface and the effect of delipidization on the frictional characteristics of the surface of the tissue. It has been noticed in an earlier study that the moisture content influences the value of contact angle between water droplets and the articular surface of cartilage, and that biological surface samples in contact with air after drying for about 1 h remained stable (van Oss et al., 1975). In the natural condition, when the joint is completely covered with synovial fluid, the surfaces of the cartilage can be seen to be superhydrophilic (around 0° contact angle) with a contact angle of zero. This condition changes with increasing time of exposure of a fresh joint to the atmosphere. The contact angle values were plotted as a function of time (Figure 6.3b).

The contact angle increased until reaching an asymptotic value of approximately 100° for air-dried samples (curve 3). This plateau region was maintained for at least 50 min. We found that, once exposed to air, the hydrophilic surfaces slowly (during around 50 min) became hydrophobic. This was established by contact angle measurements and manifested by a slowly increasing contact angle with exposure time. Using a saline interfacial energy value of 72.5 mJ/m and a contact angle of around 100°, we obtained a mean value of 22.4 mJ/m for the interfacial energy of cartilage, which is very hydrophobic for a biological surface. It can be inferred from these results that the initially very

Published by Woodhead Publishing Limited, 2013

hydrophobic surfaces became more hydrophilic (or more adhesive) when they came in contact with water. When a drop of water was placed on a dry L-α-dipalmitoylphosphatidylethanolamine (DPPE) bilayer covering a mica surface, the contact angle was 112°, a very hydrophobic surface, and $\theta \sim 10°$ and 60°, after 5 and 100 s of exposure to water, respectively (Leckband et al., 1993).

This hydrophilic → hydrophobic transition is more likely due to overturning (flip-flop) of surface phospholipid molecules, resulting in the exposure of their hydrophobic groups (Chen et al., 1989) as an aqueous fluid film is drying on the surface. At a pH of 6.9, the saline solution phosphate group ($-PO_4^{3-}$) would interact with water across the interface through dipole–dipole attraction to increase adhesion. The interpretation of the results also requires consideration of the charge density. At that pH of 6.9, the phospholipid membrane is fully charged in solution ($-PO_4^{3-}$) (hydrophilic) and begins to lose its charges in the air-dry condition, leaving the surface with more hydrophobic character, which causes an increase in the contact angle (Chen et al., 1989; Burke and Barrett, 2003a; Pawlak et al., 2010a,b). The wetting studies also indicate that the change of the surface from the hydrophobic to hydrophilic condition was much faster than the reverse hydrophilic → hydrophobic transition, probably because the surface groups became immobilized in the absence of water. When present in aqueous media, the cartilage can enhance its adhesion by exploiting the increased surface energy as a result of conformational changes in the surface phospholipids by activating hydrophilic groups (Kitano et al., 2001; Pesika et al., 2009). Figure 6.11 presents coefficient of friction v. time for the cartilage–cartilage pair for normal and delipidized surfaces. The coefficient of friction (f) values after 10 min friction increase as shown. For normal articular cartilage–articular cartilage pairs the

Published by Woodhead Publishing Limited, 2013

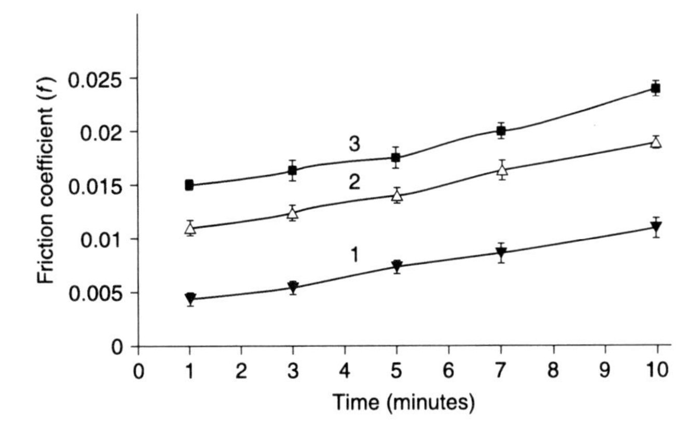

Figure 6.11 Friction coefficient v. time for the cartilage–cartilage pair of normal (curve 1) and delipidized surfaces (9 and 19 min) and measured in saline solution (curves 2 and 3, respectively) (see text for details) (n = 5, error bars = 95% confidence limit).

range of f = 0. 004–0.012, curve 1, and the range of f = 0.011–0.09 and 0.015–0.024 for the delipidized articular cartilage–articular cartilage pairs, curve 2 and 3, respectively. This reveals the significantly higher friction coefficients between articular cartilage–articular cartilage pairs in the delipidized conditions relative to those of the normal articular cartilage–articular cartilage pairs with intact contacting surfaces. The ratio of the coefficient of friction for the delipidized (articular cartilage–articular cartilage) pair/ normal (articular cartilage–articular cartilage) pair values after 5 min increased 2.3 and 3.0 times for the delipidized articular cartilage–articular cartilage pairs, curves 2 and 3, respectively. These friction tests thus confirm our hypothesis on the relation between the number of phospholipid bilayers (or hydrophobicity) and friction (Little et al., 1969; Higaki et al., 1998; Murakami et al., 1998; Ozturk et al., 2004; Trunfio-Sfarghiu et al., 2008; Pawlak et al., 2012a,b). This

Published by Woodhead Publishing Limited, 2013

hypothesis can also be extended to the molecular scale to study, for instance, the role played by the hydrophobic protein–lipid, and water-mediated, matching (Jensen and Mouritsen, 2004; Gadomski et al., 2008a).

Furthermore, it has been shown that under air-dry conditions the contact angle for the bovine patella (around 100°) is higher than that for the arthritic human knee (around 70°) (Hills and Monds, 1998a; Pawlak et al., 2010b). This can be converted into interfacial energy or the work of adhesion ($W_{adh} = \gamma_L(1 + \cos\theta)$), thereby demonstrating that this parameter is approximately 50 mJ/m^2 smaller in the arthritic human knee as compared with the bovine patella. Apart from this change in the contact angle, this reduction in interfacial energy could provide the explanation for the friction shift (Figures 6.12 and 6.13).

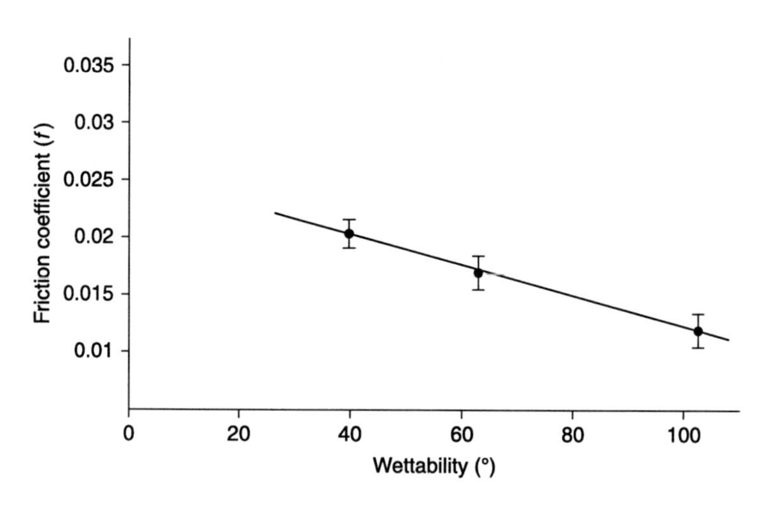

Figure 6.12 Coefficient of friction (*f*) v. wettability of normal cartilage and gradually delipidized cartilage surfaces measured in saline solution (see text for details) (n = 5, error bars = 95% confidence limit).

Published by Woodhead Publishing Limited, 2013

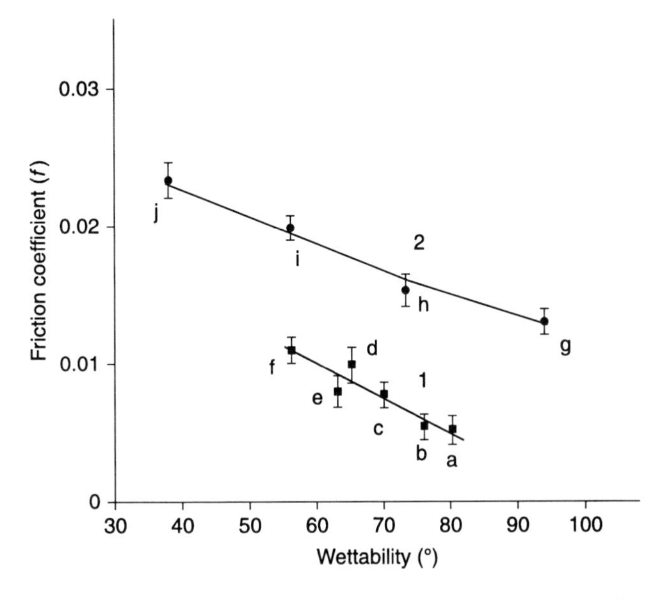

Figure 6.13 Coefficient of friction (*f*) of cartilage/cartilage pair surfaces v. wettability of various biosurfaces: normal cartilage (a, b and g) and arthritic surfaces (c–f) (curve 1) and gradually delipidized cartilage surfaces (h–j) (curve 2) (this work) in saline solution (see text for details) (n = 5, error bars = 95% confidence limit).

Figure 6.12 represents the plot of coefficient of friction (*f*) v. hydrophobicity (wettability) for normal and delipidized cartilage surface samples after 5 min of test (Figure 6.11). The frictional characteristics of this extracted cartilage were greatly increased (over 200%) as compared with the unextracted cartilage surface. Furthermore, it has been shown that phospholipid present in articular cartilage as bilayers is indeed a lubricant and supports a lubrication mechanism by lowering the friction of biosurfaces (Greene et al., 2011). Hills (2000, 1988, 1989, 1990) and other researchers (Kobayashi et al., 1995; Jurvelin et al., 1996) have revealed that the spontaneously formed SAL (*in vivo*)

Published by Woodhead Publishing Limited, 2013

consists of some phospholipid bilayers on the normal intact cartilage surface. The self-organization process involves phospholipid vesicles that are attracted to the hydrophilic cartilage surface to form a 'hybrid bilayer' (Richter et al., 2006). The results of our present study demonstrate the importance of the balance between wettability, electrostatics and lubricant composition, thereby supporting some of the previous hypotheses on the essential conditions for effective surface lubrication in a functional mammalian joint.

We have subsequently attempted to confirm our lubrication hypothesis by friction tests. Figure 6.13 presents the plot of coefficient of friction (*f*) v. hydrophobicity (wettability) for various biosurfaces: normal intact and arthritic articular cartilage surface (curve 1) and delipidized cartilage surfaces (curve 2). The articular surface contact angles of normal cartilage or arthritic surface are: articular cartilage 65° (point d), bovine patella 70° (point c), human knee 79.7° (point d), worn knee 62.9° (point e), hip 76.3° (point b), hip (arthritic) 56.3° (point f). The wettability contact angles of delipidized cartilage surfaces are: after 1 min 71°, after 3 min 56° and after 21 min 39° (points j, i and h), and normal articular cartilage was 93° (point g). The results derived from our own experiment are represented by curve 2, while curve 1 is constructed from the literature data (Chappuis et al., 1983; Hills, 1998; Hills and Monds, 1998a), for comparison.

The frictional characteristics of this extracted cartilage (f = 0.0235) were greatly increased (around 195%) as compared with those of the unextracted cartilage (f = 0.0120). The f value is comparable to that obtained by other authors (Little et al., 1969; Ballantine and Stachowiak, 2002; Ozturk et al., 2004). We therefore conclude that phospholipid present in articular cartilage as bilayers is indeed a lubricant as the SAL supports a lubrication mechanism by lowering the friction of the two biosurfaces.

Published by Woodhead Publishing Limited, 2013

A similar hypothetical illustration of the coefficient of friction (f) v. hydrophobicity (wettability) of articular cartilage was introduced recently (Pawlak and Oloyede, 2010a). This 'recliner seat'-shaped curve is presented in Figure 6.14 and it shows an inclination of around 130°. It may be justified to hypothesize that there are two regimes of phospholipid multilayer and synovial fluid intervention in joint lubrication. In an active joint, the first is the lamellar mode of the multibilayer lubrication mechanism that corresponds to frictionless lubrication by bilayer movement, which is characterized by a complete separation of the

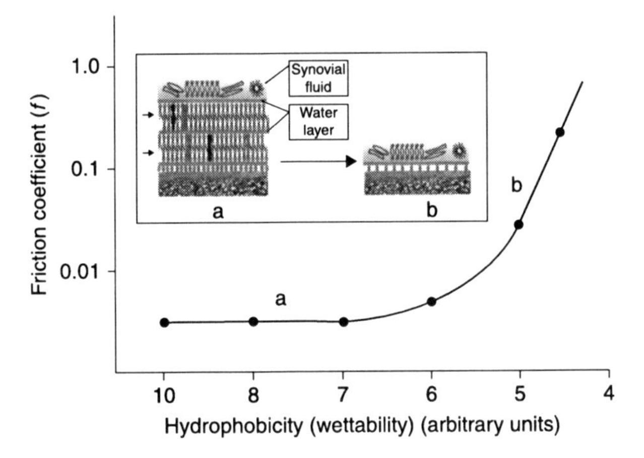

Figure 6.14 Hypothetical illustration coefficient of friction (f) v. hydrophobicity (wettability) of cartilage/cartilage tribopairs in human life. (a), Normal articular surface with wettability contact angles about 105° showing low friction coefficient. (b) Osteoarthritic articular surface with wettability contact angles of 60–70° showing a growing friction coefficient. Cartilage surface is related to a decrease in the number of phospholipid bilayers on cartilage and in wettability as well as to an increased friction coefficient.

Published by Woodhead Publishing Limited, 2013

bilayers (see Figure 6.15 below). The other mode corresponds to the biological lubrication by pressurized synovial fluid and is highly complex, involving surface topography vesicles and lamellar spheres from the synovial fluid. Figure 6.14 demonstrates that the control of SAPL surface properties, e.g. surface roughness, adhesion and hydrophilicity, is of prime importance in ensuring effective lubrication (Briscoe et al., 2006). The increase in the coefficient of friction shown might be associated with decreasing wettability of the articular surface (lower amount of articular cartilage phospholipid), which may, in turn, result in the inability of the highly hydrated three-dimensional SAL to resist compressive forces during joint loading (Hills and Thomas, 1998; Trunfio-Sfarghiu et al., 2008; Afara et al., 2011).

At this juncture, it is desirable to shed more light on the phenomenon proposed in the hypothetical mechanism that is presented in Figure 6.14. The fundamental premise is that a degree of surface hydrophobicity is required before the hydrophilic layer of the phospholipid bilayer that is necessary for lubrication can be created. Consequently, f of the contacting joint surfaces will increase dramatically with the loss of hydrophobicity. This hypothesis or 'theoretical' assertion can also be developed from an interpretation of the

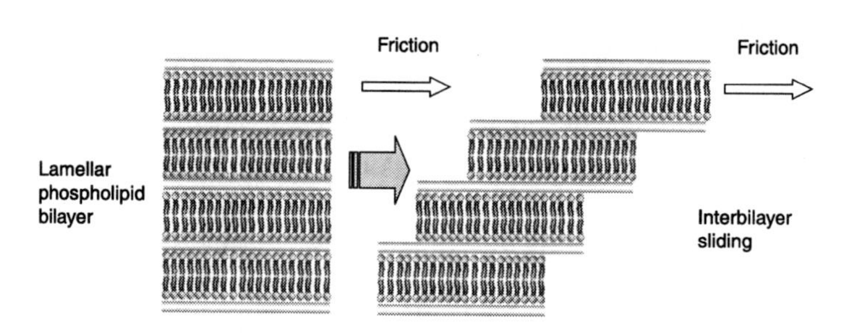

Figure 6.15 Lamellar mode of the bilayer lubrication mechanism.

Published by Woodhead Publishing Limited, 2013

results by Hills and Monds (1998a), in which the relationship between the coefficient of friction and hydrophobicity, in terms of contact angle between saline and the articular surface, was presented.

Water molecules alone, due to their inability to form a useful boundary film because of very low coefficient of viscosity and poor film-forming properties, cannot achieve the extremely low friction coefficient that is seen in natural joint systems (Schwarz and Hills, 1998; Scherge and Gorb, 2001; Hills and Crawford, 2003; Bongaerts et al., 2007). We argue that, in order to produce a highly efficient lubrication of the mammalian articular joint, a pressurized fluid film consisting of a mixture of exuded interstitial fluid (i.e. a 0.155 M aqueous electrolyte) and phospholipids held by macromolecules of glycoprotein, lubricin and hyaluronate are required. Of relevance is that osteoarthritis has been shown to deplete the phospholipids both on the surface and within the cartilage, thereby destroying this important SAL, with significant consequences for load processing and lubrication. To date, clinicians and researchers do not fully understand the biochemical basis of cartilage lipid loss, with the consequence that there is no effective treatment for the symptom (Vecchio et al., 1999; Ballantine and Stachowiak, 2002; Oloyede et al., 2004b). However, it has been demonstrated that phospholipid liposomes and lamellar spheres can resist high shear stress/strain rates and are adsorbed in less than 50 ms when near a surface (Hollinger et al., 2000; Sivan et al., 2010; Verberne et al., 2010), while it has also been shown that the injection of SAPLs relieved osteoarthritic discomfort for up to 14 weeks (Vecchio et al., 1999). It is possible to argue that the challenge in this context is how to restore the hydrophobicity of the articular cartilage surface and then rebuild the SAL (Kobayashi et al., 1995; Jurvelin et al., 1996).

6.5 Lamellar-roller-bearing joint lubrication model

The model of biological lamellar lubrication, i.e. the 'lamellar-roller-bearing joint lubrication model', is compatible with present data as well as those reported in the literature (Oloyede et al., 2004a; Trunfio-Sfarghiu et al., 2007, 2008; Pawlak et al., 2010a). Hills (1989, 1990) proposed that lubrication is provided by SAPLs that form a multibilayer structure over the articular surface of cartilage, known as the SAL. His argument and experimental evidence were based on the observations that lipid lubrication was common in the body of mammals, such as in alveoli (Stratton, 1984), pleural (Hills, 1992) and peritoneal cavities (Dobbie et al., 1988; Chen and Hills, 2000), and joints (Schwarz and Hills, 1996). Due to the presence of phospholipids on the articular surface as membranes and liposomes, and as macromolecules and lamellar spheres in synovial fluid, we propose that the mechanism of lubrication in the articulation joints is based on the model of 'fluid-lipid-assisted' lamellar lubrication.

The lubrication mechanism in joints, according to the proposed 'lamellar-roller-bearing joint lubrication' mechanism, is a bimodal process that occurs simultaneously: (i) through lamellar lubrication (Figure 6.15), which occurs when the bilayers slide over each other, and (ii) through structured synovial fluid that occurs when lamellar spheres, liposomes and macromolecules act like a roller-bearing between two cartilage surfaces in effective biological lubrication (Guerra et al, 1996; Pasquali-Ronchetti et al., 1997; Hills, 2000; Sivan et al., 2010; Verberne et al., 2010).

A tough articular cartilage surface is a vital requirement for biological lubrication. To have a good cohesion between the bilayers, Ca^{2+} ions provide cohesive plane

Published by Woodhead Publishing Limited, 2013

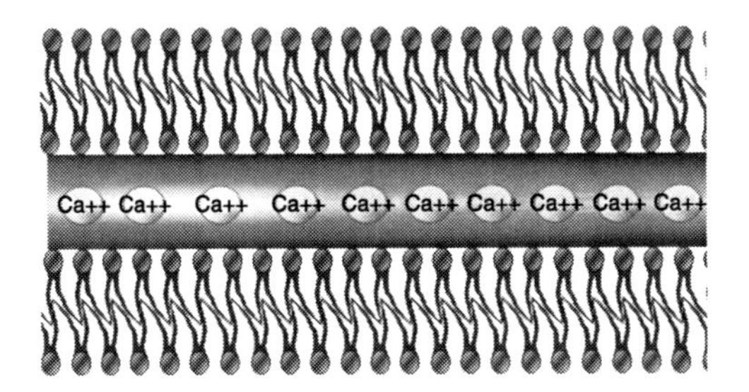

Figure 6.16 Interspersion of the mobile Ca^{2+} ions between anionic phosphate groups.

packing between phosphate groups (Figure 6.16). The calcium cations between phosphate ions pull the adsorbed phospholipid molecules into a very cohesive plane. Thus, with strong adsorption of phospholipid molecules and strong cohesion of this adsorbed lining of phospholipids, the two fundamental criteria for a high-load-bearing lubricant are satisfied (Adamson, 1976; Hills, 1988; Hills and Crawford, 2003; Wierzcholski, 2011).

The nature and composition of the aqueous fluid separating the lamellations between lipid bilayers are typically spaced at 45 Å (Hills, 2000). In the joints, one tissue plane slides over its counterface with effortless ease. The multibilayers appear to have the lamellar (lamellated solid graphite) lubrication system wherever hydrophilic surfaces slide over each other, where load bearing is either high or low. The moment the joint moves, with the action of the lamellar mode, the joint is perfectly lubricated. The phospholipid multibilayers have a greater ability to reduce friction than graphite and other lamellated solid lubricants (Figure 6.15).

Degeneration of the multibilayer is manifested in joint stiffness and adhesive wear symptoms (Gudimetla et al., 2007). The nature of cartilage degeneration and osteoarthritis has raised many questions on the possible role of the surface

Published by Woodhead Publishing Limited, 2013

and intra-matrix lipids of cartilage on its load-bearing function as different from its lubrication mechanism (Oloyede et al., 2004a,b). Presently, there are a number of studies ongoing on the characterization of the lipid bilayers of articular cartilage in joints with osteoarthritis (Hills and Monds, 1998a; Hills and Crawford, 2003; Trunfio-Sfarghiu et al., 2007, 2008; Pawlak et al., 2010a,b). Recently, we extended this study to characterize the surface of cartilage with the artificially depleted surface lipid layer (Yusuf et al., 2011). This was done by selective removal of the SAL to study the role played by the SAPLs in the function of the cartilage. It has been demonstrated that articular cartilage modeling has been controversial over the last decades (Greene et al., 2011).

Only a few of the published papers concerning the role of phospholipid bilayers in lubricating natural joints have been based on hydrophobicity (wettability) of the cartilage surface. However, other studies supporting the argument that the lubricating properties are dominated by lubricin (a glycoprotein) at the cartilage surface have been challenged and await further research. The significant contributions of phospholipids to the cartilaginous bearing appear in two issues. They supply (i) a membrane for maintaining slip plane bilayer lubricants to the joint cartilage, and (ii) liposomal synovial fluid and lamellar spheres that act also as lubricant support at the surface. They are smaller in size than hyaluronate, which is responsible for the viscosity of the fluid (Schwarz and Hills, 1996). The two contacting cartilage surfaces under pressure remain separated by a thick (greater than 0.1 μm) layer of structured synovial fluid macromolecules (lubricin and hyaluronate), lamellar phospholipid spheres and liposomes in healthy joints. The cartilage in the joint is a highly efficacious water solution tribological system that operates over a wide range of pressures, sliding speeds and shear distances (Klein, 2006; Pawlak et al., 2008c; Greene et al., 2011).

This chapter introduces a new model of biological lubrication in joints. It presents data further supporting the viewpoint that biological lubrication in joints is based on the 'lamellar-roller-bearing lubrication' system, comprised of natural articular cartilage–articular cartilage tribopairs. The model of biological lubrication according to Linn and Sokoloff (1965) – 'the secret of the low friction between the cartilage-bearing surfaces is that they never touch' – is compatible with the present data as well as those published in the literature.

One of the practical aspects of phospholipid bilayer lubrication is the initial thickness of the lubricating layer. Nature has established that three or more bilayers are needed to achieve effective biolubrication (Higaki et al., 1998; Murakami et al., 1998; Hills, 2000, 2002; Richter et al., 2006; Pawlak et al., 2012a, 2012b) at low shear stress resulting in a low coefficient of friction at the interface. Anisotropies of mechanical properties (planes of weaknesses) are characteristic of lamellar lubricants. If these lamellae are able to slide over one another at relatively low shear stress, then the lamellar solid becomes self-lubricating. This mechanism is schematically illustrated in Figures 6.15–6.17. The planes of low resistance allow relative movement between lamellae. The lamellar phospholipid molecule adheres strongly to the worn surface and the lamellar structure undergoes deformation at very low stress levels. When the phospholipid multibilayer surfaces are brought into contact, there is a weak electrostatic attraction between corresponding surfaces (Hills, 1990; Richter et al., 2006). The layered structure of phospholipids is shown in Figure 6.17, where layers about 1 μm thick are clearly visible. A lamellar crystal structure with planes and weaknesses in shear is found in some metallic compounds, such as molybdenum disulfide, molybdenum ditelluride and tungsten

Published by Woodhead Publishing Limited, 2013

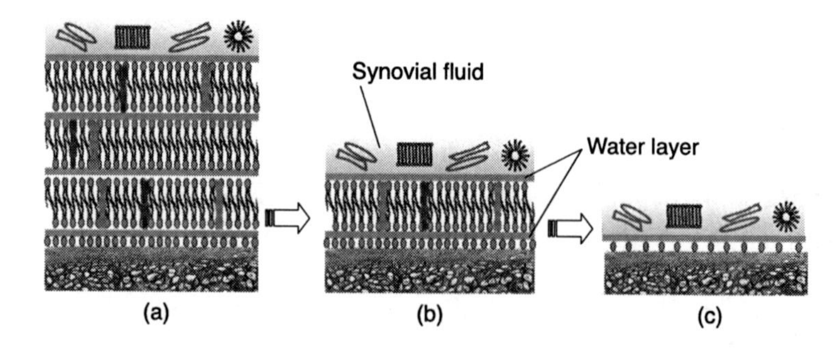

Figure 6.17 Three stages of the quality of a multibilayer structure over the articular surface of cartilage during human life: (a) normal healthy surface of articular cartilage (wettability around 103°), (b) unhealthy surface of articular cartilage (wettability around 75°) and (c) degenerated surface of articular cartilage (wettability below 60°). Note the typical interlamellar aqueous spacing of 45 Å. The lamellar spheres, liposomes and macromolecules act like a roller-bearing mechanism between two cartilage surfaces.

disulfide, as well as cadmium di-iodide and nickel di-iodide. Graphite constitutes a unique class; surface energy along cleavage planes is relatively high, and sliding between these planes is supported by the presence of a small amount of water and oxygen (Stachowiak and Batchelor, 2005). The molecules absorbed on the surface of graphite lamellae suppress bonding between lamellae. A mechanism of graphite lubrication has been suggested by Bragg (1928).

As illustrated in Figure 6.15, when the multibilamellar phospholipid lubricant present on sliding surfaces causes them to slide over one another with relative ease to provide very low friction, the interlayer share mechanism is believed to be responsible for the low friction of most lamellar solid

Published by Woodhead Publishing Limited, 2013

lubricants. As far as the excellent solid-lubricating capacities of bilayers are concerned, a region of negative electrical charge is contained within the layers. Thus, the surfaces of the phosphate groups are negatively charged, creating an electrostatic repulsion between the layers and making the interlayer slippage much easier. The relatively larger interlayer separation in phospholipid bilayers is thought to result from electrostatic repulsion between the successive atomic layers of these lipid bilayers.

The low-friction behavior of phospholipids in aqueous electrolyte is an intrinsic property of the crystal structure, where hydrophobic weak forces join and form a bilayer. A phospholipid multibilayer that displays low-friction behavior will have most of the lamellar aggregates aligned parallel with the sliding direction. The friction coefficient of bilayers, like other lamellar solids, is largely determined by the ratio of shear strength to the specific load. There is a linear relationship with contact pressure, and thus the coefficient of friction decreases with increasing contact pressure.

The friction behavior of a multibilayer coating cartilage usually follows a series of stages, shown in Figure 6.17. Typically, there is a long period of low, stable friction coefficient, with little or no apparent wear. Phospholipidic lamellar spheres, lamellae and macromolecules circulate between the contacting surfaces of articular cartilage, and can be very supportive for lubrication (Figure 6.17a).

Eventually, there is a breakthrough of the coating and degradation of the surface by biological causes. Typically, the phospholipid multibilayer undergoes deformation or fractures during the application of a load. The lamellar aggregates become reoriented so that they are parallel to the sliding direction and material transfers to the counter face. Enough liposomes and lamellar spheres can still be circulating in the system or stored in holes and troughs to 'heal' such

Published by Woodhead Publishing Limited, 2013

ruptures followed by an irreversible low-friction behavior (Figure 6.17b). Finally, when the phospholipid multibilayer structure is gone, the protection and separation between the joint surfaces are no longer in place. The tissue surface changes its structure, which eventually leads to abnormal cartilage wear and joint degeneration. The amount of structured synovial fluid is not enough to resist load and the friction rises rapidly. This behavior corresponds to the ruined joint system (Figures 6.14 and 6.17c).

A 'Biotribochemical Tree' shown in Figure 6.18 summarizes our understanding of some of the most important processes

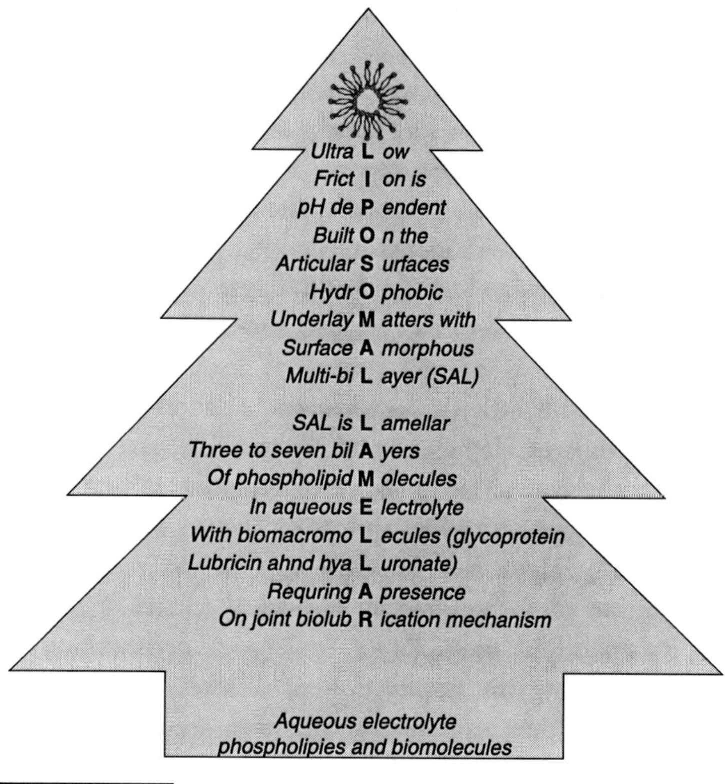

Figure 6.18 'Biotribochemical Tree'.

Source: Pawlak et al. (2010b).

Published by Woodhead Publishing Limited, 2013

occurring between natural surfaces and aqueous lubricant (Pawlak, 2003). Lubrication in nature is based on liposomes (or vesicles in nature) in synovial fluid and the lamellar SAL formed on the articular hydrophilic surface. The SAL membrane is a warranty of ultra-low friction and its disappearance is a consequence of lower phospholipid concentration in cartilage.When hydrophobicity of articular cartilage drops from 105° to about 60° it is losing power to build SAL of natural surfaces by increasing friction.

6.6 Conclusions

We report and discuss direct measurements of the local acid/base equilibrium of the phospholipid bilayer incorporated in liposomes (or vesicles) and lamellar spheres. The surface interfacial energy method has been used to address the question of how surface energy and wettability of a weak polyelectrolyte phospholipid bilayer surface influence the low friction of biosurfaces, including natural systems like articular cartilage. The lower the wettability of a surface containing phospholipid bilayers, the lower its coefficient of friction. This is consistent with the results from the study on the acid/base equilibrium of a weak polyelectrolyte hyaluronate multilayer film/poly(L-lysine). Comparing the model of weak polyelectrolytes (non-amphoteric) adsorbed on solid surfaces with our (amphoteric compound) phospholipid bilayer, we have been able to show in a semi-quantitative manner the relationship between the coefficient of friction, interfacial energy and lubricant pH on the overall joint lubrication mechanism.

We have examined natural articular surfaces covered by phospholipid bilayers, and shown the relation between wettability (hydrophobicity) and friction coefficient. AFM

Published by Woodhead Publishing Limited, 2013

imaging and characterization of the surface of normal intact and delipidized articular cartilage specimens showed greatly accelerated damage to the articular cartilage following chemical rinsing. Tests were performed to measure the nanoscopic geometry (height) of SAL wettability of intact and delipidized biosurfaces of cartilage, and the coefficients of friction of contacting cartilage surfaces. We have also demonstrated that there is a link between the coefficient of friction and hydrophobicity (wettability) or interfacial energy of lubricated biotribopairs. It has also been demonstrated that the 'smart surface' of cartilage is highly hydrophilic when wet and hydrophobic when air-dry. The surface interfacial energy of the bilayer membrane or joint surfaces in acid/base equilibrium (pH) significantly influences the effectiveness of aqueous (biological) lubrication. We have shown that surface wettability can be varied by as much as around 40° in natural joints where the surface friction can be altered by a factor of 10. It can be argued from our results that the number of phospholipid bilayers controls the wettability and surface friction, which are fundamentally important factors for joint lubrication, lending credence to the assertion of previous studies that the key to understanding the mechanism of joint lubrication lies in getting an insight into the relationships between the structure and function of surface lipids. The lamellar-roller-bearing lubrication model has been developed to incorporate a bimodal mechanism: (i) lamellar frictionless bilayer movement and (ii) roller-bearing lubrication mode through structured synovial fluid, which occurs when lamellar spheres, liposomes and macromolecules act as a roller-bearing placed between two cartilage surfaces in biological lubrication. We conclude that an understanding of the acid/base rearrangement of phospholipid surface bilayers could provide an insight into the mechanisms underlying lubrication processes in mammalian joints.

Published by Woodhead Publishing Limited, 2013

6.7 Acknowledgements

This work was supported by the Tribochemistry Consulting grant, USA.

6.8 References

Adamson A W (1976), *Physical Chemistry of Surfaces*. New York: Interscience.

Afara I O, Pawlak Z and Oloyede A (2011), 'Current state of the application of infrared optical methods for assessing articular cartilage', *Journal of Materials Science and Engineering*, **1A**: 892–898.

Ballantine G C and Stachowiak G W (2002), 'The effects of lipid depletion on osteoarthritic wear', *Wear*, **253**: 385–393.

Bole G G Jr and Peltier D F (1962), 'Synovial fluid lipids in normal individuals and patients with rheumatoid arthritis', *Arthritis and Rheumatism*, **5**: 589–601.

Bongaerts J H H, Fourtouni K and Stokes J R (2007), 'Soft-tribology: lubrication in a compliant PDMS–PDMS contact', *Tribology International*, **40**: 1531–1542.

Bragg W L (1928), *An Introduction to Crystal Analysis*. London: G. Bell & Sons.

Briscoe W H, Titmuss S, Tiberg F, Thomas R K, McGillivray D J et al. (2006), 'Boundary lubrication under water', *Nature*, **444**: 191–194.

Burke S E and Barrett C J (2003a), 'pH-responsive properties of multilayered poly(L-lysine)/hyaluronic acid surfaces', *Biomacromolecules*, **4**: 1773–1783.

Burke S E and Barrett C J (2003b), 'Acid/base equilibria of weak polyelectrolytes in multilayer thin films', *Langmuir*, **19**: 3297–3303.

Published by Woodhead Publishing Limited, 2013

Chappuis J, Sherman I A and Neumann A W (1983), 'Surface tension of animal cartilage as it relates to friction in joints', *Annals of Biomedical Engineering*, **11**: 435–449.

Chen Y and Hills BA (2000), 'Surgical adhesions: evidence for adsorption of surfactant to peritoneal mesothelium', *Australian and New Zealand Journal of Surgery*, **70**: 443–447.

Chen Y L E, Gee M L, Helm C A, Israelachvili J N and McGuiggan P M (1989), 'Effects of humidity on the structure and adhesion of amphiphilic monolayers on mica', *Journal of Physical Chemistry*, **93**: 7057–7059.

Choo J H, Spikes H A, Ratoi M, Glovnea R and Forrest A (2007), 'Friction reduction in low-load hydrodynamic lubrication with a hydrophobic surface', *Tribology International*, **40**: 154–159.

Dela Volpe C, Siboni S and Morra M (2002), 'Comments on some recent papers on interfacial tension and contact angles', *Langmuir*, **18**: 1441–1444.

Dhathathreyan A and Maheshwari R (2002), 'Surface energy, wettability, and water vapor permeability of Langmuir–Blodgett films of protein–polymer composites', *Langmuir*, **18**: 10039–10041.

Dobbie J W, Pavlina T, Lloyd J and Johnson R C (1988), 'Phosphatidylcholine synthesis by peritoneal mesothelium: its implications for peritoneal dialysis', *American Journal of Kidney Diseases*, **12**: 31–36.

Forsey R W, Fisher J, Thompson J, Stone M H, Bell C et al. (2006), 'The effect of hyaluronic acid and phospholipid based lubricants on friction within a human cartilage damage model', *Biomaterials*, **27**: 4581–4590.

Fox M F, Pawlak Z and Picken D J (1991), 'Inverse micelles and solubilization of proton donors in hydrocarbon formulations', *Tribology International*, **24**: 341–349.

Published by Woodhead Publishing Limited, 2013

Gadomski A (2008), 'Simple example of structure versus property relationship applied to a reduced-friction biosystem, a quite personal opinion', *BioSystems*, **94**: 215–217.

Gadomski A, Pawlak Z and Oloyede A (2008a), 'Directed ion transport as virtual cause of some facilitated friction-lubrication mechanism prevailing in articular cartilage: a hypothesis', *Tribology Letters*, **30**: 83–90.

Gadomski A, Santamaria-Holek I, Kruszewska N, Uher J J, Pawlak Z et al. (2008b), 'Can modern statistical mechanics unravel some practical problems encountered in model biomatter aggregations emerging in internal- & external-friction conditions?', in: Kim B-S (ed.), *Statistical Mechanics Research*, pp. 13–98. New York: Nova Science.

Gale L R, Coller R, Hargreaves D J, Hills B A and Crawford R (2007), 'The role of SALP as a boundary lubricant in prosthetic joints', *Tribology International*, **40**: 601–606.

Graindorge S, Ferrandez W, Jin Z, Ingham E, Grant C et al. (2005), 'Biphasic surface amorphous layer lubrication of articular cartilage', *Medical Engineering and Physics*, **27**: 836–844.

Grant C, Twigg P, Egan A, Moody A, Smith A et al. (2006), 'Poly(vinyl alcohol) hydrogel as a biocompatible viscoelastic mimetic for articular cartilage', *Biotechnology Progress*, **22**: 1400–1406.

Greene G W, Banquy X, Lee D W, Lowrey D D, Yu J et al. (2011), 'Adaptive mechanically controlled lubrication mechanism found in articular joints', *Proceedings of the National Academy of Sciences of the United States of America*, **108**: 5255–5259.

Gudimetla P, Crawford R and Oloyede A (2007), 'The influence of lipid-extraction method on the stiffness of articular cartilage', *Clinical Biomechanics*, **22**: 924–931.

Guerra D, Frizziero L, Losi M, Bacchelli B, Mezzadri G et al. (1996), 'Ultrastructural identification of membrane-like structure on the surface of normal articular cartilage', *Journal of Submicroscopic Cytology and Pathology*, **28**: 385–393.

Gvozdanovic D, Wright V and Dowson D (1975), 'Formation of lubricating monolayers at the cartilage surface', *Annals of Rheumatic Diseases*, **34** (Suppl. 2): 100–101.

Higaki H, Murakami T, Nakanishi Y, Miura H, Mawatari T et al. (1998), 'The lubricating ability of biomembrane models with dipalmitoyl phosphatidylcholine and γ globulin', *Proceedings of the Institution of Mechanical Engineers, Part H: Journal of Engineering in Medicine*, **212**: 337–346.

Hills B A (1988), *The Biology of Surfactant*. London: Cambridge University Press.

Hills B A (1989), 'Oligolamellar lubrication of joints by surface active phospholipid', *Journal of Rheumatology*, **16**: 82–91.

Hills B A (1990), 'Oligolamellar nature of the articular surface', *Journal of Rheumatology*, **17**: 349–356.

Hills B A (1992), 'Graphite-like lubrication of mesothelium by oligolamellar pleural surfactant', *Journal of Applied Physiology*, **73**: 1034–1039.

Hills B A (1996a), 'Synovial surfactant and the hydrophobic articular surface', *Journal of Rheumatology*, **2**: 1323–1325.

Hills B A (1996b), 'Lubrication of visceral movement and gastric motility by peritoneal surfactant', *Journal of Gastroenterology and Hepatology*, **11**: 797–803.

Hills B A (2000), 'Boundary lubrication *in vivo*', *Proceedings of the Institution of Mechanical Engineers, Part H: Journal of Engineering in Medicine*, **214**: 83–94.

Hills B A (2002), 'Surface-active phospholipid: a Pandora's box of clinical applications. Part II. Barrier and lubricating properties', *Internal Medicine Journal*, **32**: 242–251.

Hills B A and Crawford R W (2003), 'Normal and prosthetic synovial joints are lubricated by surface-active phospholipid: a hypothesis', *Journal of Arthroplasty*, **18**: 499–505.

Hills B A and Monds M K (1998a), 'Deficiency of lubricating surfactants lining the articular surfaces of replaced hips and knees', *British Journal of Rheumatology*, **37**: 143–147.

Hills B A and Monds M K (1998b), 'Enzymatic identification of the load-bearing boundary lubrication in the joint', *British Journal of Rheumatology*, **37**: 137–142.

Hills B A and Thomas K (1998), 'Joint stiffness and "articular gelling": inhibition of the fusion of articular surfaces by surfactant', *British Journal of Rheumatology*, **37**: 532–538.

Hollinger S, Georges J-M, Mazuyer D, Lorentz G, Aguerre G et al. (2000), 'High-pressure lubrication with lamellar structures in aqueous lubricant', *Tribology Letters*, **9**: 143–151.

Horvai A (2011), 'Anatomy and histology of cartilage', in: Link T M (ed.), *Cartilage Imaging: Significance, Techniques, and New Developments*, pp. 1–10. New York: Springer.

Israelachvili J N (1986), 'Measurement of the viscosity of liquids in very thin films', *Journal of Colloid and Interface Science*, **110**: 263–271.

Jeleniewicz R, Majdan M, Zwolak R, Parada-Turska J, Dryglewska M et al. (2005), 'Synovial fluid surface tension inflammatory joint disease [Napiecie powierzchniowe płynu stawowego w zapalnych schorzeniach układu ruchu]', *Reumatologia*, **43**: 331–334 (in Polish).

Published by Woodhead Publishing Limited, 2013

Jensen M O and Mouritsen O G (2004), 'Lipids do influence protein function – the hydrophobic matching hypothesis revisited', *Biochimica et Biophysica Acta – Biomembranes*, **1666**: 205–226.

Jurvelin J S, Müller D J, Wong M, Studer D, Engel A et al. (1996), 'Surface and subsurface morphology of bovine humeral articular cartilage as assessed by atomic force and transmission electron microscopy', *Journal of Structural Biology*, **117**: 45–54.

Kitano T, Ateshian G A, Mow V C, Kadoya Y and Yamano Y (2001), 'Constituents and pH changes in protein rich hyaluronan solution affect the biotribological properties of artificial articular joints', *Journal of Biomechanics*, **34**: 1031–1037.

Klein J (2006), 'Molecular mechanisms of synovial joint lubrication', *Proceedings of the Institution of Mechanical Engineers, Part J: Journal of Engineering Tribology*, **220**: 691–710.

Kobayashi S, Yonekubo S and Kurogouchi Y (1995), 'Cryoscanning electron microscopic study of the surface amorphous layer of articular cartilage', *Journal of Anatomy*, **187**: 429–444.

Kumar P, Oka M, Toguchida J, Kobayashi M, Uchida E et al. (2001), 'Role of uppermost superficial surface layer of articular cartilage in the lubrication mechanism of joints', *Journal of Anatomy*, **199**: 241–250.

Leckband D, Chen Y-L, Israelachvili J, Wickman H H, Fletcher M et al. (1993), 'Measurements of conformational changes during adhesion of lipid and protein (polylysine and S-layer) surface', *Biotechnology and Bioengineering*, **42**: 167–177.

Lee S and Spencer N D (2005), 'Aqueous lubrication of polymers: Influence of surface modification', *Tribology International*, **38**: 922–930.

Published by Woodhead Publishing Limited, 2013

Linn F C and Sokoloff L (1965), 'Movement and composition of interstitial fluid of cartilage', *Arthritis and Rheumatism*, **8**: 481–494.

Little T, Freeman M A R and Swanson S A V (1969), 'Experiments on friction in the human hip joint', in: Wright V (ed.), *Lubrication and Wear in Joints: Proceedings of a Symposium*, pp. 110–116. London: Sector Publishing.

Marti A, Haehner G and Spencer N D (1995), 'Sensitivity of frictional forces to pH on a nanometer scale: a lateral force microscopy study', *Langmuir*, **11**: 4632–4635.

Mazzucco D, Scott R and Spector M (2004), 'Composition of joint fluid in patients undergoing total knee replacement and revision arthroplasty: correlation with flow properties', *Biomaterials*, **25**: 4433–4445.

Maroudas A, Bullough P, Swanson S A V and Freeman M A R (1968), 'The permeability of articular cartilage', *Journal of Bone and Joint Surgery, British*, **50B**: 166–177.

Murakami T, Higaki H, Sawae Y, Ohtsuki N, Moriyama S et al. (1998), 'Adaptive multimode lubrication in natural synovial joints and artificial joints', *Proceedings of the Institution of Mechanical Engineers, Part H: Journal of Engineering in Medicine*, **212**: 23–35.

Oloyede A and Broom N (1994), 'The generalized consolidation of articular cartilage: an investigation of its near-physiological response to static load', *Connective Tissue Research*, **31**: 75–86.

Oloyede A, Gudimetla P, Crawford R and Hills B A (2004a), 'Consolidation responses of delipidized articular cartilage', *Clinical Biomechanics*, **19**: 534–542.

Oloyede A, Gudimetla P, Crawford R and Hills B A (2004b), 'Biomechanical responses of normal and delipidized articular cartilage subjected to varying rates of loading', *Connective Tissue Research*, **45**: 86–93.

Ozturk H E, Stoffel K K, Jones C F and Stachowiak G W (2004), 'The effect of surface-active phospholipids on the lubrication of osteoarthritic sheep knee joints: friction', *Tribology Letters*, **16**: 283–289.

Pasquali-Ronchetti I, Quaglino D, Mori G, Bacchelli B and Ghosh P (1997), 'Hyaluronan–phospholipid interaction', *Journal of Structural Biology*, **120**: 1–10.

Pawlak Z (2003), *Tribochemistry of Lubricating Oils*. Amsterdam: Elsevier.

Pawlak Z and Oloyede A (2008), 'Conceptualisation of articular cartilage as a giant reverse micelle: A hypothetical mechanism for joint biocushioning and lubrication', *BioSystems*, **94**: 193–201.

Pawlak Z, Kotynska J, Figaszewski Z A, Gadomski A, Gudaniec A et al. (2008a), 'A biochemical model for characterizing the surface-active phospholipid bilayer of articular cartilage relative to acid/base equilibrium', *Archives of Materials Science and Engineering*, **29**: 24–29.

Pawlak Z, Crawford R W and Oloyede A (2008b), 'Hypothetical model of hydrophilic lubrication in synovial joints', *Australian Journal of Mechanical Engineering*, **6**: 21–27.

Pawlak Z, Pai R, Bayrakta E, Kaldonski T and Oloyede A (2008c) 'Lamellar lubrication *in vivo* and *vitro*: friction testing of hexagonal boron nitride', *BioSystems*, **94**: 202–208.

Pawlak Z, Figaszewski Z A, Gadomski A, Urbaniak W and Oloyede A (2010a), 'The ultra low friction of the articular surface is pH-dependent and is built on a hydrophobic underlay including a hypothesis on joint lubrication mechanism', *Tribology International*, **43**: 1719–1725.

Pawlak Z, Jurvelin J S and Urbaniak W (2010b), 'Biotribochemistry of the lubrication of natural joints', *Tribologia*, **5**: 131–141.

Published by Woodhead Publishing Limited, 2013

Pawlak Z, Urbaniak W and Oloyede A (2011), 'The relationship between friction and wettability in aqueous environment', *Wear*, **271**: 1745–1749.

Pawlak Z, Petelska A D, Urbaniak W, Yusuf K Q and Oloyede A (2012a), 'Relationship between wettability and lubrication characteristics of the surfaces of contacting phospholipids-based membranes', *Cell Biochemistry and Biophysics*, doi: 10.1007/s12013-012-9437-z.

Pawlak Z, Urbaniak W, Gadomski A, Yusuf K Q, Afara I O and Oloyede A (2012b), 'The role of lamellate phospholipid bilayers in lubrication of joints', *Acta of Bioengineering and Biomechanics*, **14**: in press.

Pesika N S, Zeng H, Kristiansen K, Zhao B, Tian Y et al. (2009), 'Gecko adhesion pad: a smart surface?', *Journal of Physics: Condensed Matter*, **21**: 464132.

Petelska A D, Naumowicz M and Figaszewski Z A (2006), 'Physicochemical insights into equilibria in bilayer lipid membranes', *Advances in Planar Lipid Bilayers and Liposomes*, **3**: 125–187.

Rabinowitz J L, Gregg J R and Nixon J E (1983), 'Lipid composition of the tissues of human knee joints. II. Synovial fluid in trauma', *Clinical Orthopaedics and Related Research*, **190**: 292–298.

Richter R P, Bérat R and Brisson A R (2006), 'Formation of solid-supported lipid bilayers: an integrated view', *Langmuir*, **22**: 3497–3505.

Ropes M W and Bauer W (1953), *Synovial Fluid Changes in Joint Disease*. Cambridge, MA: Harvard University Press.

Sader J E, Chon J W M and Mulvaney P (1999), 'Calibration of rectangular atomic force microscope cantilevers', *Review of Scientific Instruments*, **70**: 3967–3969.

Scherge M and Gorb S N (2001), *Biological Micro- and Nano-Tribology*. Berlin: Springer.

Schmidt T A and Sah R L (2007), 'Effect of synovial fluid on boundary lubrication of articular cartilage', *Osteoarthritis and Cartilage*, **15**: 35–47.

Schmidt T A, Gastelum N S, Nguyen Q T, Schumacher B L and Sah R L (2007), 'Boundary lubrication of articular cartilage: role of synovial fluid constituent', *Arthritis and Rheumatism*, **56**: 882–891.

Schwarz I M and Hills B A (1998), 'Surface-active phospholipids as the lubricating component of lubricin', *British Journal of Rheumatology*, **37**: 21–26.

Schwarz I M and Hills B A (1996), 'Synovial surfactant: lamellar bodies in type B synoviocytes and proteolipid in synovial fluid and the articular lining', *British Journal of Rheumatology*, **35**: 821–827.

Siegiel D P (1984), 'Inverted micellar structures in bilayer membranes. Formation rates and half-lives', *Biophysical J*, **45**: 399–420.

Singer S J (1971), 'The molecular organization of biological membranes', in: Rothfield L I (ed.), *Structure and Function of Biological Membranes*, pp. 145–222. New York: Academic Press.

Sivan S, Schroeder A, Verberne G, Merkher Y, Diminsky D et al. (2010), 'Liposomes act as effective biolubricants for friction reduction in human synovial joints', *Langmuir*, **26**: 1107–1116.

Stachowiak G W and Batchelor A (2005), 'Solid lubrication and surface treatment', in: *Engineering Tribology (Tribology Series 24)*, pp. 485–521. Amsterdam: Elsevier/ Butterworth-Heinemann.

Stratton C J (1984), 'Morphology of surfactant producing cells and of the alveolar lining', in: Robertson B, van Golde L M G and Batenburg J J (eds.), *Pulmonary Surfactant*, pp. 68–118. Amsterdam: Elsevier.

Published by Woodhead Publishing Limited, 2013

Swann D A, Hendren R B, Radin E L and Sotman S L (1981), 'The lubricating activity of synovial fluid glycoproteins', *Arthritis and Rheumatism*, **24**: 22–30.

Szymczyk K and Jańczuk B (2008), 'Wettability of a glass surface in the presence of two nonionic surfactant mixtures', *Langmuir*, **24**: 7755–7760.

Trunfio-Sfarghiu A-M, Berthier Y, Meurisse M-H and Rieu J-P (2007), 'Multiscale analysis of the tribological role of the molecular assemblies of synovial fluid. Case of a healthy joint and implants', *Tribology International*, **40**: 1500–1515.

Trunfio-Sfarghiu A-M, Berthier Y, Meurisse M-H and Rieu J-P (2008), 'Role of nanomechanical properties in the tribological performance of phospholipid biomimetic surfaces', *Langmuir*, **24**: 8765–8771.

van Oss C J, Gillman C F and Neumann A W (1975), *Phagocytic Engulfment and Cell Adhesiveness as Cellular Surface Phenomena*. New York: Marcel Dekker.

Vecchio P, Thomas R and Hills B A (1999), 'Surfactant treatment for osteoarthritis', *British Journal of Rheumatology*, **38**: 1020–1021.

Verberne G, Schroeder A, Halperin G, Barenholz Y and Etsion I (2010), 'Liposomes as potential biolubricant additives for wear reduction in human synovial joints', *Wear*, **268**: 1037–1042.

Wierzcholski K (2011) 'Topology of calculating pressure and friction coefficients for time-dependent human hip joint lubrication', *Acta of Bioengineering and Biomechanics*, **13**: 41–56.

Wright V and Dowson D (1976), 'Lubrication and cartilage', *Journal of Anatomy*, **121**: 107–118.

Yarimitsu S, Nakashima K, Sawae Y and Murakami T (2009), 'Influences of lubricant composition on forming

Published by Woodhead Publishing Limited, 2013

boundary film composed of synovia constituents', *Tribology International*, **42**: 1615–1623.

Young T (1805), 'An essay on the cohesion of fluid', *Philosophical Transactions of the Royal Society of London*, **95**: 65–87.

Yusuf K Q, Gudimetla P, Pawlak Z and Oloyede A (2011), 'Preliminary characterization of the surface of cartilage following exposure to saturated and unsaturated synthetic lipids' in: Cowled C J L (ed.), *Proceedings of the First International Postgraduate Conference on Engineering, Designing and Developing the Built Environment for Sustainable Wellbeing*, vol. 2, pp. 347–351. Brisbane: Queensland University of Technology.

Yusuf K Q, Motta N, Pawlak Z and Oloyade A (2012), 'A microanalytical study of the surfaces of normal, delipidized and artificially "resurfaced" articular cartilage', *Connective Tissue Research*, **53**: 236–245.

Published by Woodhead Publishing Limited, 2013

7

Importance of bearing porosity in engineering and natural lubrication

Zenon Pawlak, Tribochemistry Consulting, USA and University of Economy, Poland, Wieslaw Urbaniak, University of Economy and Kazimierz Wielki University, Poland, Tadeusz Kaldonski, Military University of Technology, Poland and Adekunle Oloyede, Queensland University of Technology, Australia

DOI: 10.1533/9780857092205.311

Abstract: The multilamellar structure of phospholipids, i.e. the surface amorphous layer (SAL) that covers the natural surface of articular cartilage, and hexagonal boron nitride (h-BN) on the surface of metal porous bearings are two prominent examples of the family of layered materials that possess the ability to deliver lamellar lubrication. This chapter presents the friction study that was conducted on the surfaces of cartilage and the metal porous bearing impregnated with oil (first generation) and with oil + h-BN (second generation). The porosity of cartilage is around 75% and those of metal porous bearings were 15–28 wt%.

Published by Woodhead Publishing Limited, 2013

It is concluded that porosity is a critical factor in facilitating the excellent tribological properties of both articular cartilage and the porous metal bearings studied.

Key words: hexagonal boron nitride, phospholipid, porous cartilage, metal bearing, lamellar lubrication, friction, load, carrying capacity, porosity, permeability.

7.1 Introduction

Articular cartilage is similar to porous metal bearings in tribological applications in respect of their mutual dependence on porosity during the performance of their primary function of lubrication. Contacting cartilage surfaces, being porous and deformable with micro- to nano-scale protection by the phospholipid bilayers, enable adequate contact and molecular attachment leading to frictionless lubrication under load. In this chapter, we investigate the mechanism underlying the performance of the multiphasic fluid-like lubricant consisting of water, macromolecules and phospholipids in providing almost frictionless lubrication in the manner normally associated with porous natural bearings (around 75% porosity) under sudden or gradually applied loads (Wright and Dowson, 1976). A water-based lubricant functions well with hydrophilic layers where the surface charge provides electrostatic double-layer repulsion, in addition to the steric repulsion of the hydration layer of water molecules (Urbakh et al., 2004).

The effective porosity of porous metal bearings lies between 20 and 30% of the total weight of the bearing material – the upper limit being imposed by strength considerations that vary inversely with porosity. The main limitation of porous material bearings is that they commonly

Published by Woodhead Publishing Limited, 2013

operate with only boundary or squeeze film bearings; squeeze film occurs when two lubricated surfaces approach each other at a normal velocity and the thin film of lubricant between the two surfaces acts as a cushion preventing the surfaces from making instantaneous contact (Kumar, 1980). Hydrophilic moieties of the phospholipids coat the natural surface where they are free to interact with water molecules and ions. In more complicated systems, multicomponent, complex vesicles may be formed of two or more amphiphiles combined with other chemical entities. The vesicles self-assemble spontaneously with extraordinary ease, where the fluidity and rapidity of the process purely depend upon physical forces.

Also, the components of lamellae are commonly arranged in geometrically regular bilayers. Translocations and restructuring are common, and the statistical physics of their fluctuating surfaces is a field at a fast-moving stage of development (McPherson, 2005).

The coefficient of friction of 0.005 found in normal mammalian joints often requires a natural lubrication regime, at physiological velocities, of two orders of magnitude lower than those of engineering lubrication (Figure 7.1). The cartilage matrix can act only as a solid lubricant surfactant with the support of vesicles, lamellar spheres and macromolecules – the main components of synovial fluid (Figure 7.2). Phospholipid molecules *in vivo*, and graphite, MoS_2, WS_2 and hexagonal boron nitride (h-BN) *in vitro*, are convenient examples of frictionless, nominally solid lubricants. Phospholipids and solid materials have the ability to form multibilayer or layered structures similar to those of lamellate solids. 'Lamella' is a term for a plate-like structure appearing in multiples; these occur in various situations in biology or artificial materials. These structures are composed of fine, thin alternating layers of usually different materials

Published by Woodhead Publishing Limited, 2013

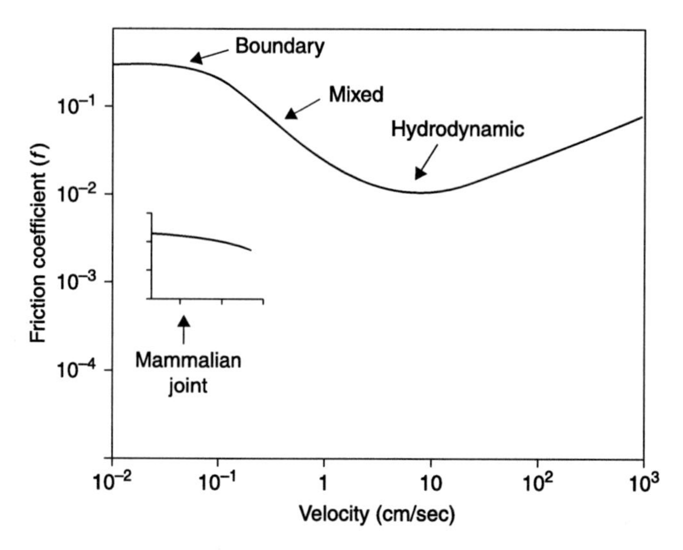

Figure 7.1 Coefficient of friction measured in the normal mammalian joint v. sliding velocities compared with the classical Stribeck engineering curve (upper).

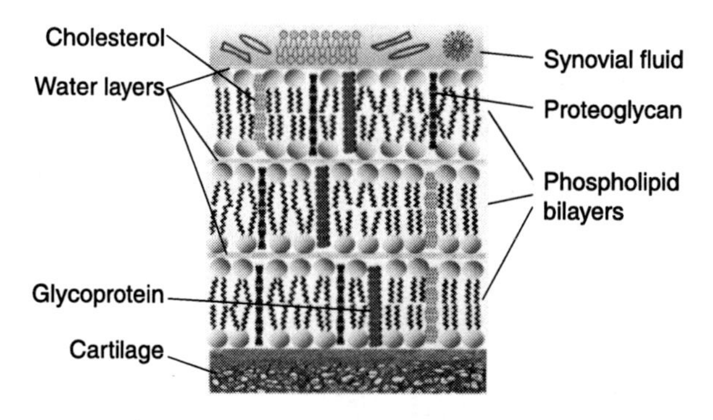

Figure 7.2 Schematic representation of a typical articular cartilage membrane showing the phospholipid SAL overlaying the articular surface. Structurally, the articular cartilage is overlaid by a thin coating of phospholipids. The three bilayers (size exaggerated) can act as a solid lubricant.

Published by Woodhead Publishing Limited, 2013

(Hills, 1989, 1992, 2002). It has been confirmed experimentally that phospholipids, as lamellar lubricants, protect the surface of joints against wear while acting as a frictionless lubricant. The ability of a solid to function as a lubricant is determined by the degree of attraction of its molecules to each other and the sliding surfaces. As a rule, solid lubricant films are superior to liquid films and provide a better surface coverage (Rabinowicz and Imai, 1995). In contacting cartilage surfaces the two multibilayers are against each other as opposing hydrophilic charged surfaces with the electric double-layers resulting in repulsive electrostatic forces, which in the presence of pressurized water and macromolecules, e.g., lubricin, are capable of lubricating with low friction forces (Figure 7.2) (Israelachvili and Wennerström, 1996).

Articular cartilage is a highly structured biological tissue and its fluid-saturated poro-elastic nature has been widely discussed. Research over the last decade has demonstrated the presence of a surface amorphous layer (SAL) overlaying the articular surface of the normal articular cartilage in the healthy joint, as illustrated in Figure 7.2 (Jurvelin et al., 1996; Kobayashi et al., 1996; Graindorge et al., 2005). The SAL has variously been claimed to comprise glycoproteins, glycosaminoglycans, proteoglycans, hyaluronic acid and phospholipids (Hills, 1989; Guerra et al., 1996). The tendency of phospholipids to form multilamellar structures, i.e. the multibilayer membrane on articular surfaces, is an important factor in enabling frictionless work under load (Hills, 1989). The articular surface is consistent with f = 0.005 that characterizes 'lamellated solid lubrication' such as that found in graphite, MoS_2, h-BN and WS_2 (Erdemir et al., 1991; Martin et al., 1992; Deacon and Goodman, 1958; Rapoport et al., 2002; Ladavière et al., 2003; Pawlak et al., 2008).

Published by Woodhead Publishing Limited, 2013

A lamellar solid material, h-BN, has a layered structure in which the bonds between the layers are much weaker than the interlayer bonding. The individual plate-like crystallites, consisting of several thousands of atomic layers, align themselves parallel to the direction of relative motion and slide over one another. Recent experiments with porous bearings, in which h-BN was used as an additive, have demonstrated this very low friction coefficient, low wear rate mechanism (Pawlak et al., 2007). It is well-known that h-BN is a softer phase bonded through localized graphite-like sp^2 hybridization in the hexagonal plane and delocalized weak π orbitals (Mosuang and Lowther, 2002). The structure of h-BN is constructed from layers consisting of a flat or nearly flat network of B_3N_3 hexagons with the layers stacked one over the other along the (001) direction.

Interest in nano- and microparticle lubricants and their applications has grown rapidly during the past decade (Gunsel and Friberg, 1992). Novel lubricants and additives containing boron compounds have received extensive attention in recent years (Bhushan and Gupta, 1991; Westergård et al., 1998; Pawlak, 2003). Boron additives have several useful characteristics, such as wear resistance, friction-reducing ability, oxidation inhibition, compatibility with mating pairs and producing negligible quantities of harmful elements to catalytic converters (Culley et al., 1996; Perry and Tysoe, 2005). The borate molecules are broken down during the rubbing process, resulting in the formation of h-BN (190.3 eV) (Junbin, 1997). The layered structures of boric acid with a particle size ranging from 0.2 to 40 μm can easily slide over one another to ensure low friction. It has been reported that the addition of 10 wt% of boric acid to mineral oils (wear test 52100 steel/alumina) can reduce the friction coefficient from 0.16 to 0.03 and wear rate from 1.1×10^{-4} to 2.0×10^{-6} mm^3/m (Erdemir, 1995; Ladavière et al., 2003).

Published by Woodhead Publishing Limited, 2013

Self-lubricating porous sliding (or plain) bearings have commonly been used over a long period of time (Neale, 1973; Yoshimoto et al., 2003; Pawlak et al., 2008). The reason for their selection is that there is no need for an external supply of lubricant, low operating cost and the capacity to operate effectively in applications where contamination from oil leakage is undesirable, e.g. in the textile and food industries. Other applications include water pump bearings and domestic applications, e.g. in washing machines, vacuum cleaners, lawn mowers and electronic equipment (Neale, 1973; Elsharkawy and Guedouar, 2001; Lawrowski, 2006). Due to the presence of capillary channels, the structure of porous bearings resembles that of a metal sponge. The porous structure is obtained by pressing-in appropriate powder followed by sintering the mold at an appropriate temperature. Considering the strength of the material and active pores, the optimal porosity range is 20–30% of the weight of such bearings. The porous self-lubricated bearing becomes saturated with oil either during the impregnation procedure in hot oil or under vacuum (Neale, 1973; Lawrowski, 2006). The mechanism of outflow of the oil from the porous wall is principally based on the difference between the thermal expansion of the oil and that of the metallic sleeve (Gururajan and Prakash, 2003). At the beginning of the lubrication process, elastic deformation of the material takes place under the pressure of the tube neck resulting in squeezing the oil from the pores (so-called first-generation bearings) (Neale, 1973; Stachowiak and Batchelor, 2005; Saha and Majumdar, 2002). Further progress in improving performance of the porous bearing would be selection of a formulation (oil + solid additive) with a variety of additives, e.g. h-BN or WS_2, to suppress friction and increase the load-carrying capacity (LCC), especially at low speeds (so-called second-generation bearings) (Kaldonski, 1997; Rapoport et al., 2002; Nikas and Sayles, 2008).

Published by Woodhead Publishing Limited, 2013

Porous bearings, in which pores are impregnated with oil or oil + nanoparticle additives, e.g. h-BN, MoS_2 and WS_2, are used in industrial applications (Rapoport et al., 2002; Erdemir, 2005). Oil-impregnated porous bearings operate under hydrodynamic conditions in the initial stages when the pores are full of lubricant. The bearings operate under boundary lubrication conditions during starting and stopping, and when the lubricant in the pores has been exhausted or the bearing is in the transition to seizure. In the case of seizure, severe plastic deformation of the metal surface takes place.

In practice, porous bearings work without any such additional oil supply. However, a substantial increase in coefficient of friction was noted when the oil content was reduced to about 50% of the original oil content (Raman and Vinod-Babu, 1984; Pawlak et al., 2009). Experiments conducted under high speed (around 69 000 r.p.m.) and light load conditions showed that porous bearings could work under hydrodynamic conditions even under these speeds (Quan et al., 1985). Recent experiments, in which h-BN was used as an oil additive, showed these h-BN nanoparticles exhibit a very low friction coefficient and slow wear rate (Pawlak et al., 2007a,b). In some conditions, we can expect the transition to seizure of operated bearings. The seizure process usually occurs when the contact surface is deprived of lubricants, with plastic deformation of the metal and increased friction coefficient and temperature. h-BN differs from the graphite type. It is white in color and is an insulating material, while graphite is black and an electrical conductor (Moauang and Lowther, 2002). These are two prominent members of the family of layered materials possessing a hexagonal lattice structure (Hod, 2012).

Porous media are typically characterized by two physical quantities: porosity and permeability. Porosity (ϕ), or void

Published by Woodhead Publishing Limited, 2013

fraction, is a measure of the void (i.e. 'empty') spaces in a material and is the fraction of the volume of voids V_V over the total volume V_T of material, $\phi = V_V/V_T$. Permeability is a measure of the ease with which a fluid filtrates through a solid. Permeability is part of the proportionality constant in Darcy's law, which relates discharge (flow rate) and the fluid's physical properties (e.g. viscosity) to a pressure gradient applied to the porous medium. The permeability of articular cartilage depends on the packing density of the proteoglycans, and the volumetric fraction and orientation of the collagen fiber. The current model (Federico and Herzog, 2008) of articular cartilage and experimental results (Maroudas and Bullough, 1968; Oloyede and Broom, 1994) explaining the increase in permeability from the deep to the middle zone 0.13 to 0.39×10^{-3} mm^4/Ns, and the decrease to 0.28×10^{-3} mm^4/Ns in the superficial zone, demonstrate this characteristic of the tissue.

Under compression, the volume of cartilage is decreased while its intramatrix pressure is increased. The tissue's permeability varies non-linearly, decreasing with increasing deformation/time, in a pattern that is greater in the radial (parallel to the horizontal plane) than the axial (perpendicular) direction. Under compression, porosity is reduced and the density of the negative charge contribution is increased due to the increased concentration of proteoglycans. Both the decreased porosity and the increase in the negative charge density make it harder for water to exit the cartilage matrix, leading to an increase in its stiffness or load-bearing capacity (Mirzayan, 2006).

The primary purpose of our studies was to evaluate the second-generation porous bearings impregnated with the two-phase fluid (oil + h-BN) and compare the results relative to lamellar lubrication and porosity to articular cartilage, a natural bearing surface and a well-known porous bearing

Published by Woodhead Publishing Limited, 2013

saturated with oil + h-BN. The h-BN additive has been found to contribute to the reduction of the friction coefficient and to increase the LCC, which can prevent early transition to seizure. Specifically, we examined the influence of the h-BN additive under sliding conditions on friction, bearing temperature and transition to seizure under different velocities and loadings. A recent fundamental study explores the possibility of increasing the LCC of porous bearings by external delivery of two-phase fluid into porous bearings.

7.2 Experimental

7.2.1 Experimental conditions, apparatus and procedure

BN was prepared in the laboratory; the process for synthesizing h-BN as an oil additive was previously described by Kaldonski (2006). The porous material was impregnated under vacuum with a well-mixed suspension of the oil with h-BN additive. The characteristics of the porous bushes and bearings used are collected in Table 7.1.

The porous bushes of composition indicated in Table 7.1 were compressed and sintered below the melting point of

Table 7.1 Characteristics of the porous bushes

Description	Values
Porous material (iron + copper powder)	97.5 + 2.5 (wt%)
Bush sizes (mm)	25/36 (diameter) × 20; 6/7.5 (diameter) × 8
Mean density (g/cm^3)	5.62–5.68
Open porosity (%)	15.5, 22.0, 27.8
Mean mass content of oil (wt%)	3.2–3.5
Permeability coefficient, k (m^2)	5.0–6.5 × 10^{-14}

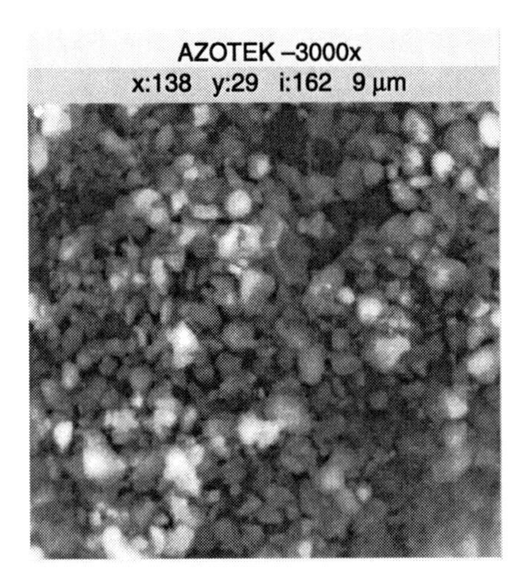

Figure 7.3 Scanning electron micrograph of boron nitride (×3000). The particle diameter of the boron nitride was less than 2 μm (1 cm bar = 9.0 μm).

Source: Kaldonski (2006).

copper. Their density was 5.6 g/cm^3. Particles of h-BN with a size ranging between 0.5 and 2.0 μm in diameter (Figure 7.3) were added as an additive to naphthenic mineral oil (Table 7.2). For the experiments, the bushes were run at sliding velocities of 1.0, 1.5 and 2.0 m/s, and impregnated with:

- Oil only and the two-phase fluid: 0.5 and 2.0 wt% h-BN.
- Oil only and the two-phase fluid: 0.2, 0.5, 1.0 and 2.0 wt% h-BN. Additionally, the oil only and the two-phase

Table 7.2 Physical properties of transformer oil, naphthenic oil and Vaseline

Parameter	Transformer oil	Naphthenic oil	Vaseline
Density (g/cm^3 at 15 °C)	0.888	0.870 (20 °C)	0.877
Viscosity (cSt at 40 °C)	9.6	11.65	Melting point at 36 °C
Viscosity (cSt at 100 °C)	2.3	NA	NA

Published by Woodhead Publishing Limited, 2013

fluid were externally delivered to the bushes at a rate of 1.9–2.5 cm^3/min.

Friction tests were carried out on a tribotester that was purpose-built at the Warsaw University of Technology, Warsaw, Poland (Krzeminski, 2002). The characteristics of the porous bush were determined with the test apparatus (Figure 7.4).

The dimensions of the porous bushes were 6/7.5 (diameter) × 8 and 6/9 (diameter) × 6 mm, and an NC6 grade steel with a hardness of 62 HRC and diameter 24.95 mm. The friction experiments were performed by subjecting the bearings to loads of 0.5–2.5 MPa at sliding velocities of 1 and 2 m/s. The load was increased by steps of 50–200 N to avoid seizure. The temperature of the block was measured by a resistor placed at a distance of 0.5 mm from the bearing surface.

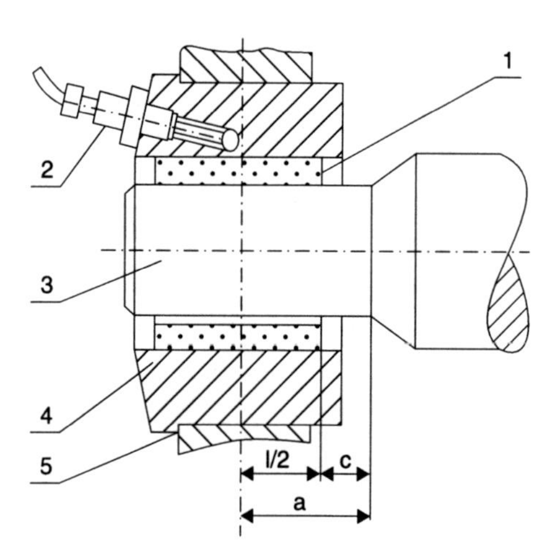

Figure 7.4 Schematic diagram of the test apparatus showing the locations of its key components: porous bush (1), thermocouple (2), steel journal (3), clamping (4) and rolling bearing (5).

Source: Kaldonski (2006).

Published by Woodhead Publishing Limited, 2013

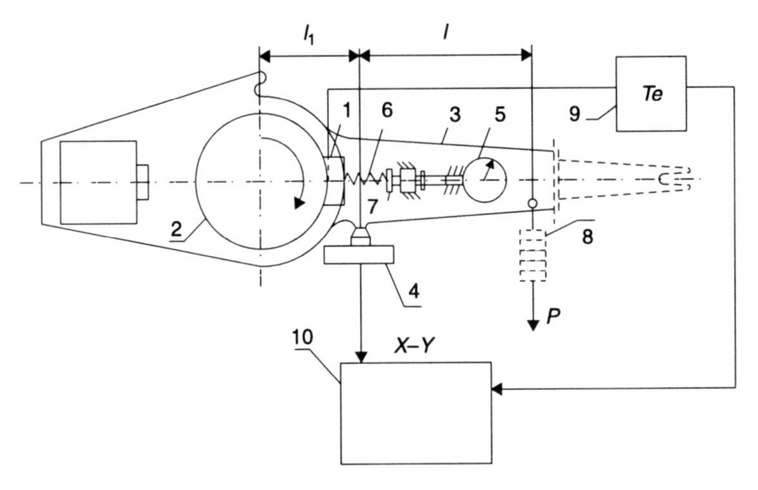

Figure 7.5 Tribotester KEWAT-6 for assessment of friction coefficient: sample (1), antisample (2), rocking lever (3), dynamometer indicator (4), dial indicator (5), set spring (6), adjustment screw (7), weight bobs (8), temperature gauge (9) and *x–y* recorder (10)

Friction tests were carried out on a KEWAT-6 tribotester (made at the Military University of Technology, Warsaw, Poland) (Figure 7.5). A porous bearings test was used to measure the characteristics, e.g. impregnation, friction coefficient and transition time to seizure.

7.3 Results and discussion

7.3.1 Two generations of porous bearings: load, temperature and seizure characteristics

The effect of the load (1.1, 1.35 and 1.60 MPa) on the transition time to seizure and temperature characteristics of porous bearings is shown in Figure 7.6. The curves are

Published by Woodhead Publishing Limited, 2013

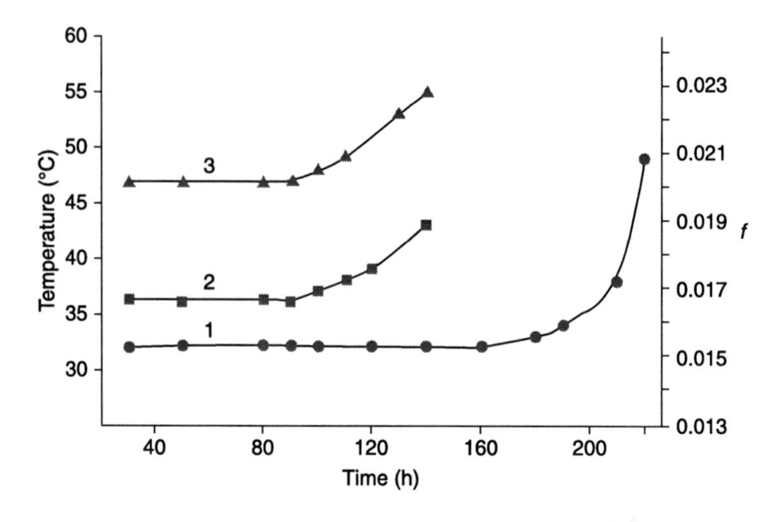

Figure 7.6 Effect of load (MPa), 1.2 (curve 1), 1.35 (curve 2) and 1.60 (curve 3), on transition time to seizure and temperature characteristics of porous bushes (6/7.5 (diameter) × 8 mm) impregnated by transformer oil + 2% h-BN. Mean open porosity 22%. Velocity V = 2.5 m/s.

Source: Kaldonski (2006).

typical for all the impregnated porous bushes. The tribotest results of the three porous bushes of 6/7.5 × 8 mm with transformer oil + 2% h-BN for velocity V = 2.5m/s are shown with a transition time to seizure of 181, 89 and 97 min.

It has been noticed that the transition to seizure occurs when the wear debris accumulates in the pores on the surface of the bushes. The temperature of the rolling bearing was measured by a thermocouple, which was placed at a distance of 0.5 mm from the contact surface of the porous bush. The temperature and the friction coefficient increased significantly, indicating transition to seizure of the mating metal pair (Figure 7.6).

The effect of the load on the temperature characteristics of porous bushes impregnated with transformer oil + 2% h-BN (the six porous bushes) is shown in Figure 7.7. It was found

Published by Woodhead Publishing Limited, 2013

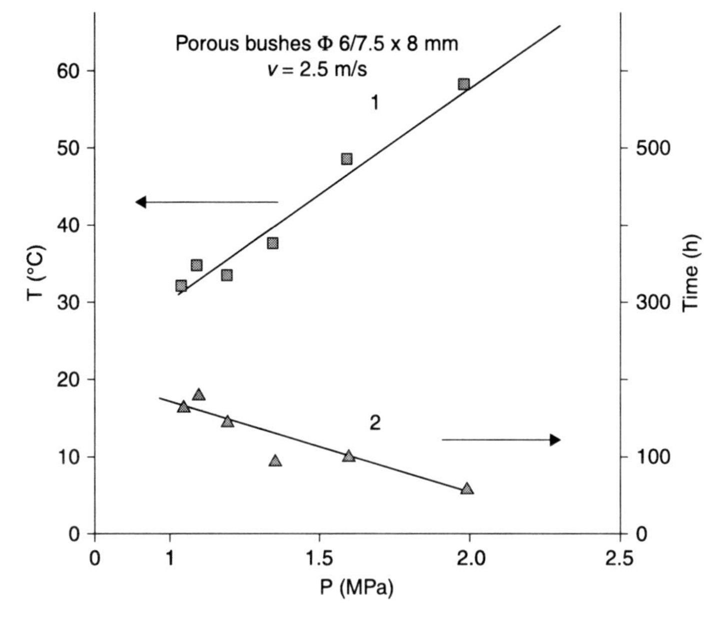

Figure 7.7 Effect of load on the seizure time (curve 2) and the temperature characteristics (curve 1) for porous bushes impregnated by transformer oil + 2% h-BN. Porosity 22%.

that under the load of 1.05 and 2.0 MPa the temperature increased from 21 to 31 and 47°C, respectively. Porous bushes impregnated with Mobil DTE-BB oil without h-BN exhibited transition to seizure at a temperature higher (32°C) than that of the porous bushes impregnated with transformer oil + 2% h-BN, statistically higher by a factor of around 1.5 (Pawlak et al., 2009).

The conditions adopted in the test were as follows: the porous bushes were impregnated with oil without h-BN nanoparticles and repeated runs were carried out for each test. Each porous bush was under different load, with a constant velocity of 2.5 m/s, and the oil content of impregnated oil was measured after a seizure. Obviously, such an effect can be attributed to addition of the h-BN to

Published by Woodhead Publishing Limited, 2013

the lubricating oil. This test demonstrates that h-BN is as effective as porous bearings in reducing friction during lubrication.

Figure 7.7 shows the effect of load on the transition time to seizure for porous bearings, with bushes impregnated with transformer oil + 2% h-BN. It was found that under a load range of 1.05–2.0 MPa the porous bearings impregnated with Mobil DTE-BB lubricant exhibited a much longer transition time to seizure than those impregnated with transformer oil + h-BN, statistically longer by a factor of around 2.4 (Pawlak et al., 2009).

The impregnation of Fe–Cu porous bushes with h-BN lubricant leads to improvement in some properties, such as a very low friction coefficient and lower temperature during operation, but the transition time to seizure is shorter than that of Mobil DTE-BB professional lubricant. The effect of the *PV* (pressure–velocity) parameter on the transition time to seizure for porous bearings made of bronze–graphite, iron–graphite and iron–nickel–graphite impregnated with WS_2 + oil results in a very efficient lubrication ($f \sim 0.06$) under a much higher parameter ($PV = 84$ MPa.m/s) conditions the transition to seizure (Raman and Vinod-Babu, 1984; Rapoport et al., 2001, 2002). In our studies, porous bearings impregnated with h-BN microparticles also provide efficient lubrication with a friction coefficient less than $f \sim 0.03$ and $PV \sim 6$ MPam/s (Pawlak et al., 2009). The friction coefficient reported by Lelonis et al. (2003) of solid lubricant powders is 0.17 for h-BN, while for comparison that for graphite is 0.28, for Teflon is 0.60 and for MoS_2 is 0.73.

Very recent studies have shown that h-BN coatings can impart tribologically higher wear than graphite, while a comparable friction coefficient was measured for both. The effects of graphite and h-BN on the tribological properties of Cu-based composites were investigated by Chen et al. (2008).

Published by Woodhead Publishing Limited, 2013

The wear rate of Cu-based composites containing 10% h-BN is three times higher than that of Cu-based composites containing 10 wt% graphite, while the friction coefficients are similar. The interplanar spacing of h-BN is smaller than that of graphite, e.g., the distances between the adjacent interlayers of h-BN and graphite are 3.33 and 3.35 Å, respectively (Pease, 1952; Klein et al., 1993). Due to the weaker interlayer bonding of graphite (0.02 Å), it can more easily shear along the basal plane of the crystalline structures as compared with h-BN, which may result in the better performance of graphite.

Figure 7.8 shows the results for impregnation with naphthenic oil and the two-phase fluid for sintered porous Fe–Cu bearings under sliding speeds of 2 m/s and the load ranging from 0.4 to 1.25 MPa during 10 h. Impregnation of the h-BN micro-particles into the pores improved friction coefficient and LCC. A low friction coefficient and surface

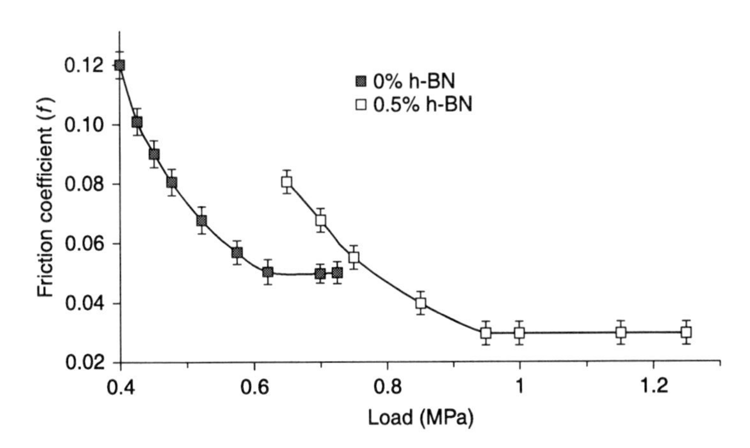

Figure 7.8 Coefficient of friction (*f*) v. load for porous sliding bearings impregnated with naphthenic oil only (curve 1) and oil + 0.5% h-BN fluid (curve 2). The velocity was 2 m/s during a 10-h run. Porosity 25%.

temperature (around 60 °C) were noticed over 6 h and under the LCC exceeding the pressure of 1 MPa.

The results have shown that the porous bearings impregnated with the diphase fluid had the friction coefficient reduced by a factor of 2 (Figure 7.8). The author's earlier studies showed (Pawlak et al., 2009) that a small amount of h-BN is required to substantially decrease the coefficient of friction of the porous bearings.

7.3.2 Advantages of the diphase fluid as a lamellar lubricant

The second part of our tests was run with bushes impregnated with the naphthenic oil and with the diphase fluid, and additionally lubricated with the naphthenic oil and the diphase fluid supplied externally, at a velocity of 1.0 m/s. The h-BN concentration in the fluid was 0.0 and 0.5 wt%, as shown in Figure 7.9.

Typical experimental data are shown in Figure 7.9: the measured coefficient of friction and temperature under increasing load for bushes impregnated with oil and with the diphase fluid. It was found that over the load range of 0.5–1.25 MPa, for bushes impregnated with oil, the friction coefficient decreased from 0.12 to 0.06 (mean SD ± 5%) and the temperature increased from 21 to 43 °C during the 140-min run. The results for porous bushes impregnated and externally lubricated with the oil + 0.5% h-BN fluid over the load range of 0.8–2.5 MPa were as follows: the friction coefficient was below 0.02 (mean SD ± 5%) and the temperature increased from 20 to 42 °C during a 140-min run. The experiment revealed the effective lubrication of the porous bearing with the diphase fluid as demonstrated by reducing the friction coefficient by a factor of 3.

Published by Woodhead Publishing Limited, 2013

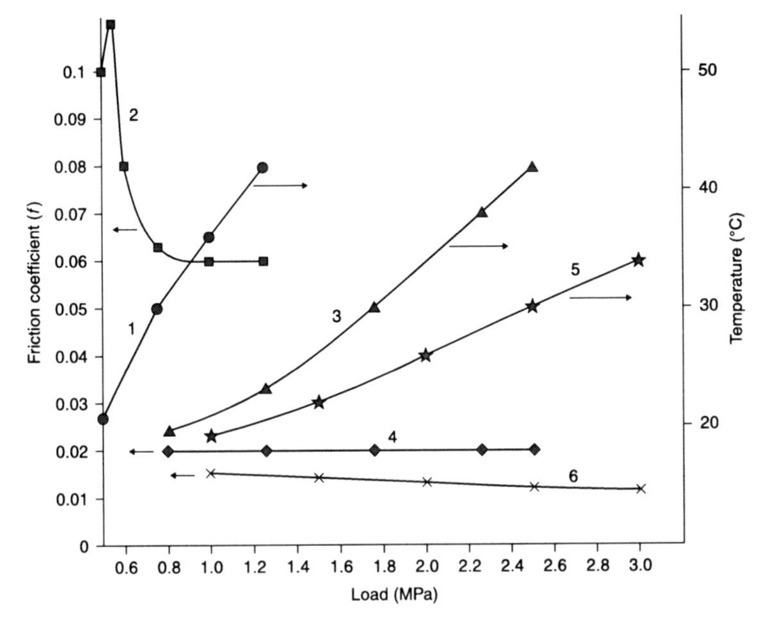

Figure 7.9 Coefficient of friction and temperature under increasing load for impregnated porous bushes and externally lubricated with oil (curves 1 and 2), oil + 0.5% h-BN (curves 3 and 4) and oil + 2.0% h-BN (curves 5 and 6) during 140-min test. Velocity $V = 1$ m/s.

The effect of the h-BN concentration on the LCC is presented in Figure 7.10. The LCC is expressed by a ratio of maximum load with 0.25, 0.50, 1.0 and 2.0% h-BN/ maximum load with 0% h-BN for two sets of bushes run at a velocity of 1 and 2 m/s. It was found that at the velocity of 1 m/s and 0.5% h-BN concentration the LCC increased about twice as compared with that of ordinary porous bearings lubricated with oil only. The lower curve representing the higher velocity shows a lesser effect. This may be due to shifting of the particulate phase and upsetting the even distribution on the bearing surface. The test results showed that the LCC was enhanced with increasing concentration of

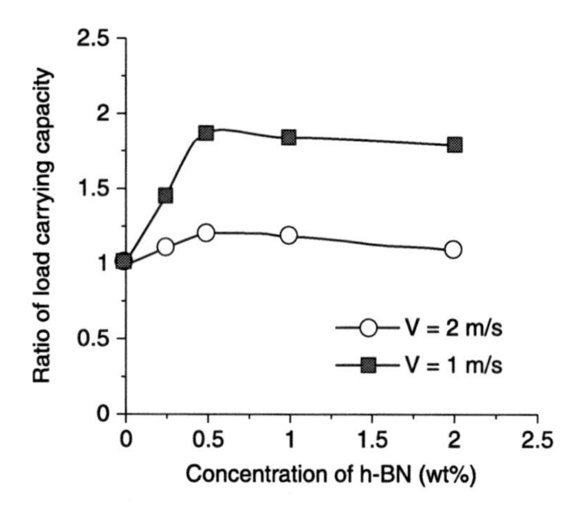

Figure 7.10 **Ratio of LCC v. h-BN wt% for porous sliding bearings at a velocity of 1 and 2 m/s lubricated with external supply of the biphase fluid (oil + h-BN). Porosity 25%.**

Source: Kaldonski (2006).

the additive up to 0.5% h-BN, and the velocity was set to around 1 and 2 m/s.

Figure 7.11 shows the variation of the mean LCC with bearing velocity for bushes impregnated with oil and the diphase fluid, compared with that of the bearings lubricated by external supply of the two fluids to the bushes.

It can be seen that, for a given increase in velocity, LCC increases for bushes lubricated with oil (Figure 7.11a) and LCC decreases for those lubricated with the diphase fluid (Figure 7.11b), indicating some differences in the mechanism of bearings impregnated with the two lubricants. In addition, it can be noticed that the bushes lubricated by external supply of the fluids have almost twice as high LCC as compared with those lubricated only by impregnation.

The lubrication of the porous bearings impregnated with oil hinges on the principle that oil is squeezed out of the

Published by Woodhead Publishing Limited, 2013

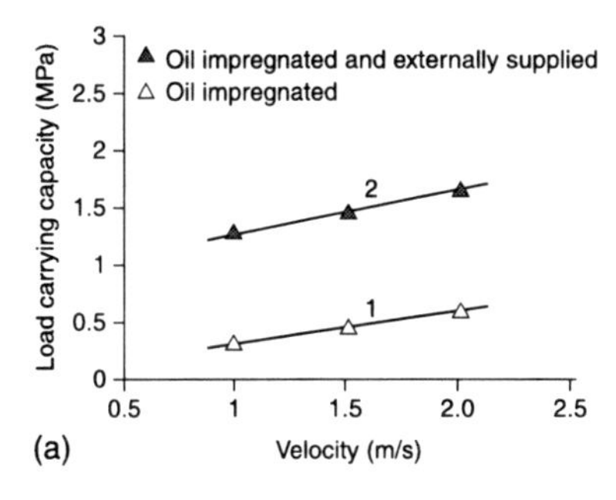

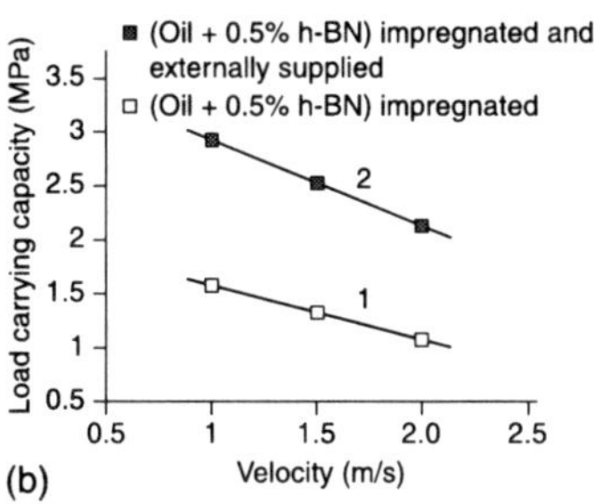

Figure 7.11 **Effect of velocity on the LCC of porous bushes impregnated with (a) naphthenic oil and (b) diphase fluid (oil + 0.5% h-BN). Curves (1) impregnated bushes and curves (2) impregnated and additionally lubricated by externally supplied oil and the oil + 0.5% h-BN fluid during the test. Porosity 25%.**

unloaded part of the bearing by suction before being partially returned to the bearing in the loaded area by the developed hydrodynamic pressure (Stachowiak and Batchelor, 2005). The mechanism of the outflow of oil from the porous wall is mainly based on the difference of thermal expansion of the oil and the metal skeleton sleeve. At the beginning of the movement, it could also be argued that the tube neck plays a role in elastic deformation of material under pressure, resulting in squeezing oil out of the pores (Lawrowski, 2006).

The LCC v. velocity of the bushes impregnated with the diphase fluid (Figure 7.11b) and those impregnated with oil showed a reverse trend. The particulate (h-BN) phase added to lubricant, as explained above, acts as a one-way valve on the pores, blocking and unblocking them. The LCC can be doubled as a result of the innovative lubrication with the diphase fluid. External supply of the fluid increased the LCC through delivering an additional amount of the lubricant, additionally intensifying about twice the cooling process (Figure 7.9). Figure 7.11 shows a bearing impregnated with the diphase fluid that has a three times higher LCC as compared with that of the oil-impregnated one, and the critical load for transition to seizure would be substantially higher. The concept to improve LCC by using diphase fluids works well when the concentration of the particulate phase is around 0.5% h-BN and the velocity about 1 m/s (Figure 7.10).

To enhance the lubrication of porous bearings, the introduced mechanism involving the diphase fluid showed an advantage over that of self-lubricating porous bearings impregnated with oil. The h-BN lamella (platelet)-forming particles have a thickness comparable to the film thickness and diameter larger than the average pore size of the porous material. A possible lubrication mechanism with polymer particles (platelets) + oil for a tailor-made test rig for a marine engine was examined experimentally and the concept was proven theoretically (Nikas and Sayles, 2008). The intention was to enhance lubrication of big-end bearings typically found in marine engines and other applications such as constant velocity ball joints.

The concept of enhancing lubrication under certain conditions by utilizing lamellar crystallites is examined in this study. The h-BN particles dispersed in oil and acting as one-way valves in porous media during the loading and unloading cycles are involved in the mechanism of lubrication on porous sliding surfaces. When the load is decreased, the lamellae obstruct oil flow into the pores of the porous bearing surfaces owing to hydrodynamic suction. The lamellae acting as one-way valves would prevent oil seeping back into the reservoir when the pressure on the outer bearing is increased. When the load is increased, the pores are uncovered and oil stored in the pores is released due to the positive pressure of the oil stored in the bearing material (Nikas and Sayles, 2008). The additional oil released from the pores could also be transferred by adhesion to other contacts. The proposed lubrication mechanism in our experiment was examined under different operating conditions: loads (0.5–2.50 MPa), velocities (1 and 2 m/s) and increasing concentration (h-BN wt%: 0.25, 0.5, 1.0 and 2.0) of the solid lubricant (Figure 7.6).

The studies have shown that the diphase fluid can be beneficial to lubrication, especially for porous bearing materials as a very effective hydrodynamic lubricant under load (Figures 7.7 and 7.8). These results indicate that h-BN could facilitate deposition of the plate-like crystallites. We therefore claim that adapting this knowledge for machine operation would lead to a significant reduction in maintenance cost and extend the lifespan of machine parts, leading to substantial economic gain for industry. The LCC of lubricated sliding surfaces is determined mainly by the lubrication conditions, including the properties of the lubricant, the nature of rubbing elements and the operating conditions. Their properties and the concentration of h-BN determine the LCC of porous sliding bearings. The formation of surface layers of the lamellar particles of h-BN, graphite and MoS_2 on metal surfaces gives rise to plate-like crystallites.

7.3.3 Porosity of natural and engineering bearings in lamellar lubrication

In 1989, Hills discovered the lubricating capabilities of phospholipids in synovial fluid and on the articular cartilage surface, which is rendered particularly hydrophobic by its adsorption (Hills, 1989). This hydrophobicity is attributed to phospholipids adsorbed to the underlying proteoglycan matrix in articular cartilage, which is otherwise hydrophilic. Hydrophobicity can be determined in terms of the contact angle, where a large value indicates strong adsorption (normal human articular cartilage value of over 90° and less than half this value for osteoarthritic cartilage).

Published by Woodhead Publishing Limited, 2013

The effect of the porosity of bearings on the friction coefficient for Vaseline + 5% h-BN samples is shown in Figure 7.12. It was found that journal bearings with low porosity (15.5 wt%) and impregnated with h-BN + Vaseline have much higher friction coefficient (Figure 7.12) than samples with 22 and 27.8 wt% porosity. Also, the friction and temperature increase abruptly, leading finally to seizure. It was established that impregnation of Vaseline + h-BN macroparticles porous non-full journal bearings with 27.8 wt% porosity by provides very efficient lubrication at temperatures over 100 °C. The experimental results clearly show that decreasing the porosity of engineering bearings from 28% to 15% increases both friction and temperature.

The friction coefficients of Vaseline + 5% h-BN compared with the graphite grease and cartilage–cartilage tribopair are shown in Figure 7.13. It can be seen that h-BN with Vaseline

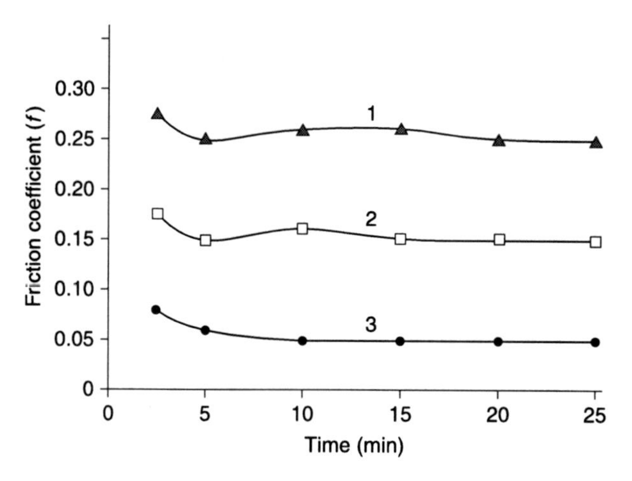

Figure 7.12 Effect of porosity on the friction coefficient of the porous sliding bearings impregnated by Vaseline + 5% h-BN during a 25-min test, load = 0.64 MPa, velocity V = 6.0 m/s, porosity 15.5% (curve 1), 22% (curve 2) and 27.8% (curve 3).

Published by Woodhead Publishing Limited, 2013

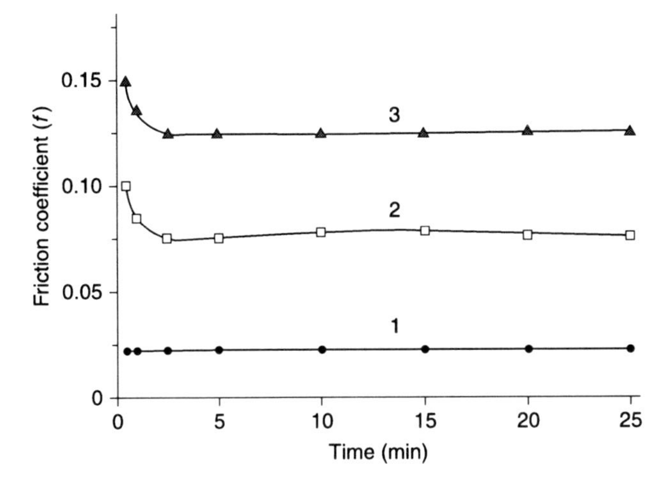

Figure 7.13 Friction coefficient as a function of time for impregnated porous journal bearings of the Vaseline + 5% h-BN (curve 2) and graphite grease (curve 3) during 25-min friction time, load = 0.64 MPa, velocity V = 6.0 m/s, bearing porosity 27.8%, compared with cartilage–cartilage pair from bovine knee (porosity around 75%) measured in saline solution (curve 1).

gives a lower friction coefficient relative to the graphite grease additives. The ability of hydrophobic articular cartilage to strongly adsorb phospholipids until it has built up multiple layers was discovered (Hills, 1989) and is represented as shown in Figure 7.14.

The bilayers of the lamellar phase can extend over large distances (commonly of the order of micrometers or more), and have properties of being strong under load and able to slide over each other as a lubricant (Fuller et al., 1995).

The formation of the lamellar solid of h-BN (Figure 7.15) gives rise to plate-like crystallites that lie flat with relatively low surface energy. The low adhesion between the crystallites allows them to become oriented in their most favorable

Published by Woodhead Publishing Limited, 2013

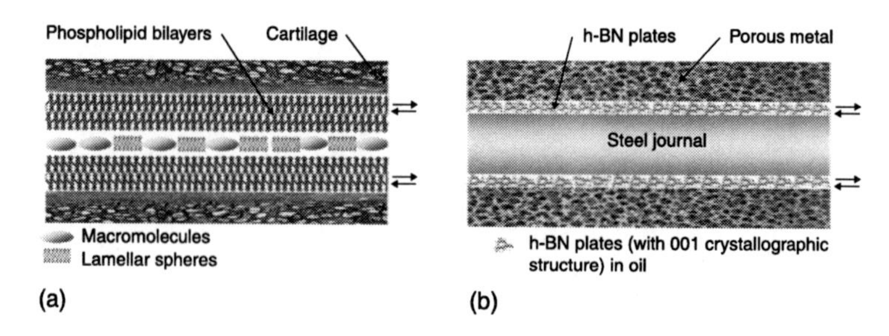

Figure 7.14 Schematic representation of the lamellar lubrication: (a) articular cartilage and (b) porous journal bearing. (a) The composition of phospholipid bilayers (or surface morphous layer) and synovial fluid appears to consist of macromolecules (hyaluronate, proteins and glycoprotein) and lamellar spheres. (b) Porous bearing impregnated with oil + h-BN macroparticles.

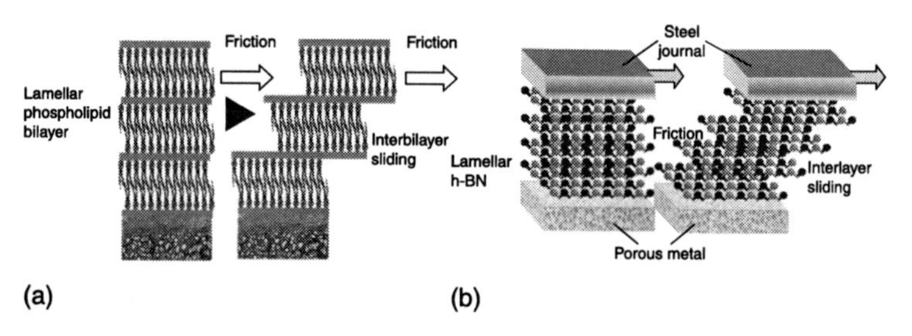

Figure 7.15 Lamellar mode of the phospholipid bilayer friction mechanism (a) and h-BN lamellate solid lubricant during friction mode (b). The lamellar bilayers and phases have a layer structure, which has directional order giving LCC and localized layer disorder giving low resistance to shear.

position and independently causes the friction to be low (Adams et al., 2001; Pawlak, 2003).

A multilamellar structure of phospholipids has the capability of lubricating intact joints *in vivo*. This has been termed the superficial layer of articular cartilage (Jurvelin et al., 1996; Yusuf et al., 2012) or the SAL (Pickard et al., 1998; Graindorge et al., 2005; Naka et al., 2005). The SAL was revealed as being acellular and non-fibrous, i.e. amorphous. Schematic representations of the lamellar lubrication for articular cartilage (a) and journal bearings (b) are presented in Figures 7.14 and 7.15. Dark arrows indicate the direction of the relative magnitude of weak friction between phospholipid layers (a) and weak interaction in each plate h-BN layer. The SAL covering the articular cartilage as multibilayers has a hydrophilic surface and appears remarkably similar to the structure of graphite, which is known as a 'lamellated solid' lubricant (Jurvelin et al., 1996; Kobayashi et al., 1996).

For h-BN and graphite, lubrication occurs by shearing between molecular plates, giving a low friction coefficient under high load leading to the characteristic boundary lubrication. The lamellar lubrication of h-BN and graphite is compatible with the multilamellar structure of the phospholipid lubricant that overlays cartilage in the joints (Table 7.3).

The effect of porosity on the coefficient of friction and stiffness is presented in Figure 7.16. It was found that, for engineering porous bearings over the range of 15–28.7% porosity, the friction coefficient decreased sharply (curve 1) and for cartilage bearings the porosity showed a similar trend (curve 2). It can be seen that, for a given increase in porosity, the cartilage stiffness increases (curve 3) (Oloyede at al., 2004).

Published by Woodhead Publishing Limited, 2013

Table 7.3 Friction coefficient on biological and engineering material surfaces during lamellar lubrication

Biological or material engineering surfaces	Type of surface	Friction coefficient (f)
Biological surfaces		
Natural articular cartilage[a] with surface layer (SAL[b])	Hydrophilic	<0.025
Natural (articular cartilage) (SAL was washed or wiped)	Hydrophilic	Increased 14%
Natural (articular cartilage) (protein washed from SAL)	Hydrophobic	Increased 35%
Natural (articular cartilage) (lipids washed from SAL)	Hydrophobic	Increased 22%
Material engineering surfaces		
Mica (model of (–) charged surface + LUB[c] (or rinsed))	Hydrophilic	0.038 (0.22)
Mica (monolayer (+) charged poly-lysine + LUB)	Hydrophilic	0.16
Gold (monolayer with hexadecanethiol + LUB)	Hydrophobic	0.39
Porous bearings (transformer oil + h-BN)	Hydrophobic	0.015
Porous non-full journal bearing (Vaseline + h-BN)	Hydrophobic	0.030
Silicone elastomer (poly(dimethylsiloxane)) in water	Hydrophobic	>1.0
Ox-silicone elastomer (ox-poly(dimethylsiloxane)) in water	Hydrophilic	<0.1

[a] Articular cartilage (wt%): collagen 10–30, proteoglycans 3–10, water and mineral salts 60–87 with small quantities of proteins, glycoproteins and lipids.
[b] SAL ($\mu g/cm^2$): lipids 54.5, proteins 68.1, glycosaminoglycans 61.4 (SAL is non-collagenous and acellular).
[c] Lubricin glycoprotein with $M_w = 2.3 \times 10^5$ g/mol at pH 7.2–7.6 has a positive charge.

Source: Pickard et al., 1998; Lee and Spencer, 2005; Bongaerts et al., 2007; Zappone et al., 2007; Pawlak et al., 2008.

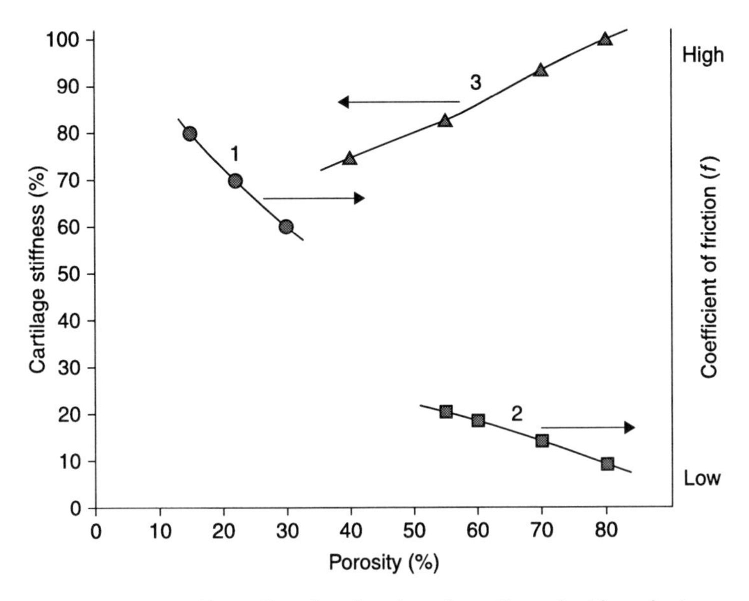

Figure 7.16 Porosity of natural and engineering bearing v. cartilage stiffness (normal and delipidized, curve 3) and coefficient of friction (f = 0.27–0.05, engineering bearing curve 1) and (f = 0.005–0.02, articular cartilage natural bearing curve 2).

The articular cartilage surface is covered by a superficial multibilayer mainly composed of phospholipids, which act as a lubricant and control fluid shift across the surface of the tissue. Unfortunately, any changes in the superficial zone, e.g. the removal of lipid bilayers, lowers by about 25% the stiffness of articular cartilage in comparison to normal tissue at physiological rates of loading (Oloyede et al., 2004). Reduction of compressive stiffness of articular cartilage has been reported as one of the first signs of cartilage degeneration (Franz et al., 2001). The surface quality would contribute to effective lubrication and other parameters will change, e.g. friction coefficient, wettability, porosity, surface energy and permeability of the matrix (Pawlak et al., 2012; Setton et al., 1993).

Published by Woodhead Publishing Limited, 2013

Cartilage tissue is highly porous (porosity in the range of 75–80%) with a pore size in the range of 2.0–6.5 nm and very low permeability values in the range 10^{-15} to 10^{-16} m^4/Ns (Mow and Ateshian, 1997). In a human joint, the effect of interstitial flow water on lubrication is small because hydraulic permeability of the cartilage is low and the porosity of articular cartilage is mainly responsible for fluid film generation (Jil et al, 1992). A friction study has shown that an osteoarthritic and delipidized cartilage surface raised the coefficient of friction (Katta et al., 2008). This increase in friction may be due to a reduction in the fluid load support.

7.3.4 Natural lubrication v. engineering porous bearing lubrication

The articular cartilage is polar and porous and contains 4–10% (dry weight) of phospholipids. Their polar groups ($-PO_4^-$, $-NH_3^+$) are adsorbed on the articular surface with close-packed fatty acid hydrocarbon chains that render them highly hydrophobic with a contact angle of 103°. Such a surface is very susceptible to direct bonding of an initial or foundation phospholipid layer and subsequent formation of two additional phospholipidic bilayers (Hills, 1989). The charged ends of phospholipid molecules allow formation of an interface of a hydrophilic–hydrophilic biopair model based on lamellar biolubrication. In this respect, in normal joints boundary or hydrodynamic lubrication is not feasible (Pawlak and Oloyede, 2007). This biomembrane of phospholipids would act similarly to a lamellated-solid lubricant, being frictionless and wearless. However, if hydrophobicity becomes lower than normal, such as occurs in osteoarthritis, wear of the articular cartilage will result. It was demonstrated that lipid depletion on the surface of

Published by Woodhead Publishing Limited, 2013

articular cartilage is a key factor in the development of osteoarthritis (Hills and Monds, 1998; Ballantine and Stachowiak, 2002).

Total joint replacement has evolved into a successful technique, as evidenced by the number of artificial knees/hips being implanted. The artificial joints consist commonly of a Co–Cr or titanium alloy component bearing against high-molecular-weight polyethylene. The articulating surfaces of the joint prostheses come into contact and operate under boundary lubrication processes; wear debris will occur (Ingham and Fisher, 2000). One of the major concerns relating to the long-term clinical performance of joint replacement is the generation of polyethylene wear debris. An adverse tissue reaction to wear debris can result in poor implant performance. To imitate articular cartilage, current research into biomaterials is focused on designing and fabricating an elastomeric material that is coated with a lipid-attracting copolymer (William et al., 1995) or using a biomaterial, e.g. pyrolytic carbon (PC), with a very high potential of adsorption of phospholipids (Gale et al., 2007). Strong evidence for the formation of phospholipid bilayers was demonstrated with poly(polymer-*block*-styrene) (Kojima et al., 1991). The presence of the articular cartilage surface phospholipid layer and orthopedic cushion bearings in prosthetic synovial joints might play the same lubricating role in normal and prosthetic joints. The development of porous metal and coatings has revolutionized the field of orthopedics. The open-cell structure of these materials presents several intriguing properties, such as high porosity (60–80%), low modulus of elasticity and high fractional characteristics of 0.53–0.88. Subsequent short- to mid-term follow-up has provided excellent results for both primary and revision total hip and knee arthroplasty (Levine et al., 2006, Levine, 2008; Meneghini et al., 2008). Nevertheless,

Published by Woodhead Publishing Limited, 2013

longer-term clinical data is necessary to validate these exciting new applications in orthopedic surgery.

Many models of joint lubrication have been based on a fluid film in order to explain the very low coefficient of friction in the biological joints. Originally, Hills (1989) discovered the lubricating properties of phospholipids and their ability to adsorb to tissue surfaces. Additionally, biological surfaces have the ability to form a bilayer of phospholipids on articular cartilage or other tissues where biolubrication is taking place. Adsorption of phospholipids on metals or polyethylene surfaces is energetically very weak, without the ability to form a bilayer phospholipid membrane. The inability to form such a structure on the surface of the engineering materials that are used in human joints makes them susceptible to boundary friction. Much evidence supports the hypothesis that elastomeric or porous material synthesized similarly to biological tissue structure and with biological hydrophobicity can make prosthetic joints comparable to biological ones (Hills, 1995; William et al., 1995).

The fact that layered phospholipids are lamellar solid lubricants comparable to graphite, h-BN or MoS_2 in terms of their macromolecular structure is supportive of our hypothesis to construct prosthetic joints based on the principles used in the design of porous journal bearings, combining a high porosity material and lamellar nanolubricant, which would be more similar to biological tissues. Hydrogel lamellar polymeric materials are used in many capacities in the human body. Hydrogels are polymer networks that contain substantial fractions of water and they are typically hydrophilic, e.g. poly(2-hydroxyethylmethacrylate); ox-poly(dimethylsiloxane) is the primary material for human use (Dunn et al., 2008). Two new polymer surfactants consisting of a polysiloxane backbone and the formation of multilamellar vesicles (onions) at intermediate shear rates (Burgemeister and Schmidt, 2002) have also been proposed.

This recent study, with previous testing of porous bearings impregnated with oily solvent + lamellar nanoparticles lubricant (Pawlak et al., 2007a,b, 2008), has demonstrated the ability to achieve a very low friction coefficient over standard bearings. Lamellar-type lubrication is a key factor in reducing the coefficient of friction. Self-lubricating porous sliding (or plain) bearings have been commonly used over a long period of time. The reason for their selection is because there is no need for an external supply of lubricant for running in, low cost of operation and their usefulness in applications where contamination from oil leakage cannot be tolerated, such as in the textile or food industry. Other application areas include water pump bearings and domestic applications, e.g. washing machines, vacuum cleaners and lawn mowers.

7.4 Conclusions

The impregnation of the Fe–Cu porous bearings (15–30 wt% porosity) with oil (first generation) or oil + h-BN (second generation) allows us to improve all of the tribological properties, such as wear scar diameter, friction coefficient and load. The mechanism of friction and wear for h-BN microparticles on porous surfaces can be explained by the slow release of oil and macroparticles from the open pores to the contact surface to prevent the straight contact of two surfaces. Also, h-BN is a layered compound like graphite, being soft and lubricious. These results indicate that h-BN could facilitate the deposition of the lining of h-BN providing efficient boundary lubrication. The

Published by Woodhead Publishing Limited, 2013

formation of the lamellar solid of h-BN gives rise to plate-like crystallites that lie flat with relatively low surface energy. The low adhesion between the crystallites allows them to become oriented in their most favorable position and independently causes the friction to be low. It was found that journal bearings with low porosity (15 wt%) and impregnated with oil + h-BN have a much higher friction coefficient than samples with a 27.8 wt% porosity. Also, the friction and temperature increase abruptly, leading finally to a seizure.

The results have shown that the friction coefficient and transition time to seizure were affected by load and *PV* parameters. Important conclusions obtained from this work can be summarized as follows. (i) Porous bearings (Fe–Cu) impregnated with h-BN microparticles have shown a very low friction coefficient (0.02–0.03), twice as low as those impregnated with oil only (first-generation bearings). (ii) In the bench test, porous bearings have demonstrated that impregnation with oil + h-BN would satisfy 100 000 h of clutch operation in a real engine.

The novel lubrication mechanism of second-generation porous bearings involving diphase fluids is capable of providing a low friction coefficient and high LCC. The porous bearings impregnated with the diphase fluid were run additionally with external lubricant and the results of the experiment led to the following conclusions: (i) porous materials externally lubricated with the diphase fluid at a h-BN concentration of 0.5 wt% double the LCC; (ii) velocities of 1–2 m/s gave a good indication that the concept based on the blocking/unblocking of pores works well at low velocities; (iii) particulates of porous bearings impregnated with the diphase fluid act as one-way valves on the pores, blocking and unblocking them. Phospholipid molecules (phospholipids) *in vivo* and h-BN *in vitro* are excellent examples of frictionless lubricants. Phospholipids and h-BN have the ability to form layered structures similar to those of lamellate solids. It has been confirmed experimentally that lamellar lubricants protect the surface of natural and engineering tribopairs.

7.5 Acknowledgements

This work was supported by the Tribochemistry Consulting grant, USA.

7.6 References

Adams J B, Hector Jr L G, Siegel D J, Yu H and Zhong J (2001), 'Adhesion, lubrication and wear on the atomic scale', *Surface and Interface Analysis*, **31**: 619–626.

Ballantine G C and Stachowiak G W (2002), 'The effects of lipid depletion on osteoarthritic wear', *Wear*, **253**: 385–393.

Bhushan B and Gupta B K (1991), *Handbook of Tribology: Materials, Coatings, and Surface Treatments*. New York: McGraw-Hill.

Bongaerts J H H, Fourtouni K and Stokes J R (2007), 'Soft-tribology: lubrication in a compliant PDMS–PDMS contact', *Tribology International*, **40**: 1531–1542.

Burgemeister D and Schmidt C (2002), 'Shear flow of lamellar polymer surfactants', *Progress in Colloid & Polymer Science*, **121**: 95–100.

Chen B, Bi Q, Yang J, Xia Y and Hao J (2008), 'Tribological properties of solid lubricants (graphite, H-BN), for Cu-based P/M friction composition', *Tribology International*, **41**: 1145–1152.

Published by Woodhead Publishing Limited, 2013

Culley S A, McDonnell T F, Ball D J, Kirby C W and Hawes S W (1996), 'The impact of passenger car motor oil phosphorus levels on automotive emission control systems', *SAE International Technical Paper Series*, **961898**, 13–20.

Deacon R F and Goodman J F (1958), 'Lubrication by lamellar solids', *Proceedings of the Royal Society of London, Series A: Mathematical, Physical and Engineering Sciences*, **423**: 464–482.

Dunn A C, Cobb J A, Kantzios A N, Lee S J, Sarntinoranont M et al. (2008), 'Friction coefficient measurement of hydrogel materials on living epithelial cells', *Tribology Letters*, **30**: 13–19.

Elsharkawy A A and Guedouar L H (2001), 'Hydrodynamic lubrication of porous journal bearings using a modified Brinkman-extended Darcy model', *Tribology International*, **34**: 767–777.

Erdemir A (1991), 'Tribological properties of boric acid and boric acid-forming surfaces. Part I: crystal chemistry and mechanism of self-lubrication of boric acid', *Lubrication Engineering*, **47**: 168–173.

Erdemir A (1995), Lubrication from mixture of boric acid with oils and greases. US Patent 5,431,830.

Erdemir A (2005), 'Review of engineered tribological interfaces for improved boundary lubrication', *Tribology International*, **38**: 249–256.

Erdemir A, Fenske G R, Erck R A and Nichols F A (1991), 'Tribological properties of boric acid and boric acid-forming surfaces. Part II: mechanisms of formation and self-lubrication of boric acid films on boron- and boric oxide-containing surfaces', *Lubrication Engineering*, **47**: 179–184.

Federico S and Herzog W (2008), 'On the anisotropy and inhomogeneity of permeability in articular cartilage',

Published by Woodhead Publishing Limited, 2013

Biomechanics and Modeling in Mechanobiology, 7: 367–378.

Franz T, Hasler E M, Hagg R, Weiler C, Jakob R P et al. (2001), '*In situ* compressive stiffness, biochemical composition, and structural integrity of articular cartilage of the human knee joint', *Osteoarthritis and Cartilage*, 9: 582–592.

Fuller S, Li Y, Gordon J T T, Wyn-Jones E and Arnell R D (1995), 'Formulation of lyotropic lamellar phases of surfactants as novel lubricants', *Langmuir*, **11**: 1980–1983.

Gale L R, Coller R, Hargreaves D J, Hills B A and Crawford R (2007), 'The role of SALP as a boundary lubricant in prosthetic joints', *Tribology International*, **40**: 601–606.

Graindorge S, Ferrandez W, Jin Z, Ingham E, Grant C et al. (2005), 'Biphasic surface amorphous layer lubrication of articular cartilage', *Medical Engineering and Physics*, **27**: 836–844.

Guerra D, Frizziero L, Losi M, Bacchelli B, Mezzadri G et al. (1996), 'Ultrastructural identification of membrane-like structure on the surface of normal articular cartilage', *Journal of Submicroscopic Cytology and Pathology*, **28**: 385–393.

Gunsel S, Yu B and Friberg S E (1992), 'A liquid crystal lubricant with partial polymerisation', *Lubrication Science*, **4**: 191–199.

Gururajan, K. and Prakash, J. (2003), 'Effect of velocity slip in a narrow rough porous journal bearing', *Proceedings of the Institution of Mechanical Engineers, Part J: Journal of Engineering Tribology*, **217**: 59–70.

Hills B A (1989), 'Oligolamellar lubrication of joints by surface active phospholipid', *Journal of Rheumatology*, **16**: 82–91.

Hills B A (1992), 'Graphite-like lubrication of mesothelium by oligolamellar pleural surfactant', *Journal of Applied Physiology*, **73**: 1034–1039.

Hills B A (1995), 'Remarkable anti-wear properties of joint surfactant', *Annals of Biomedical Engineering*, **23**: 112–115.

Hills B A (2002), 'Surface-active phospholipid: a Pandora's box of clinical applications. Part II. Barrier and lubricating properties', *Internal Medicine Journal*, **32**: 242–251.

Hills B A and Monds M K (1998), 'Deficiency of lubricating surfactants lining the articular surfaces of replaced hips and knees', *British Journal of Rheumatology*, **37**: 143–147.

Hod O (2012), 'Graphite and hexagonal boron-nitride have the same interlayer distance. Why?', *Journal of Chemical Theory and Computation*, **8**: 1360–1369.

Ingham E and Fisher J (2000), 'Biological reactions to wear debris in total joint replacement', *Proceedings of the Institution of Mechanical Engineers, Part H: Journal of Engineering in Medicine*, **214**: 21–37.

Israelachvili J and Wennerström H (1996), 'Role of hydration and water structure in biological and colloidal interactions', *Nature*, **379**: 219–225.

Jin Z M, Dowson D and Fisher J (1992), 'The effect of porosity of articular cartilage on the lubrication of a normal human hip joint', *Proceedings of the Institution of Mechanical Engineers, Part H: Journal of Engineering in Medicine*, **206**: 117–124.

Junbin Y (1997), 'Antiwear function and mechanism of borate containing nitrogen', *Tribology International*, **30**: 387–389.

Jurvelin J S, Müller D J, Wong M, Studer D, Engel A et al. (1996), 'Surface and subsurface morphology of bovine humeral articular cartilage as assessed by atomic force and transmission electron microscopy', *Journal of Structural Biology*, **117**: 45–54.

Published by Woodhead Publishing Limited, 2013

Kaldonski T (1997), 'Complex self-lubrication mechanism of porous bearing–two models', *Tribologia*, **28**: 653–657 (in Polish).

Kaldonski T (2006), *Tribological Application of Boron Nitride*. Warsaw: WAT (in Polish).

Katta J, Jin Z, Ingham E and Fisher J (2008), 'Biotribology of articular cartilage – a review of the recent advances', *Medical Engineering and Physics*, **30**: 1349–1363.

Klein C, Hurlbut C S and Dana J D (1993), *Manual of Mineralogy*, 21th edn. New York: Wiley.

Kobayashi S, Yonekubo S and Kurogouchi Y (1996), 'Cryoscanning electron microscopy of loaded articular cartilage with special reference to the surface amorphous layer', *Journal of Anatomy*, **188**: 311–322.

Kojima M, Ishihara K, Watanabe A and Nakabayashi N (1991), 'Interaction between phospholipids and biocompatible polymers containing a phosphorylcholine moiety', *Biomaterials*, **12**: 121–124.

Krzeminski K (2002), *Plain of the Gradient Properties Bush*. Warsaw: Oficyna Wydawnicza Politechniki Warszawskiej (in Polish).

Kumar V (1980), 'Porous metal bearings – a critical review', *Wear*, **63**: 271–287.

Ladavière R, Martin J M, Le Mogne T, Vacher B, Constans B et al. (2003), 'Tribochemistry: friction-induced lamellar solids from lubricant additives', *Tribology Series*, **41**: 15–22.

Lawrowski Z (2006), *Maintenance-Free Plain Bearings*. Warsaw: Oficyna Wydawnicza Politechniki Warszawskiej (in Polish).

Lee S and Spencer N D (2005), 'Aqueous lubrication of polymers: influence of surface modification', *Tribology International*, **38**: 922–930.

Lelonis D A, Tereshko J W and Andersen C M (2003), 'Boron nitride powder – a high performance alternative for solid

Published by Woodhead Publishing Limited, 2013

lubrication', *General Electric Advanced Ceramics*, **81506**: 1–4.

Levine B (2008), 'A new era in porous metals: applications in orthopaedics', *Advanced Engineering Materials*, **10**: 788–792.

Levine B, Della Valle C J and Jacobs J J (2006), 'Applications of porous tantalum in total hip arthroplasty', *Journal of the American Academy of Orthopedic Surgeons*, **14**: 646–655.

McPherson A (2005), 'Micelle formation and crystallization as paradigms for virus assembly', *BioEssays*, **27**: 447–458.

Martin J M, Le Mogne Th, Chassagnette C and Gardos M N (1992), 'Friction of hexagonal boron nitride in various environments', *Tribology Transactions*, **35**: 462–472.

Meneghini M, Lewallen D G and Hanssen A D (2008), 'Use of porous tantalum metaphyseal cones for severe tibial bone loss during revision total knee replacement', *Journal of Bone and Joint Surgery, American*, **90**: 78–84.

Maroudas A, Bullough P, Swanson S A V and Freeman M A R (1968), 'The permeability of articular cartilage', *Journal of Bone and Joint Surgery, British*, **50B**: 166–177.

Mirzayan R (2006), *Cartilage Injury in the Athlete*. New York: Thieme.

Mosuang T E and Lowther J E (2002), 'Relative stability of cubic and different hexagonal forms of boron nitride', *Journal of Physics and Chemistry of Solids*, **63**: 363–368.

Mow V C and Ateshian G A (1997), 'Friction, lubrication and wear of diarthrodial joints', in: Mow V C and Hayes W C (eds), *Basic Orthopaedic Biomechanics*, pp. 275–315. Philadelphia, PA: Lippincott-Raven.

Naka M H, Morita Y and Ikeuchi K (2005), 'Influence of proteoglycan and of tissue hydration on the fractional characteristics of articular cartilage', *Proceedings of the Institution of Mechanical Engineers, Part H: Journal of Engineering in Medicine*, **219**: 175–182.

Neale M J (1973), *Tribology Handbook*. London: Butterworths.

Nikas G K and Sayles R S (2008), 'A study of lubrication mechanisms using two-phase fluids with porous bearing materials', *Proceedings of the Institution of Mechanical Engineers, Part J: Journal of Engineering Tribology*, **222**: 771–783.

Oloyede A and Broom N (1994), 'The generalized consolidation of articular cartilage: an investigation of its near-physiological response to static load', *Connective Tissue Research*, **31**: 75–86.

Oloyede A, Gudimetla P, Crawford R and Hills B A (2004), 'Biomechanical responses of normal and delipidized articular cartilage subjected to varying rates of loading', *Connective Tissue Research*, **45**: 86–93.

Pawlak Z (2003), *Tribochemistry of Lubricating Oils*. Amsterdam: Elsevier.

Pawlak Z and Oloyede A (2007), 'Articular cartilage as a giant reverse micelle – a new perspective on biocushioning as the basic of joint lubrication', in: *Proceedings of the International Conference on Advances in Manufacturing Engineering*, Manipal, India, paper keynote #4.

Pawlak Z, Kotynska J, Figaszewski Z A, Oloyede A, Gadomski A et al. (2007a), 'Impact of the charge density of phospholipid bilayers on lubrication of articular cartilage surfaces', *Journal of Achievements in Materials and Manufacturing Engineering*, **23**: 47–50.

Pawlak Z, Kaldonski T, Praveen P and Oloyede A (2007b), 'Boron nitride as a lamellar lubricant in self-lubricated porous film sliding bearing', *Proceedings of the 4th International Conference on Leading Edge Manufacturing in the 21st Century*, Fukuoka, Japan, pp. 913–918.

Pawlak Z, Pai R, Bayraktar E, Kaldonski T and Oloyede A (2008), 'Lamellar lubrication *in vivo* and *vitro*:

friction testing of hexagonal boron nitride', *BioSystems*, **94**: 202–208.

Pawlak Z, Kaldonski T, Pai R, Bayraktar E and Oloyede A (2009), 'A comparative study on the tribological behaviour of the hexagonal boron nitride (h-BN), as lubricating micro-particles – an additive in porous sliding bearing for a car clutch', *Wear*, **267**: 1198–1202.

Pawlak Z, Petelska A D, Urbaniak W, Yusuf K Q and Oloyede A (2012), 'Relationship between wettability and lubrication characteristics of the surfaces of contacting phospholipid-based membranes', *Cell Biochemistry and Biophysics*, doi: 10.1007/s12013-012-9437-z.

Pease R S (1952), 'An X-ray study of boron nitride', *Acta Crystallographica*, **5**: 356–361.

Perry S S and Tysoe W T (2005), 'Frontiers of fundamental tribological research', *Tribology Letters*, **19**: 151–161.

Pickard J E, Fisher J, Ingham E and Egans J (1998), 'Investigation into the effects of proteins and lipids on the frictional properties of articular cartilage', *Biomaterials*, **19**: 1807–1812.

Quan Y-X, Ma J, Tian Y-G, Zhou G-R, Shi G-Y et al. (1985), 'Investigation of sintered bronze bearings under high-speed conditions', *Tribology International*, **18**: 75–80.

Rabinowicz E and Imai M (1964), 'Frictional properties of pyrolytic boron nitride and graphite', *Wear*, **7**: 298–300.

Raman R and Vinod-Babu L (1984), 'Test on sintered bearings with reduced oil contents', *Wear*, **95**: 263–269.

Rapoport L, Lvovsky M, Lapsker I, Leshchinsky W, Volovik Y et al. (2001), 'Friction and wear of bronze powder composites including fullerene-like WS_2 nanoparticle', *Wear*, **249**: 149–156.

Rapoport L, Leshchinsky V, Lvovsky M, Lapsker I, Volovik Y et al. (2002), 'Load bearing capacity of

Published by Woodhead Publishing Limited, 2013

bronze, iron and iron–nickel powder composites containing fullerene-like WS_2 nanoparticles', *Tribology International*, **35**: 47–53.

Saha N and Majumdar B C (2002), 'Study of externally-pressurized gas-lubricated two-layered porous journal bearings: a steady state analysis', *Proceedings of the Institution of Mechanical Engineers, Part J: Journal of Engineering Tribology*, **216**: 151–158.

Setton L A, Zhu W and Mow V C (1993), 'The biphasic poroviscoelastic behavior of articular cartilage: role of the surface zone in governing the compressive behavior', *Journal of Biomechanics*, **26**: 581–592.

Stachowiak G W and Batchelor A W (2005), *Engineering Tribology*. Amsterdam: Elsevier/Butterworth-Heinemann.

Urbakh M, Klafte J, Gourdon D and Israelachvili J (2004), 'The nonlinear nature of friction', *Nature*, **430**: 525–528.

Westergård R, Åhlin A, Axén N and Hogmark S (1998), 'Sliding wear and friction of Si_3N_4-SiC-based ceramic composites containing hexagonal boron nitride', *Proceedings of the Institution of Mechanical Engineers, Part J: Journal of Engineering Tribology*, **212**: 381–387.

William III P F, Powell G L, Love B, Ishihara K, Nakabayashi N et al. (1995), 'Fabrication and characterization of dipalmitoylphosphatidylcholine-attracting elastomeric material for joint replacements', *Biomaterials*, **16**: 1169–1174.

Wright V and Dowson D (1976), 'Lubrication and cartilage', *Journal of Anatomy*, **121**: 107–118.

Yoshimoto S, Tozuka H and Dambara S (2003), 'Static characteristics of aerostatic porous journal bearings with a surface-restricted layer', *Proceedings of the Institution of Mechanical Engineers, Part J: Journal of Engineering Tribology*, **217**: 125–132.

Published by Woodhead Publishing Limited, 2013

Yusuf K Q, Motta N, Pawlak Z and Oloyade A (2012), 'A microanalytical study of the surfaces of normal, delipidized and artificially "resurfaced" articular cartilage', *Connective Tissue Research*, 53: 236–245.

Zappone B, Ruths M, Greene G W, Joy G D and Israelachvili J N (2007), 'Adsorption, lubrication, and wear of lubricin on model surfaces: polymer brush-like behavior of a glycoprotein', *Biophysical Journal*, 92: 1693–1708.

Published by Woodhead Publishing Limited, 2013

8

Tribological characterization of human tooth enamel

E. Sajewicz, Bialystok University of Technology, Poland

DOI: 10.1533/9780857092205.355

Abstract: This chapter describes the influence of some factors on the tribological behavior of human tooth enamel. Experimental results of the influence of the type of loading, enamel microhardness and material of the counterbody on the tribological performance of tooth enamel are presented.

Key words: tooth enamel, friction, wear, loading, microhardness.

8.1 Introduction

Nowadays tooth enamel, the hardest tissue of the human body, is becoming an object of increasing interest of the tribological community. This interest comes from the fact that enamel presents unique tribological behavior; its fine resistance to wear is certainly the most important. The latter statement is justified despite quite poor working conditions from a tribological point of view, i.e. widely ranging cyclic

Published by Woodhead Publishing Limited, 2013

load, complex movements of the contacting tooth surfaces, temperature shocks caused by consumed food and presence of chemically active food components.

Tooth tribology is part of a new biotribological direction called 'oral tribology' (Zhou and Zheng, 2006). There are a few main goals of the investigations being conducted in this area:

(i) Similarly to any scientific studies, we want to find out 'how it is', i.e. researchers pursue a cognitive aim.

(ii) Although sound tooth enamel still presents good wear resistance, some circumstances accompanying modern life may lead to unsatisfactory tribological durability of human teeth. Among them are increasing life expectancy and new nutrition habits, including increasing intake of soft drinks, smoking and others. Furthermore, there are some clinical abnormalities manifested in oral environments leading to pathological tooth wear, e.g. poor saliva secretion (xerostomia, Sjögren's syndrome) or bruxism. A better understanding of tribological processes occurring within the oral cavity can protect us from excessive tooth wear.

(iii) Knowledge of the tribological behavior of human teeth is indispensable in the context of dental materials. On the one hand, it is possible to fabricate better dental materials by applying biomimetic principles, i.e. utilizing information regarding structure and properties of hard tooth tissues; on the other hand, it is expected that new dental materials possessing good tribological characteristics will not lead to excessive wear of opposing natural teeth.

Published by Woodhead Publishing Limited, 2013

8.2 Structure and properties of tooth enamel

Human dentition, as well as dentition of other vertebrates, is mainly a mechanical device enabling food processing during mastication. The simplest description of the tooth, being the elementary part of the dentition, covers the crown located externally to the body and the internal root. The tooth has three hard tissues – enamel of thickness 2–3 mm covering the crown, dentine lying beneath the enamel and cementum covering the root. The most important tissue from the tribological point of view is enamel, as this is the part of the tooth directly contacting with a food bolus or with opposing teeth. However, dentine also plays an important role, as a more elastic tissue compared with enamel, and furthermore it is capable of spreading the stress in the tooth. Moreover, when excessive wear of enamel occurs uncovered dentine takes over the enamel's role.

Enamel is an example of a biological multiscale structure, designed in a hierarchical manner that gives the enamel its unique mechanical properties. Other examples of multiscale natural structures with a similar biological organization are long bones, collagen in tendons, proteins in hair and cellulose in wood (Rho et al., 1998; Vincent, 2006). These structures can also be considered as multifunctional (multipurpose) materials if we take into account the fact that their inner design is aimed at achieving mechanical anisotropy (Weiner et al., 2000). A multipurpose function of tooth enamel is realized as a response of the material to the following requirements: the enamel should be resistant to normal loading while the food is being crushed and also resistant to shear stresses arising while grinding the food bolus to reduce

Published by Woodhead Publishing Limited, 2013

its size. Moreover, friction forces produced during mastication should be high enough to avoid sliding of food particles and, simultaneously, the enamel should be resistant to tribological wear in spite of the presence of relatively high friction. Although some of the requirements listed above are in opposition, it is obvious that all of them have to be fulfilled at the same time. Tooth enamel is characterized by a great functionality not only due to its specific microstructure, but also due to its mineralized form; in particular, mineralization gives the enamel extraordinary hardness.

Tooth enamel can be considered as a biological ceramic that is approximately 95% inorganic by weight and predominantly formed of hydroxyapatite ($Ca_{10}(PO_4)_6(OH)_2$). The remaining components are water and organic materials (Sakae et al., 1997). The basic structural units of tooth enamel are the so-called 'prisms' – aligned rods with an average width of 3–5 μm (Skobe and Stern, 1980). The prisms are bundles of hydroxyapatite crystallites that extend from the dentine–enamel junction to the outer enamel surface without interruption (Sander, 1997). The hexagonal crystallites are tightly packed within the prisms and have approximately uniform size with average dimensions of the cross-sections: 89 (width) and 50 nm (thickness). The length of the crystallites ranges from 100 to 150 nm (Brès and Hutchison, 2002). The interfacial area between prisms is filled by an interprismatic protein-rich substance containing hydroxyapatite crystallites of sizes smaller than those in the area of the prism.

The enamel structure shown at different levels is presented in Figure 8.1. At a relatively small magnification it is possible to see alternating dark and light bands on the longitudinal cross-section of a tooth (Figure 8.1a). These bands are an effect of a spatial decussation of the prisms, which are decussated in bands, in such a way that some of them are perpendicular to the section plane, whereas the others are set-up parallel. This is clearly seen in Figure 8.1(b). The bands, called Hunter–Schreger bands, have a thickness varying from one to 30 prisms (Koenigswald and Sander, 1997). The prisms oriented perpendicularly to the plane of a section are arranged in a specific array and, as can be seen in Figure 8.1(c), typically shaped in a keyhole pattern. Biological

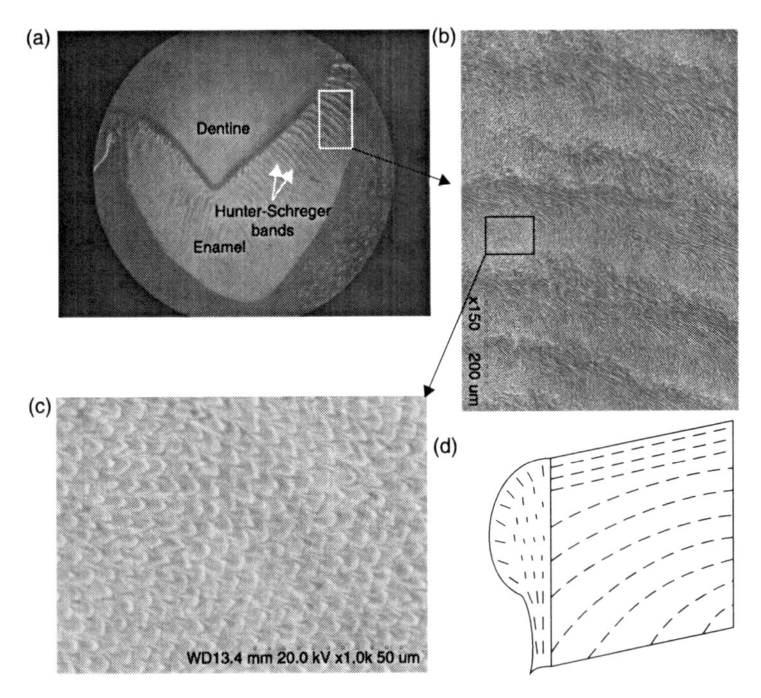

Figure 8.1 Enamel structure of a human molar shown at different scales of observation. (a) Hunter–Schreger bands (light microscopy; original magnification ×20). (b) Different orientation of the prisms in Hunter–Schreger bands (SEM; original magnification ×150). (c) Keyhole pattern of the prisms (SEM; original magnification ×1000). (d) Sectioned single enamel prism with marked orientation of hydroxyapatite crystallites – model representation.

Published by Woodhead Publishing Limited, 2013

organization of the enamel structure is not incidental, but emerges as a response to the enamel's expected functions. In particular, due to the spatial decussation, each Hunter–Schreger band inhibits the propagation of cracks within bulk enamel. In this way brittle properties, typical for any engineering ceramic, are substantially limited with regard to tooth enamel being a biological ceramic.

In order to fulfill the complex functions of the whole masticatory system the tooth enamel must possess sufficient mechanical, physical and chemical properties. The most essential properties are listed in Table 8.1. Characteristically, the majority of the properties presented in Table 8.1 show a wide range of variability. There are at least several causes of that variability, but the diversity of techniques and methodologies of measurements used to determine enamel properties seems to be the most influential.

Properties of tooth enamel are not constant in the bulk material, but their values are crucially dependent on the location in the tooth. Apart from the structural diversity, the enamel also has a different chemical composition in different locations. Comprehensive studies performed by Cuy et al.

Table 8.1 Selected properties of the tooth enamel (values summarized from Sajewicz, 2007b)

Property	Value
Hardness	3.0–4.6 GPa
Young's modulus	9.65–131 GPa
Tensile strength	10–42.2 MPa
Compressive strength	95–400 MPa
Shear strength	64–95 MPa
Density	2.9 g/cm^3
Thermal conductivity	0.88 W/mK
Thermal expansion	11.4 p.p.m./°C
Electrical resistance	2.5–10 × 10^6 Ω

Published by Woodhead Publishing Limited, 2013

(2002) showed that in the outer layer of the enamel the concentration of CaO and P_2O_4 is less than in the deeper layers, whereas the concentration of Na_2O and MgO is higher near dentine than at the surface of enamel. They also reported that both hardness and Young's modulus exhibit decreasing values towards dentine. That fact has been confirmed by other authors (Zheng et al., 2003; Low, 2004).

8.3 Factors influencing tribological behavior of tooth enamel: general remarks

During mastication the teeth taking part in this process are subjected to complex tribological action. Frictional resistance and wear of teeth are functions of a number of factors, which often vary over a wide range in the oral environment. In general, these factors can be divided into two groups: enamel properties (intrinsic factors), and input parameters, properties of the oral environment and properties of the food subjected to mastication (extrinsic factors). The factors influencing the tribology of teeth are shown schematically in Figure 8.2. In addition to the tooth–tooth interactions there are other tribological interactions in the oral cavity, e.g. those incorporating soft tissues. However, in this section our attention will be focused on the tribology of the tooth enamel, as it is crucial for the durability of the whole masticatory system.

The complexity of tribological processes occurring in the oral cavity is not only due to a set of influencing factors (the majority of which are listed in Figure 8.2), but the complexity also comes from the fact that there are intricate interplays among these factors. All of this has to be taken into account when designing tribological tests. A good example is an

Published by Woodhead Publishing Limited, 2013

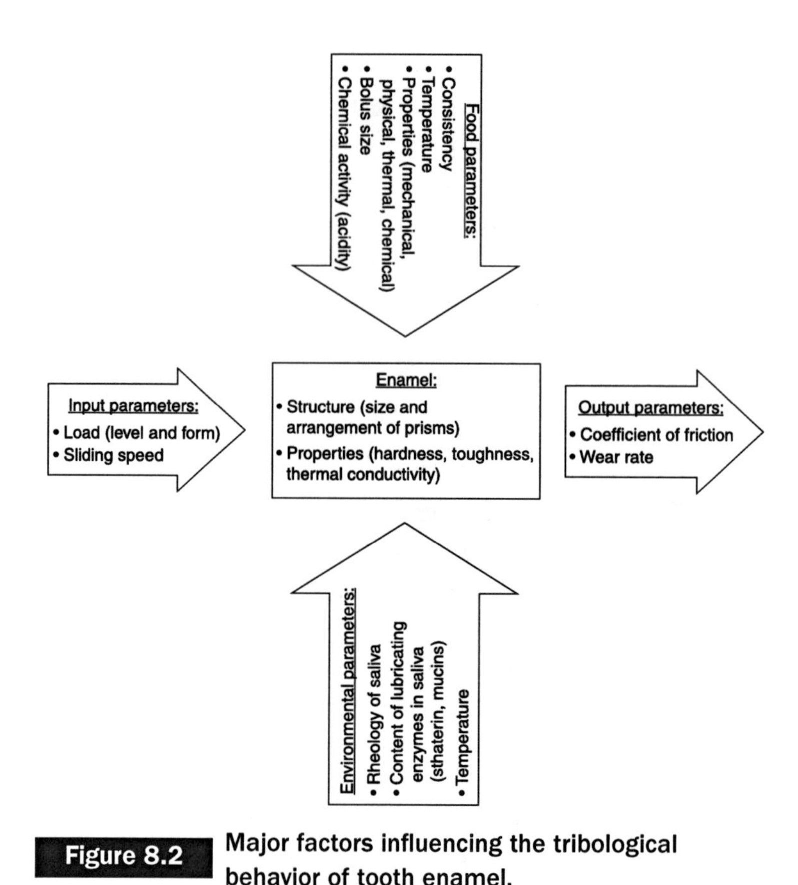

Figure 8.2 Major factors influencing the tribological behavior of tooth enamel.

investigation carried out by Eisenburger et al. (2003), who performed tribological tests in an acidic environment (simultaneous chemical and mechanical actions) and obtained a sufficiently higher wear rate of enamel compared with that obtained during alternating chemical and mechanical action. Another example is that shown by Sajewicz (2009), who studied the effect of saliva containing hard particles on tribological characteristics of tooth enamel and obtained different results dependent on saliva viscosity. Namely, after experiments with saliva containing A_2O_3 particles a significant increase of wear rate at low viscosity was observed when compared with the results found using the same saliva without alumina particles. At higher values of the viscosity the difference turned out not to be statistically significant. Those results mean that the simultaneous influence of saliva viscosity and the hard particles on wear rate of enamel occurs only at low values of viscosity. In other words, saliva having sufficiently high viscosity is capable of protecting tooth enamel against environmental abrasiveness.

One of the distinguishing features of tooth enamel in relation to tribological behavior is that the enamel manifests anisotropy of tribological parameters at the micro(nano) scale. So far, however, that problem has rarely been studied and described in the literature. One of the first comprehensive works related to the anisotropy of tribological properties of tooth enamel was published by Shimizu et al. (2005). On the basis of detailed analysis of a single enamel prism structure, i.e. an analysis of crystal orientation inside a prism, and by using the finite element method (FEM) the authors showed that the tensile stress induced by friction forces depends on the prism orientation in relation to the enamel surface. Namely, it was found that the stresses were lowest when the prisms approached the surface at low angles (more obliquely cut prisms) and highest when the prisms approached the surface at 60° (less obliquely cut prisms). Assuming that wear rate positively correlates with stresses, the authors concluded that their findings imply greater wear resistance at the intercuspal region of the tooth and less wear resistance at the lateral enamel at midcrown. Some conclusions drawn by the authors were recently confirmed by Zheng et al. (2011), who published the results of investigations performed by using nanoscratch testing. The experimental results indicated that the microtribological behavior of enamel was closely associated with the orientation of enamel prisms in the longitudinal section of the enamel. The scratch-induced damage was anisotropic on the longitudinal section of tooth enamel, i.e. it was weaker along the direction parallel to the enamel prism axis than along the vertical axis. However, unlike Shimizu et al. (2005), Zheng et al. (2011) hypothesize that greater wear resistance of the tooth enamel in the direction parallel to the prism axis is connected to the buffering effect of the interprismatic enamel.

In light of the results presented above it becomes clear that global behavior of the whole enamel strongly depends on its local properties, i.e. the enamel microstructure. Micro(nano) tribology of teeth seems to be very promising, and it is expected that employing new experimental techniques, such as atomic force microscopy (AFM) equipped with an add-on nanoindentation device used by Guidoni et al. (2009), should give us new results and, consequently, a better understanding of the tribological behavior of enamel as well as the whole dentition.

Although some attempts have been made in order to theoretically explain the influence of selected factors on the tribological behavior of the tooth enamel, most of the works concerning that problem still have an experimental character. Two experimental approaches are possible: the first performed in the oral environment (*in vivo* experiments), and the other performed by using test machines (tribometers) (*in vitro* experiments). It would seem that the first approach based on experiments carried out in the oral environment should be preferred, as it takes into account the influence of clinical (real) conditions. This approach has unquestionable advantages; however, there are also certain difficulties, as clinical investigations are time-consuming and, more importantly, the control of influencing factors is not possible. A wide variety of these factors makes it often impossible to assess the impact of an individual factor. This is why *in vitro* tests are widely used to determine tribological characteristics

Published by Woodhead Publishing Limited, 2013

of tooth enamel. Some results of *in vitro* experimental studies performed by the author are presented in Section 8.4.

8.4 Experimental studies of selected factors influencing the tribological behavior of human enamel

8.4.1 Test machine

It is now commonly accepted that tribological investigations of hard dental tissues should be performed in a way that simulates the complexity of intra-oral conditions as much as possible. This means that both the methodology of tribological testing of hard tooth tissues and the apparatus designed for these purposes should incorporate the main oral features in terms of tribology. In order to meet these requirements some authors try to design new test machines taking into account some of 'the most probable' oral conditions. Most functioning oral simulators have been constructed on the basis of that assumption. In particular, considerable attention has been focused on the kinematics to replicate the physiological pattern of teeth motion (DeLong and Douglas, 1991; Yap et al., 1999). However, the main problem is that there is no one 'most probable pattern'. Oral conditions vary widely due to the stochastic nature of oral processes, depending, among others, on the kind of food subjected to mastication. Thus, the actual pattern of the mandible movements is food-dependent; moreover, it is specific for each individual. According to the literature sources (Yamashita et al., 1999) there are at least seven basic masticatory patterns. Therefore, it is reasonable to utilize an apparatus with the possibility of wide control of key parameters rather than an apparatus with a fixed

Published by Woodhead Publishing Limited, 2013

'most probable' set of parameters, allowing us to carry out more fundamental studies instead of simple wear evaluation after testing.

In order to perform advanced studies of the tribological behavior of tooth enamel a new tribometer has been designed (Sajewicz and Kulesza, 2007). The device is capable of simulating oral kinematic conditions as well as loading produced during the mastication process. The tribometer has the following main features:

- cyclic loading of test samples;
- oscillating movement of test samples with separation of the contacting surfaces during backward motion (unidirectional movement is also possible);
- appropriate force-movement timing;
- controlled ambient conditions;
- possibility of measurement and recording of normal loading and frictional force.

One of the unique features of the tribometer is the manner in which the loading is coupled with sample movement. Typically, a half-sine cyclic loading is used, i.e. due to the symmetrical shape of loading the maximal force corresponds to the middle of the sliding stroke. However, as reported by Kohyama et al. (2004), during mastication the force curve is asymmetric and the maximum force is reached at 59–67% of the whole occlusion time. That finding corresponds with the results obtained by Condone and Ferracane (1997), who found that the chewing force is increased at the end of the chewing stroke. An important consequence is that different mechanisms of wear can be observed along the contact tooth area. In the presented tribometer, due to programmable loading, appropriate force-movement timing is possible, i.e. test conditions are close to the oral conditions.

Published by Woodhead Publishing Limited, 2013

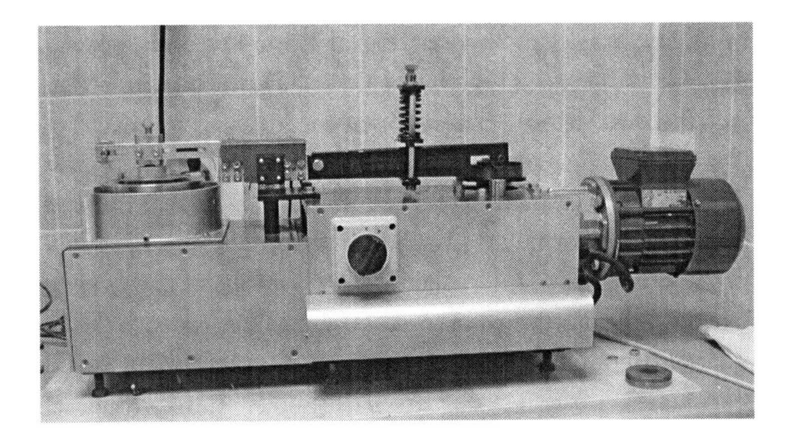

Figure 8.3 General view of the tribometer.

More details referring to the tribometer utilized for friction and wear studies of human tooth enamel presented in this chapter are available in the author's previous publication (Sajewicz and Kulesza, 2007). A general view of the tribometer is shown in Figure 8.3.

8.4.2 Effect of loading mode

During friction a locally acting load varies due to the irregularity of contacting surfaces at the micro scale. Thus, despite the constant value of the load at the macro scale, locally variable loading occurs. This, in turn, leads to fatigue effects causing crack nucleation, its propagation and finally the appearance of wear debris. Some authors consider fatigue wear as a principal mechanism of wear occurring at moderate frictional conditions (Kragelski et al., 1982).

Fatigue wear effects accompanying friction become intensified when the external loading of a frictional couple has a cyclic form. Tribological experiments performed on various materials at cyclic loading showed that the wear rate

Published by Woodhead Publishing Limited, 2013

in this case was much higher than the rate revealed at steady load (Barbour et al., 1997; Hu et al., 1999). So far comparative studies of the tribological behavior of tooth enamel under different modes of loading have not been carried out, because it is generally assumed that cyclic loading intensifies the wear of enamel, as is the case for other materials (biomaterials). On the other hand, microscopic observations of the occlusal surfaces of human teeth do not show up symptoms of fatigue wear, although pits similar to those characterizing pitting wear, i.e. the fatigue wear occurring at rolling friction, are sometimes observed. However, it has been proved unequivocally in the literature (Teaford and Walker, 1984; Bonis and Virot, 2002; Organ et al., 2005) that the pits are of dietary origin. According to the above-mentioned literature sources, the pits are caused by hard particles present in consumed food.

This section presents the results of investigations regarding the influence of the loading mode on the tribological behavior of human tooth enamel. The study was performed using the tribometer described above. Enamel samples shaped into truncated cones were subjected to frictional action with disc countersamples made of amalgam. Detailed information concerning the preparation of the enamel samples and countersamples was given elsewhere (Sajewiczb, 2007). The main parameters of the investigations are presented in Table 8.2. The loading parameters were chosen on the basis of clinical data.

The results of the experiments are shown in Figure 8.4. The volume wear of enamel samples is expressed as a function of the applied initial contact pressure. Here, the contact pressure is used in order to normalize the load due to some differences in initial diameters of the enamel samples. The relationships between the initial contact pressure and the wear are described in an exponential model for the steady

Published by Woodhead Publishing Limited, 2013

Table 8.2 **Conditions for investigation on the influence of loading mode on the tribological behavior of human enamel**

Enamel samples	Shape	Truncated cone
	Quantity	54
Countersample	Shape	Disc
	Material	Dispersalloy amalgam
Parameters	Countersample movement	Unidirectional rotation
	Frictional radius	5 mm
	Sliding speed	5.2 mm/s
	Cyclic loading contact pressure	Mean: 8.5–47.4 MPa
	Steady load contact pressure	6.5–43.3 MPa
	Duration of a single measurement	3 h
Environment	Type	Physiologic saline
	Temperature	Room temperature (20–22 °C)

loading mode and in a linear model for cyclic loading. On the basis of the results obtained from the regression analysis, it can be stated that the load explains 54% of the variability of the enamel wear (the coefficient of determination R^2 = 0.54, attained significance level $p < 0.05$) when steady loading is applied and only 8.5% when cyclic loading is used.

An important conclusion can be drawn on the basis of the obtained experimental results – for the assumed range of contact pressure, i.e. up to nearly 50 MPa, unlike the wear at steady loading, the wear at cyclic loading practically does not depend on the value of the contact pressure. This means that the tooth enamel better 'accepts' cyclic loading than steady loading. This finding is unexpected because for the majority of materials subjected to friction it is the opposite. On the other hand, typically, oral loading conditions have a cyclic form and thus the results can be treated as a proof of

Published by Woodhead Publishing Limited, 2013

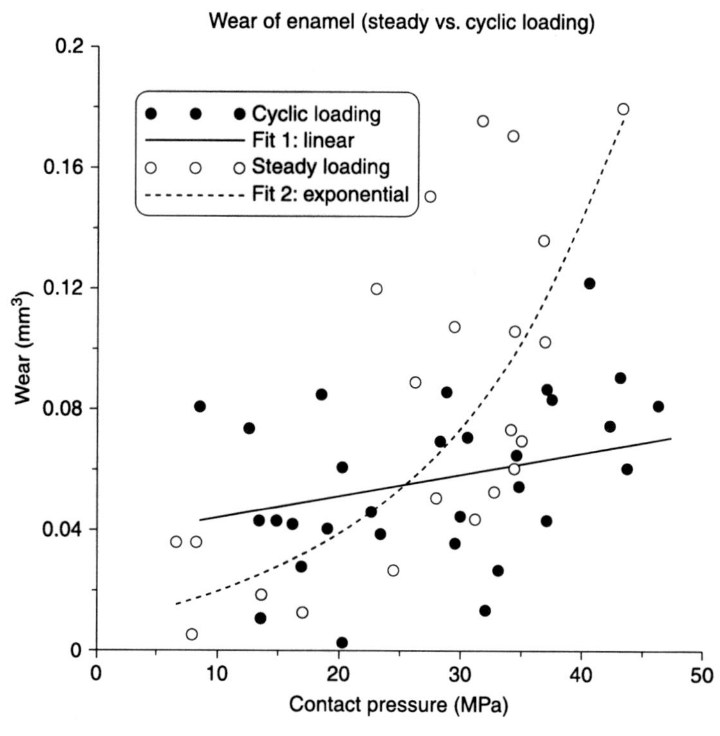

Figure 8.4 **Volume wear of enamel obtained at steady and cycling loading (mean values of the contact pressure are given for cyclic loading).**

the adaptation of enamel to the oral conditions. In other words, tooth enamel appears to fulfill a tailor-made material function (Weiner et al, 2000).

For a better understanding of the processes occurring on enamel surfaces during sliding, scanning electron microscopy (SEM) examinations of worn surfaces for both steady and cyclic loading have been performed (Figure 8.5). The micrographs show some typical surface topography formed during the wear experiments. However, the differences are not evident and thus it can be stated that the loading form does not affect the wear mechanism. Energy dispersive X-ray spectroscopy (EDS) spectra of the enamel surfaces (not

Published by Woodhead Publishing Limited, 2013

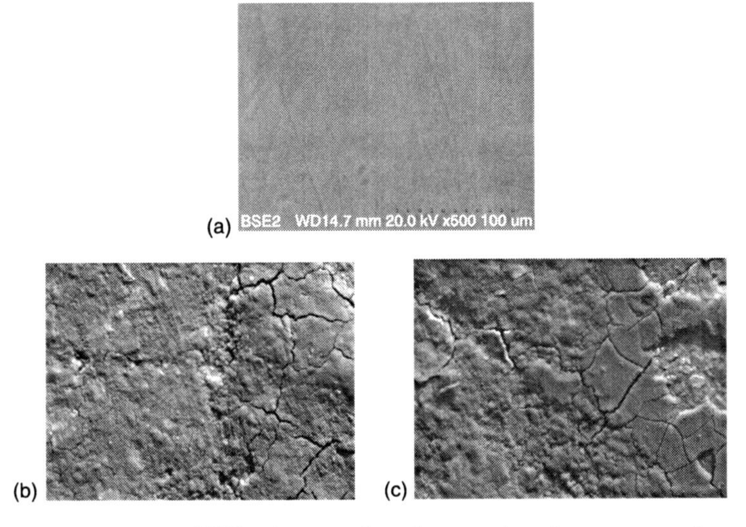

Figure 8.5 SEM micrographs of enamel surfaces worn at different loading modes: (a) before testing (original magnification ×500), (b) after testing at steady loading (original magnification ×800) and (c) after testing at cyclic loading (original magnification ×800).

presented here) did not show differences in the chemical constitution of surface layers obtained for both forms of loading. Hence, the nature of the tribological behavior of the tooth enamel at different loading forms remains an open question.

8.4.3 Effect of enamel microhardness

Hardness is one of the principal quantities characterizing the mechanical properties of any material and because of this it is also often analyzed in tribological studies. Microhardness, i.e. hardness measured at the micro scale, is widely examined in tribological experiments performed to study problems analyzed by the dental community. For instance, in many

Published by Woodhead Publishing Limited, 2013

studies concerning dental materials it is assumed that their mechanical properties should be close to those possessed by tooth hard tissues and microhardness appears to be the key parameter determining resistance to wear of those materials. However, available data are often contradictory, since some authors obtained a strong correlation between the wear resistance and hardness of restorative materials (Mandikos et al., 2001; Zheng et al., 2005), whereas other authors indicated the lack of the correlation (Chadwick et al., 1990; Yap et al., 1999).

The role of hardness in the tribological behavior of the enamel has rarely been studied. However, the ambiguity of opinions regarding tooth enamel and dental materials likewise is clearly visible. The problem is even more complicated due to inhomogeneity of enamel, which causes microhardness values dependent on a measurement location. As a result, different conclusions are presented by different authors. Furthermore, even the same authors sometimes present diverse opinions in their different publications. Among others, Zhou and Zheng (2006a) concluded that the wear resistance of tooth enamel decreases towards dentine and related that fact to the decreasing hardness of enamel in that direction. On the other hand, in another work (Zhou and Zheng, 2006b) the same authors formulated their conclusion less radically, namely: 'It is implied that microhardness is not the only influencing factor on the friction and wear behavior of human teeth.'

Analyzing the literature data referring to the influence of hardness on the tribology of tooth enamel, it is clearly seen that the wear and friction behavior in this case is mostly dependent on the conditions under which tribological processes occur. In this section that opinion is verified by comparing the results obtained during two types of investigations: the first was carried out without induced

Published by Woodhead Publishing Limited, 2013

abrasive wear and the other was performed under abrasive wear conditions. The enamel samples were obtained from freshly extracted human premolars of orthodontic patients. Two kinds of enamel samples were prepared from the extracted teeth. For the first type of the experiments the samples were shaped into truncated cones, whereas for the second type the extracted teeth were embedded in plastic rings using bone cement, and both cusps of each tooth were ground flat and polished down to approximately 0.5 mm. Figure 8.6 shows an enamel sample and a diamond bur used as a countersample prepared for the second type of experiment.

Microhardness of the enamel samples was measured after completing tribological tests and six measurements for each cusp were carried out close to the wear track. The mean values were then calculated. The main parameters and conditions of the experiments are presented in Tables 8.3 and 8.4.

The results of the investigations are presented in Figures 8.7 and 8.8. It is clearly seen that no dependence exists between the Vickers microhardness of enamel and its wear when a non-abrasive mechanism of enamel wear dominates. This

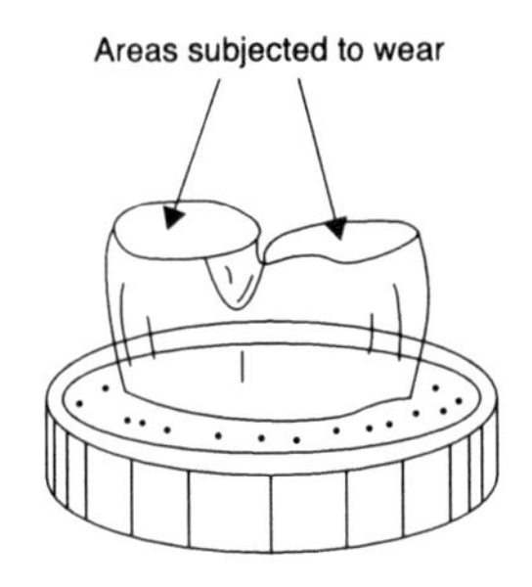

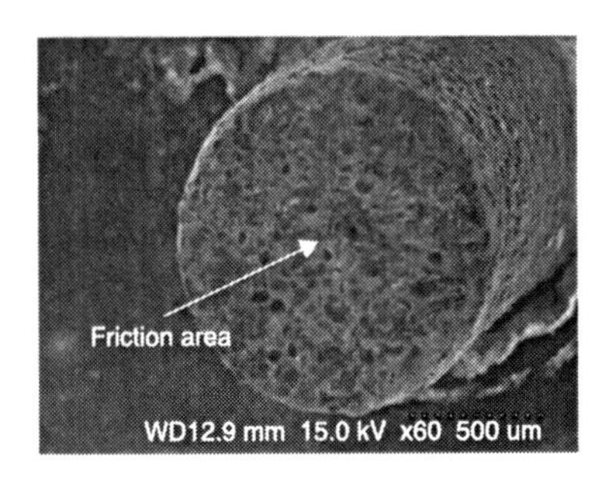

Figure 8.6 Drawing of an enamel sample prepared for tribological tests and photograph of a diamond dental bur as a countersample.

Published by Woodhead Publishing Limited, 2013

Table 8.3 **Conditions for investigation of the influence of microhardness of enamel on its tribological behavior – non-abrasive wear**

Enamel samples	Shape	Truncated cone
	Quantity	31
Countersample	Shape	Disc
	Material	Dispersalloy amalgam
Parameters	Countersample movement	Unidirectional rotation
	Radius of friction	5 mm
	Sliding speed	5.2 mm/s
	Loading	Cyclic sine loading
	Contact pressure	Mean: 9.0 MPa
	Duration of a single test	3 h
Environment	Media	Physiologic saline
	Temperature	Room temperature (20–22 °C)

Table 8.4 **Conditions for investigation of the influence of microhardness of the enamel on its tribological behavior – abrasive wear**

Enamel samples	Shape	According to Figure 8.6
Countersample	Quantity	11
	Shape	Diamond dental bur of diameter 1 mm
Parameters	Countersample movement	Oscillating
	Length of a wear track	~ 2 mm
	Sliding speed	Mean: 3.3 mm/s
	Loading	Cyclic half-sine loading
	Contact pressure	0–50 MPa
	Duration of a single test	5 min (500 cycles)
Environment	Media	Human saliva; viscosity: 3.0 mPas
	Temperature	Room temperature (20–22 °C)

Published by Woodhead Publishing Limited, 2013

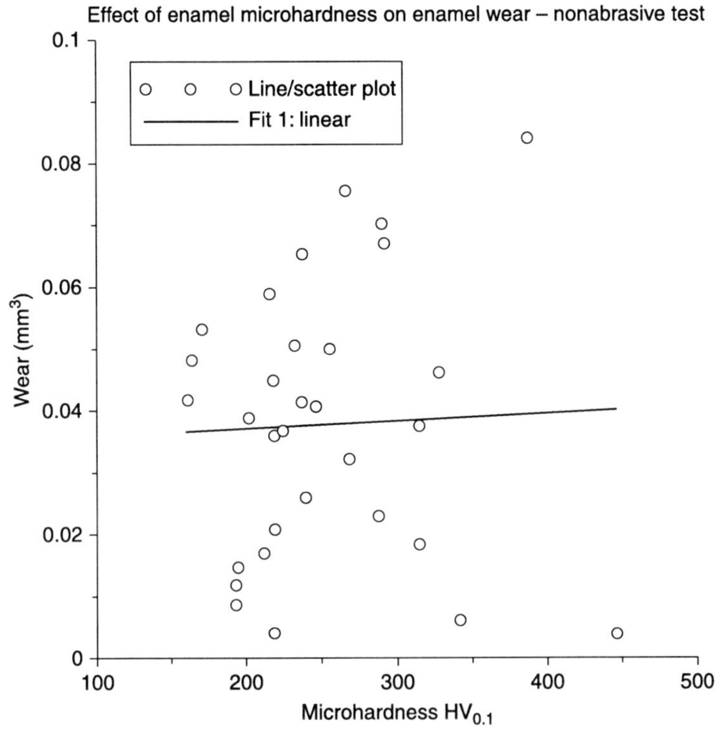

Figure 8.7 **Effect of enamel microhardness on enamel wear – non-abrasive test.**

fact is also confirmed by the results of statistical analysis, i.e. the coefficient of determination calculated for the linear regression model showed $R^2 = 0.0015$.

The results obtained after completion of the tests using the diamond bur indicate a strong correlation between the enamel wear and its hardness. A polynomial regression line was the best fit to the wear v. hardness data. The coefficient of determination was $R^2 = 0.68$ at a significance level $p < 0.05$.

In order to help interpret the results of the tribological tests, SEM observations and elemental mapping of the enamel surfaces were performed (Figures 8.9 and 8.10). The

Published by Woodhead Publishing Limited, 2013

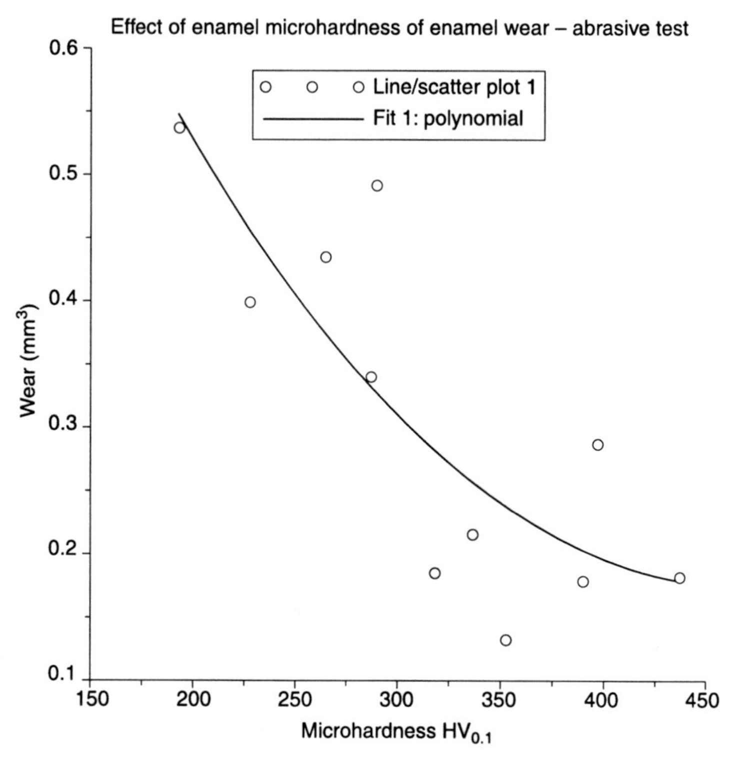

Figure 8.8 Effect of enamel microhardness on enamel wear – abrasive test.

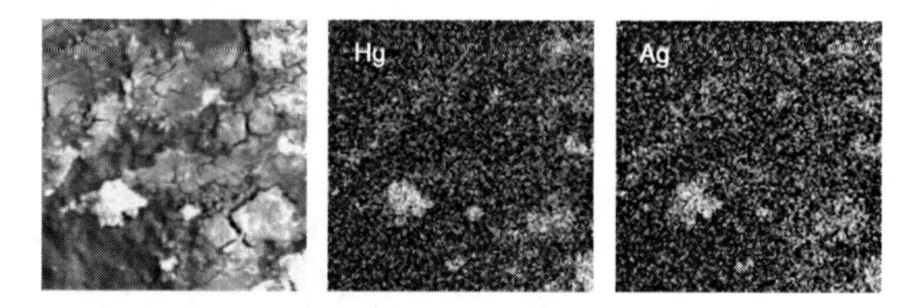

Figure 8.9 SEM microphotographs of enamel topography formed during non-abrasive wear (original magnification ×800) and distribution of amalgam elements on worn surface.

Published by Woodhead Publishing Limited, 2013

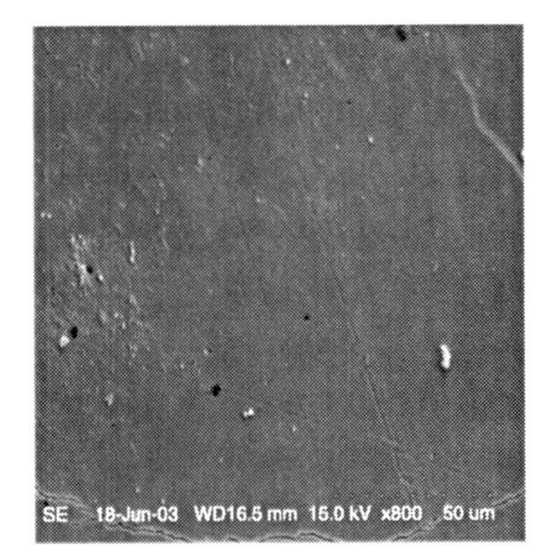

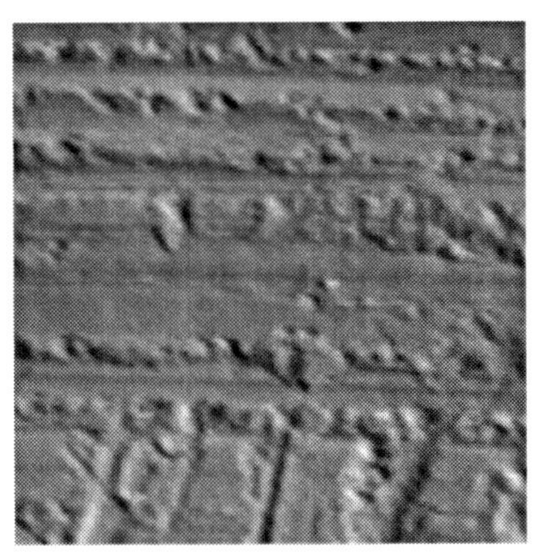

Figure 8.10 SEM microphotographs of enamel topography before tribological tests (left) and after abrasive wear (right) (original magnification ×800).

SEM micrographs show substantial differences in the surface topography constituted during different tribological experiments. The typical surface topography formed during the first type of experiments (nonabrasive wear) is characterized by thin superficial layers and uncovered intact enamel from where the layers have been detached (Figure 8.9). Furthermore, the elemental mapping showed increased concentrations of Hg and Ag, i.e. elements of amalgam composition. This means that mass transfer from the countersample occurs, and thus the superficial layers are formed with the participation of countersample matter in that process. A microphotograph of the enamel surface taken after the abrasive test is presented in Figure 8.10. Deep scratches characterizing intense destruction of the enamel are visible. Additional EDS examinations (not presented here) showed no changes in chemical composition of the outer layers of the enamel samples.

Summarizing the results, it can be stated that the influence of enamel microhardness on its wear essentially depends on the wear mechanism, which in turn depends mainly on

Published by Woodhead Publishing Limited, 2013

external conditions of the tribological investigation. If there are no hard abrasive particles in the friction area, transformed enamel superficial layers will appear. Hence, the tribological behavior of tooth enamel depends on the properties of those layers and the initial enamel microhardness plays a minor role. However, if abrasive wear occurs there are no possibilities to form protective superficial layers. As a result, material loss has a mechanical nature with no participation of physical and chemical processes. Thus, in this case bulk enamel properties are decisive – the wear depends on enamel microhardness. This statement is not only valid for tooth enamel, but it was also confirmed for other materials (Zum Gahr, 1998).

8.4.4 Effect of counterbody material

It is well known that material aspects may play a fundamental role in the course of tribological processes. Although friction and wear are not directly correlated with the properties of bulk material, materials-related aspects may influence the tribological behavior considerably (Chichos et al., 1995). The above means that tribological behavior of any material depends also on the material association of the friction pair. It is valid in relation to both engineering and biological materials. Thus, due to the system's dependence, tribological behavior of tooth enamel should also be determined by the material of a contacting body. During tribological testing of the tooth enamel the countersamples made of different materials are used up, so that it is reasonable to pay more attention to this problem.

Frictional interactions may cause substantial changes in the outer layers of enamel, which can be examined *post factum* by means of different analytical methods, providing us with information useful to reconstruct the course of tribological processes. Further, principal changes induced

Published by Woodhead Publishing Limited, 2013

during these processes in the superficial layer of the enamel associated with different materials are described. The material presented here has been extracted from different studies performed by the author. Additional information regarding the methodology of experiments conducted is available in another work by the author (Sajewicz, 2007b).

Enamel–enamel pair

Microscopic images of changes in the surface topography of tooth enamel induced under oral conditions (*in vivo*) are quite often presented in the literature. Most of the publications are located in the paleontological literature and are related to analysis of so-called 'microwear'. This term refers to pits and scratches created on tooth surfaces during oral food processing. The microwear analysis is used mostly for examinations of extinct and extant species (King et al., 1999). On the basis of the results obtained during such studies it is possible, among others, to reconstruct a diet. The surface studies of natural teeth are usually restricted to morphological analyses and hardly ever refer to chemical or physical features. Much more comprehensive studies of tooth surfaces are possible after *in vitro* tribological testing. Unlike *in vivo* conditions the parameters of *in vitro* testing can be controlled, which offers researchers an opportunity to associate the observations of changes induced in the superficial tooth layer with the general conditions of the tribological investigations.

Figure 8.11 presents examples of the enamel surface topography constituted in the course of *in vitro* testing of enamel–enamel connections using two lubricating media, i.e. human and artificial saliva. Although both enamel surfaces were formed after contacting with enamel countersamples, the differences in the topographies are evident. The surface displayed in Figure 8.11(a) is smoother and the enamel prisms

Published by Woodhead Publishing Limited, 2013

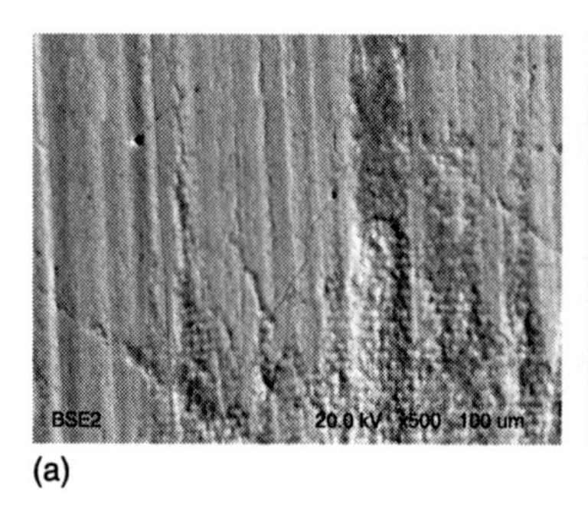

(a)

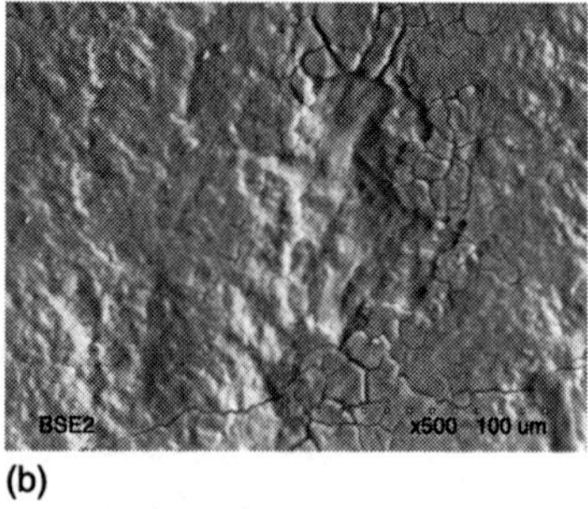

(b)

Figure 8.11 SEM micrographs of enamel surfaces formed after testing of an enamel–enamel frictional pair: (a) after testing in human saliva and (b) after testing in artificial saliva (original magnification ×500).

are clearly seen. Similar images are sometimes visible when tooth surface topography formed in the oral environment is observed (Ungar et al., 2006). When artificial saliva is utilized as a lubricating medium the different surface topography of enamel can be seen (Figure 8.11b), i.e. the enamel surface is covered by a surface thin film containing a network of cracks. The images presented in Figure 8.11 suggest that the presence of natural saliva in a tribological contact area leads to the predominance of plastic properties of the formed superficial enamel layers, whereas artificial saliva causes the formation of more brittle enamel surface layers.

EDS spectra acquired from the worn surfaces provides interesting additional information. It is surprising that no differences in the chemical composition of the outer surface of enamel are found while comparing the spectra obtained before and after tribological testing in the human saliva environment (Figure 8.12). In contrast, some demineralization of enamel occurs during testing in an artificial saliva environment, as the EDS spectra indicate a decrease of Ca and P contents (Figure 8.13).

Published by Woodhead Publishing Limited, 2013

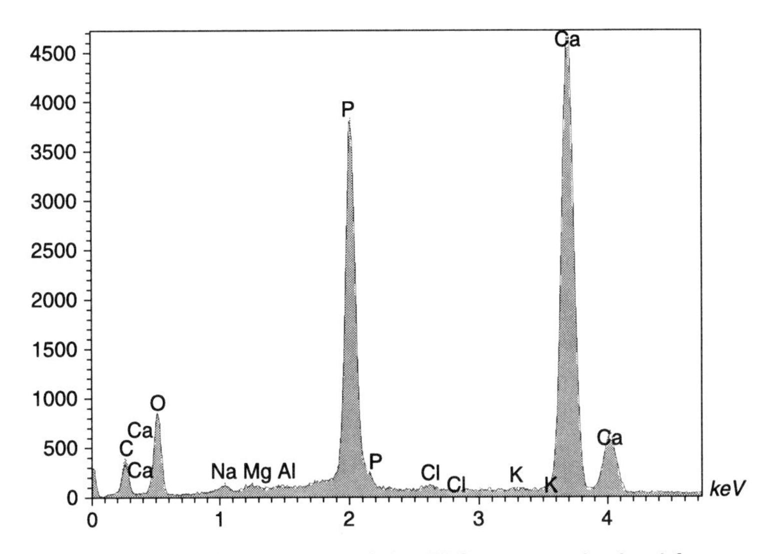

Figure 8.12 Comparison of the EDS spectra obtained from the enamel surface before (filled spectrum) and after (line) tribological testing in human saliva environment.

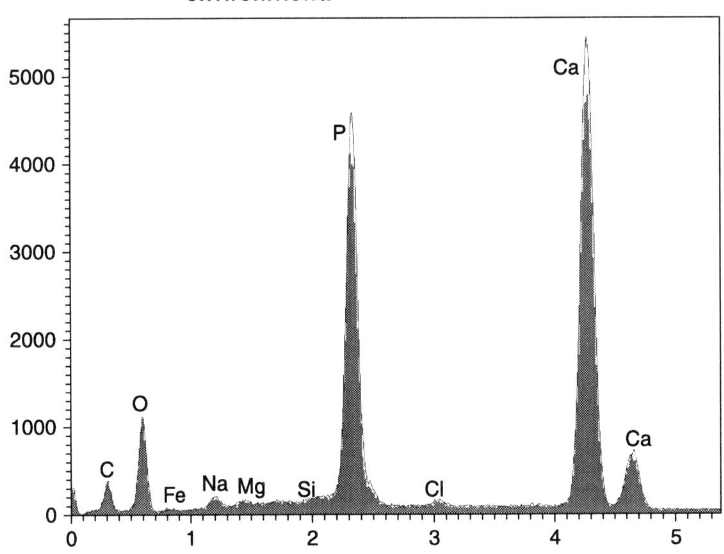

Figure 8.13 Comparison of the EDS spectra obtained from the enamel surface before (line) and after (filled spectrum) tribological testing in artificial saliva environment.

Published by Woodhead Publishing Limited, 2013

Enamel–steel pair

Metallic countersamples are quite often utilized for tribological testing of the tooth enamel. A Ti ball was used by Zheng et al. (2003) to investigate the influence of microstructure orientation of tooth enamel on its tribological behavior. The same methodology was also used by Zheng and Zhou (2006b) to study friction and wear behavior of enamel samples collected from donors of different ages, and to investigate the tribological behavior of tooth enamel in the presence of food particles in the friction area (Zheng and Zhou, 2007). Steel countersamples were used by some researchers for tribological characterization of tooth enamel (De Gee and Pallav, 1994; Willems et al., 1992; Li and Zhou, 2002; Shortall et al., 2002). In some approaches the choice of steel as a countersample material is valid if one takes into account that stainless steel is used to fabricate orthodontic and prosthodontic devices contacting directly with teeth, unlike Ti.

Figure 8.14 shows SEM images of worn enamel surfaces after testing with 316 LVM steel countersamples obtained at

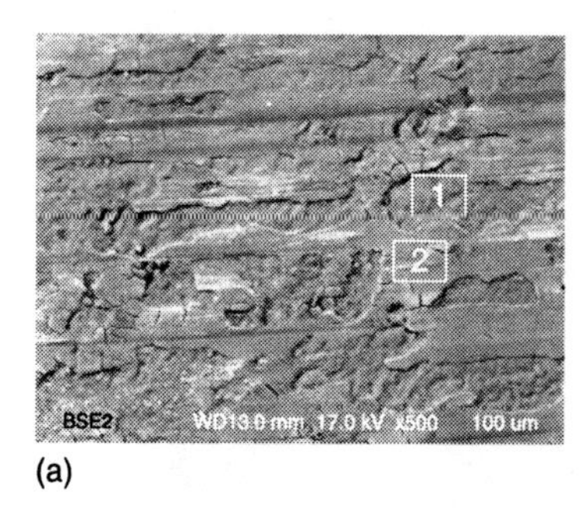

(a)

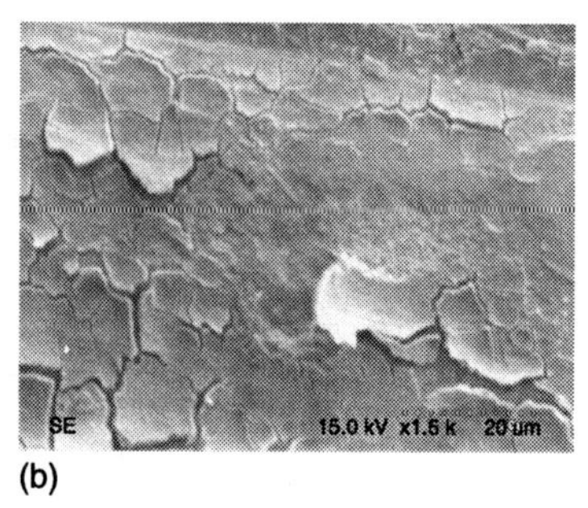

(b)

Figure 8.14 SEM micrographs of enamel surfaces obtained after testing an enamel–stainless steel pair: (a) magnification ×500 (numbers indicate the areas where EDS examination was performed) and (b) magnification ×1500.

Published by Woodhead Publishing Limited, 2013

different magnifications. A typical surface topography formed during the tests shows a thin superficial film and locally uncovered intact enamel from where the film has been detached. It is evident that some transformation of the outer enamel occurs when sliding against the stainless steel countersample and a new structure emerges. Further delamination of the film proceeds and finally, after its defragmentation, wear debris is produced.

The comparative EDS analysis (Figure 8.15) of different regions of the worn enamel surfaces revealed substantial differences between those regions, i.e. presence of Cr, Fe, increased concentration of O, and decreased concentrations of Ca and P in superficial thin film (denoted 2 in Figure 8.14) compared with uncovered intact enamel (denoted 1 in Figure 8.14). This means that material transfer from the metallic countersample towards the enamel samples and simultaneous demineralization of the enamel occur.

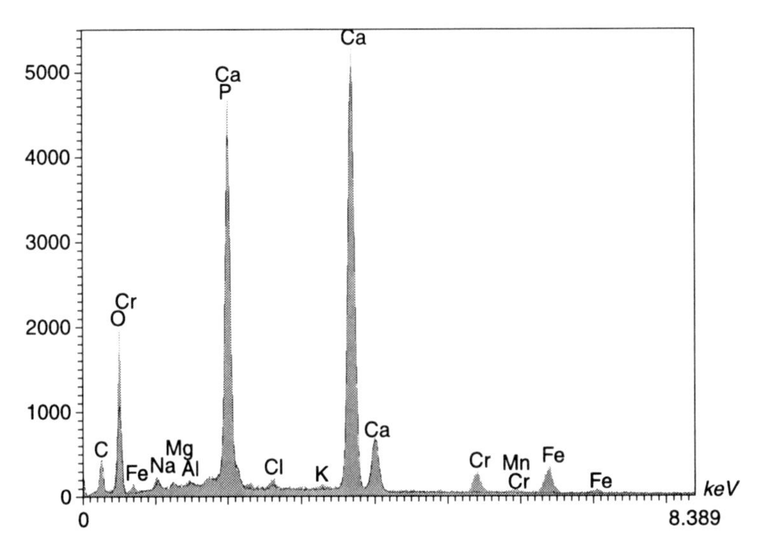

Figure 8.15 Comparison of the EDS spectra obtained from area denoted 1 (line) and 2 (filled spectrum) in Figure 8.14.

Published by Woodhead Publishing Limited, 2013

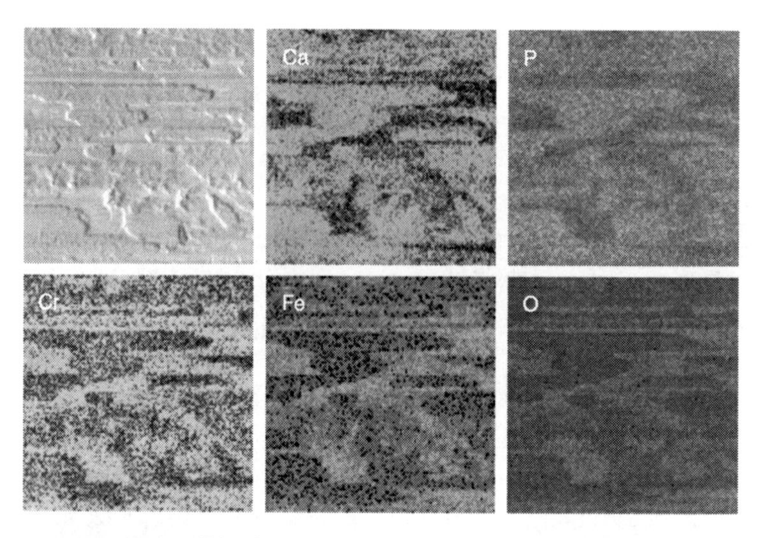

Figure 8.16 Distribution of elements on worn enamel surface obtained after sliding enamel against stainless steel.

The elemental mapping (Figure 8.16) confirmed the aforementioned finding. However, image inversion is noticeable, i.e. areas with increased contents of O, Fe and Cr (bright regions) correspond to decreased content of Ca and P (dark regions). Furthermore, increased O content in the film indicates possible oxidation of the tribologically transformed layers.

Enamel–dental composite pair

Nowadays, restorative dentistry appears to be one of the most developing areas of medical care, principally connected with the commonness of dental caries. The most popular materials for restoring cavities are light-curing composite resins. Dental composites are still being improved and it is commonly accepted that their properties should match those of tooth enamel. It is expected that restorative composites

Published by Woodhead Publishing Limited, 2013

should not only enable us to make highly wear-resistant occluding surfaces, but should not cause simultaneous excessive wear or corrosion-wear on the opposing structures (Lambrechts et al., 2006).

Tooth enamel–dental material connection is often the subject of tribological investigations; enamel is used mainly as a physiological standard with which composite resins are compared (Lambrechts et al., 2006). However, the influence of dental composites on the tribological behavior of tooth enamel is not frequently studied. Here, some results of SEM and EDS analysis of enamel surfaces previously subjected to wear in contact with several dental resins are presented. The exemplary SEM micrographs are shown in Figure 8.17. The enamel surface topographies are very similar despite some

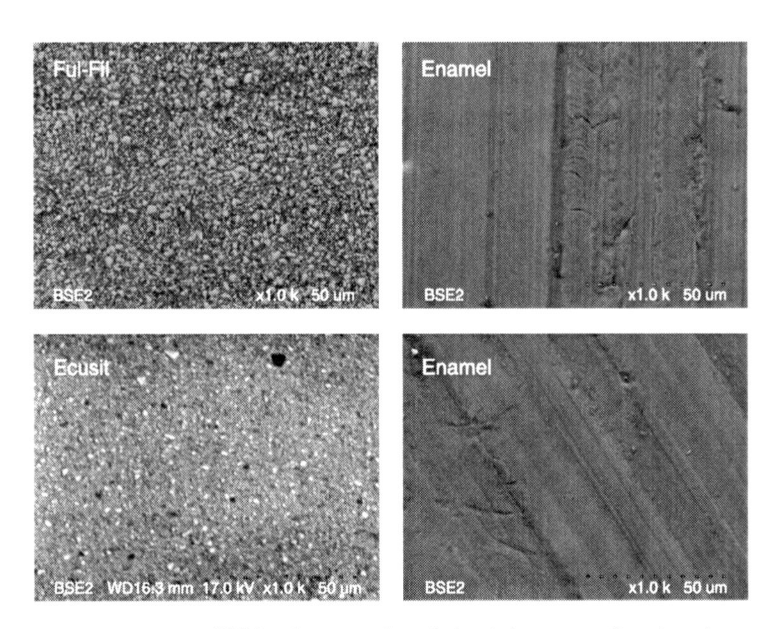

Figure 8.17 SEM micrographs of dental composite structure and surface topographies of the worn enamel samples used in the study (original magnification ×1000).

Published by Woodhead Publishing Limited, 2013

structural differences between composite materials used. Namely, Ful-Fil (Caulk/Dentsply, USA) restorative material has filler sizes in the range of 0.04–5.0 μm whilst filler sizes of Ecusite composite (DMG, Germany) range from 0.02 to 1.5 μm. Furthermore, microscratches similar to those obtained after sliding against enamel countersamples (Figure 8.11a) are seen on both enamel surfaces. No surface films are visible on the enamel surfaces.

EDS spectra were taken from the enamel surfaces after testing in order to acquire additional information about the changes that occurred in superficial enamel layers. Basically, no changes in chemical composition of the outer enamel layer are observed regardless of the type of the composite materials used. Figure 8.18 presents one of the EDS spectra.

The whole experimental material presented above demonstrates the variety of the changes occurring in tooth

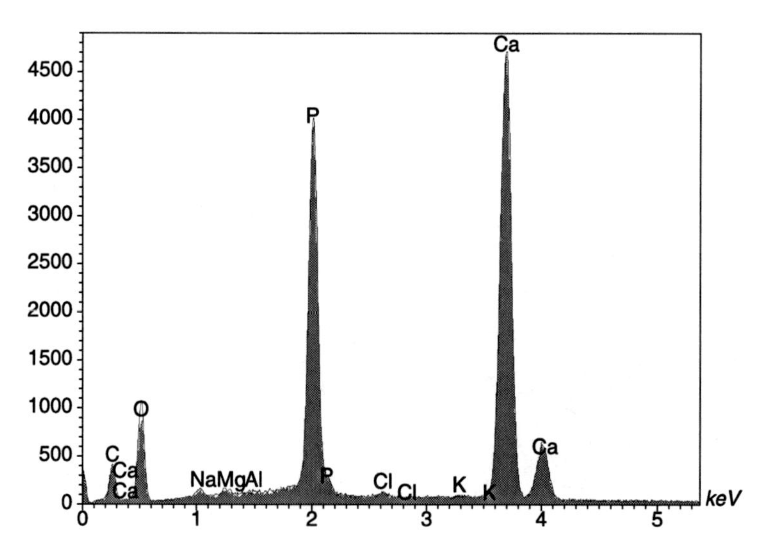

Figure 8.18 Comparison of the EDS spectra obtained from the enamel surface before (filled spectrum) and after (line) sliding against Ful-Fil composite material.

Published by Woodhead Publishing Limited, 2013

enamel that underwent frictional interactions. It is reasonable to expect that there are significant associations between the types of the mentioned changes and tribological parameters such as the coefficient of friction (friction force) and the wear rate. The relevant tribological data are presented in Table 8.5. Some explanation is indispensable here before studying the data included in Table 8.5. As tribological experiments described in this chapter were performed under different conditions, e.g. load, sliding speed, sample contact area, etc., and were different in separate investigations, some normalization of the data obtained is required. In the author's papers (Sajewicz, 2006, 2010) it was shown that the specific wear energy, i.e. the friction dissipated energy referred to the wear, can be successfully used to evaluate wear resistance of hard tooth tissues and dental materials. The energy approach also allows us to describe the tribological behavior of the tested material more comprehensively, as the specific wear energy is a parameter including contemporaneously frictional and wear components of a tribological process.

Comparison of the calculated values of specific wear energy showed their dependence on conditions under which the tests were performed. The results also confirmed a general principle – there are no 'tribological properties of a material'

Table 8.5 **Specific wear energy calculated for tooth enamel tested on different materials**

Frictional pair	Environment	Specific wear energy (J/mm^3)
Enamel–enamel	Human saliva	$0.6–1.2 \times 10^5$
Enamel–enamel	Artificial saliva	3.2×10^5
Enamel–dental restorative material	Artificial saliva	$0.7–3.2 \times 10^4$
Enamel–steel 316 LVM	Artificial saliva	5.0×10^4
Enamel–diamond dental bur	Human saliva	1.8×10^1

Source: On the basis of data published by Sajewicz, 2007b.

because tribological behavior of any material is in fact 'a systems property', which should be referred to the system structure, i.e. elements with their properties and the relations between them. Taking the above-mentioned into account, it can be stated that much more energy is needed to remove a volume unit of the enamel surface while testing the enamel–enamel couple in the human saliva environment than for other systems used in the study. Thus, we can conclude that the natural system composed of the enamel–enamel couple and the saliva lubricant is optimally matched with regard to tribology behavior.

It is clearly seen when analyzing the results that the intensity of the wear process can be associated with the wear mechanism; however, such connections are not trivial. For instance, when EDS analysis is used in order to recognize specificity of the wear process, similar results are obtained for two tests. However, the calculated values of specific wear energy for these tests can be substantially different, e.g. when comparing the results obtained for enamel coupled with enamel and with a diamond dental bur tested in human saliva. Thus, more sensitive tools are required for a better understanding of the processes occurring on enamel surfaces. Preliminary investigations of a worn enamel surface performed by the author have brought encouraging results. It was shown by using X-ray diffraction that a 2-μm thick superficial enamel layer constituted after sliding against enamel contained defragmented hydroxyapatite crystallites with a specific privileged orientation (Sajewicz, 2007b).

8.5 Concluding remarks

Friction and wear behavior of tooth enamel is very complex and that complexity depends on many factors, such as the

Published by Woodhead Publishing Limited, 2013

structure and properties of the enamel, input parameters (load, sliding speed, temperature), properties of the counterbody, content and properties of the environment, etc. Characteristically, in the oral environment the ranges of the parameters influencing friction and wear of enamel are broad, and a huge variety of parameter combinations is present. It can be presumed that perfect tribological behavior of enamel under these complex conditions is linked to its particular adaptive properties. Some aspects of the adaptive behavior of tooth enamel have been described in this work.

The tribological response of tooth enamel to certain conditions is often very specific, which was ascertained, among others, while studying the effect of loading mode on the wear rate of enamel. Lower wear rate obtained at cycling loading compared with steady loading confirms the adaptive properties of enamel, as cycling loading is dominant in oral conditions.

A lack of dependence between enamel hardness and its wear resistance, which holds true under 'normal conditions', shows another example of enamel adaptability, as this tissue still presents good wear resistance even at decreased hardness.

Adaptability of tribological systems is well known (Kostetsky, 1992). One of the main features of the adaptability is the creation of the so-called 'dissipative structures' on friction surfaces. These structures contain transformed original material that is a result of conversion of the external friction energy into the energy of internal processes. The most often observed dissipative structures contain components of the counterbodies and/or components of the environment. Such structures were probably observed after enamel sliding against the metal or the amalgam countersamples. On the other hand, from a tribological

Published by Woodhead Publishing Limited, 2013

point of view, the most effective structures formed on the enamel surface were found while testing the enamel–enamel couple and the structures contained no external components. It can be hypothesized that enamel is able to form unique dissipative structures and that the formation is based on the changes of its crystalline structures. Further studies are indispensible to confirm that hypothesis.

8.6 References

Barbour P S M, Barton D C and Fisher J (1997), 'The influence of stress conditions on the wear of UHMWPE', *J. Mater. Sci. Mater. Med.*, **8**: 603–611.

Bonis L and Virot L (2002), 'Teeth and paleoanthropology', *Connect. Tissue Res.*, **43**: 87–93.

Brès E F and Hutchison J L (2002), 'Surface structure study of biological calcium phosphate apatite crystals from human tooth enamel', *J. Biomed. Mater. Res. (Appl. Biomater.)*, **63**: 433–440.

Chadwick R G, McCabe J F and Walls A W G (1990), 'The effect of storage media upon of surface microhardness and abrasion resistance of three composites', *Dent. Mater.*, **6**: 123–128.

Chichos H, Klaffke D, Santner E and Woydt M (1995), 'Advances in tribology: material point of view', *Wear*, **190**: 155–161.

Condone J R and Ferracane J L (1997), '*In vitro* wear of composite with varied cure, filler level, and filler treatment', *J. Dent. Res.*, **76**: 1405–1411.

Cuy J L, Mann A B, Livi K J, Teaford M F and Weihs T P (2002), 'Nanoindentation mapping of the mechanical properties of human molar tooth enamel', *Arch. Oral Biol.*, **47**: 281–291.

Published by Woodhead Publishing Limited, 2013

DeGee A J and Pallav P (1994), 'Occlusal wear simulation with ACTA wear machine', *J. Dent.*, **22** (suppl. 1): S21–S27.

DeLong R and Douglas W H (1991), 'An artificial oral environment for testing dental materials', *IEEE Trans. Biomed. Eng.*, **38**: 339–345.

Eisenburger M, Shellis R P and Addy M (2003), 'Comparative studies of wear of enamel induced by alternating and simultaneous combination of abrasion and erosion *in vitro*', *Caries Res.*, **37**: 450–455.

Guidoni G M, Swain M V and Jäger I (2009), 'Wear behavior of dental enamel at the nanoscale with a sharp and blunt indenter tip', *Wear*, **266**: 60–68.

Hu X, Harrington E, Marquis P M and Shortall A C (1999), 'The influence of cyclic loading on the wear of a dental composite', *Biomaterials*, **20**: 206–212.

King T, Aiello L C and Andrews P (1999), 'Dental microwear of *Griphopitecus alpani*', *J. Hum. Evol.*, **36**: 3–31.

Koenigswald W v and Sander P M (1997), 'Glossary of terms used for enamel microstructures', in: Koenigswald W v and Sander P M (eds), *Tooth Enamel Microstructure*, pp. 267–280. Rotterdam: Balkema.

Kohyama K, Hatakeyama E, Sasaki T, Haruka D, Azuma T et al. (2004), 'Effects of sample hardness on human chewing force; a model study using silicone rubber', *Arch. Oral Biol.*, **49**: 805–816.

Kostetsky B I (1992), 'The structural-energetic concept in theory friction and wear (synergism and self-organization)', *Wear*, **159**: 1–15.

Kragelski I V, Dobychin M N and Kombalov V S (1982), *Friction and Wear – Calculation Methods*. Oxford: Pergamon.

Lambrechts P, Goovaerts K, Bharadwaj D, De Munck J, Bergmans L et al. (2006), 'Degradation of tooth

Published by Woodhead Publishing Limited, 2013

structure and restorative materials: a review', *Wear*, **261**: 980–986.

Li H, Zhou Z R (2002), 'Wear behaviour of human teeth in dry and artificial saliva conditions', *Wear*, **249**: 980–984.

Low I-M (2004), 'Depth-profiling of crystal structure, texture, and microhardness in a functionally graded tooth enamel', *J. Am. Ceram. Soc.*, **87**: 2125–2131.

Mandikos M N, McGivney G P, Davis E, Bush P J and Carter J M (2001), 'A comparison of the wear resistance and hardness of indirect composite resins', *J. Prosthet. Dent.*, **85**: 386–395.

Organ J M, Teaford M F and Larson C S (2005), 'Dietary inferences from dental occlusion microwear at mission San Luis de Apalachee', *Am. J. Phys. Anthrop.*, **128**: 801–811.

Rho J-Y, Kuhn-Spearing L and Zioupos P (1998), 'Mechanical properties and the hierarchical structure of bone', *Med. Eng. Phys.*, **20**: 92–102.

Sajewicz E (2006), 'On evaluation of wear resistance of tooth enamel and dental materials', *Wear*, **260**: 1256–1261.

Sajewicz E (2007a), 'Tribological behavior of human enamel in red wine and apple juice environments', *Wear*, **262**: 308–315.

Sajewicz E (2007b), *Tribological Approach to Human Organ Behavior*. Bialystok: Bialystok University of Technology (in Polish).

Sajewicz E (2009), 'Effect of saliva viscosity on tribological behavior of tooth enamel', *Tribol. Int.*, **42**: 327–332.

Sajewicz E (2010), 'A comparative study of tribological behavior of dental composites and tooth enamel: an energy approach', *Proc. IMechE J.*, **224**: 559–568.

Sajewicz E and Kulesza Z (2007), 'A new tribometer for friction and wear studies of dental materials and hard tooth tissues', *Tribol. Int.*, **40**: 885–895.

Published by Woodhead Publishing Limited, 2013

Sakae T, Suzuki K and Kozawa Y (1997), 'A short review of studies on chemical and physical properties of enamel crystallites', in: Koenigswald W v and Sander P M (eds), *Tooth Enamel Microstructure*, pp. 31–40. Rotterdam: Balkema.

Sander P M (1997), 'Non-mammalian synapsid enamel and the origin of mammalian enamel prisms: the bottom-up perspective', in: Koenigswald W v and Sander P M (eds), *Tooth Enamel Microstructure*, pp. 41–62. Rotterdam: Balkema.

Shimizu D, Macho G A and Spears I R (2005), 'Effect of prism orientation and loading direction on contact stresses in prismatic enamel of primates: implications for interpreting wear patterns', *Am. J. Phys. Anthropol.*, **126**: 427–434.

Shortall A C, Hu X Q, Marquis P M (2002), 'Potential countersample materials for in vitro simulation wear testing', *Dent Mater.*, **18**: 246–54.

Skobe Z and Stern S (1980), 'The pathway of enamel rods at the base of cusps of human enamel', *J. Dent. Res.*, **59**: 1026–1032.

Teaford M F and Walker C A (1984), 'A review of dental microwear and diet in modern mammals', *Scan. Microsc.*, **2**: 204–207.

Ungar P S, Grine P, Teaford M F and Zaatari S E (2006), 'Dental microwear and diets of African early *Homo*', *J. Hum. Evol.*, **50**: 78–95.

Vincent J F V (2006), 'Making a mechanical organism', *J. Bion. Eng.*, **3**: 43–58.

Weiner S, Addadi L and Wagner H D (2000), 'Materials design in biology', *Mater. Sci. Eng. C*, **11**: 1–8.

Willems G, Celis J P, Lambrechts P, Braem M, Roos J R, Vanherle G (1992) 'In vitro vibrational wear under small displacements of dental materials opposed to annealed chromium-steel counterbodies', *Dent Mater.*, **8**: 338–344.

Published by Woodhead Publishing Limited, 2013

Yamashita S, Hatch J P and Rugh J D (1999), 'Does chewing performance depend upon a specific masticatory pattern?', *J. Oral Rehabil.*, **26**: 547–553.

Yap A U J, Ong L F K L, Teoh S H and Hassings G W (1999), 'Comparative wear ranking of dental restorative material with the BIOMET wear simulator', *J. Oral Rehabil.*, **26**: 228–235.

Zheng J and Zhou Z R (2006a), 'Effect of age on the friction and wear behaviors of human teeth', *Tribol. Int.*, **39**: 266–273.

Zheng J and Zhou Z R (2006b), 'Oral tribology', *Proc. IMechE J.*, **220**: 739–754.

Zheng J and Zhou Z R (2007), 'Friction and wear behavior of human teeth under various wear conditions', *Tribol. Int.*, **40**: 278–284.

Zheng J, Sato Y, Ohkubo C and Hosoi T (2005), '*In vitro* wear of three types of composite resin denture teeth', *J. Prosthet. Dent.*, **94**: 453–457.

Zheng J, Zhou Z R, Hang H, Li H and Yu H Y (2003), 'On friction and wear behavior of human enamel and dentine', *Wear*, **255**: 967–974.

Zheng S Y, Zheng J, Gao S S, Yu B J, Yu H Y et al. (2011), 'Investigation on the microtribological behavior of human tooth enamel by nanoscratch', *Wear*, **271**: 2290–2296.

Zum Gahr K-H (1998), 'Wear by hard particles', *Tribol. Int.*, **31**: 587–596.

Published by Woodhead Publishing Limited, 2013

9

Liposome-based carrier systems and devices used for pulmonary drug delivery

Iftikhar Khan, Abdelbary Elhissi, Mahmood Shah, Mohamed Albed Alhnan and Waqar Ahmed, University of Central Lancashire, UK

DOI: 10.1533/9780857092205.395

Abstract: Liposomes are spherical lipid carrier vesicles that vary in size (typically in the range of 20 nm to 20 μm), and are composed of single or multi-concentric bilayers, and have the ability to entrap both hydrophilic therapeutic agents within their central aqueous core or lipophilic drugs within their bilayer compartment. These carriers can transport drugs to particular sites of action within the pulmonary system by employing specially designed delivery devices. These devices work through specific mechanisms and their performance depends upon the formulation. Dry powder inhalers deliver dry powdered formulations. By contrast, pressurized metered dose inhalers deliver liquid formulations when an appropriate liquefied propellant is included. However, nebulizers are capable of delivering aqueous suspensions or solutions with no need for inclusion of a propellant. Liposomes were first reported in 1965 and since then significant

Published by Woodhead Publishing Limited, 2013

developments in liposome research have emerged. Liposomes are now well established as carrier systems that accommodate therapeutic agents and deliver them to various sites in the body. Liposomes can sustain the release of the entrapped therapeutic materials, hence enhancing the therapeutic outcome. Liposome carrier systems have been studied extensively for prophylaxis against and the treatment of pulmonary diseases.

Key words: liposome, drug delivery, pulmonary disease, niosome, dry powder inhaler, pressurized meter dose inhaler, nebulizer

9.1 Introduction

The developments of new technologies and techniques in the field of pharmaceuticals and biotechnology have caused revolutionary changes over the last 10 years through the introduction of new therapeutic agents or drugs. However, most of these technologies are still being investigated for suitable application in drug delivery (Sharma and Sharma 1997). Scientists are trying to improve and invent novel methodologies and techniques for delivering drugs through the use of macromolecules (Johnson 1997). Respiratory diseases have been targeted by certain medicines to act locally, but these may also diffuse into the systemic circulation via the lungs, causing systemic adverse effects.

A survey on 40 diabetic patients was performed for self-injection of insulin and 75% of the patients showed anxiety during self-injection (Bashoff and Beaser 1995). Therefore, drug delivery systems that replace the need for needles are desirable, and these should be safe, reproducible and show

Published by Woodhead Publishing Limited, 2013

high bioavailability after administration (Johnson 1997). Although the oral route is possibly the most patient-friendly route, its prime limitation is the poor bioavailability of some drugs. This is due to first-pass hepatic inactivation, or degradation by enzymes or the pH environment within the gastrointestinal tract (GIT). To overcome the degradation in GIT, the lungs are one of the best options for drug delivery. The lung has a large surface area for drug absorption (i.e. the normal human adult lung has a surface area of more than $100\,m^2$) (Todo et al. 2004). Deposition of particles in the periphery of the tracheo-bronchial tree (TBT) may follow impaction, interception or sedimentation, depending on particle size and physiological conditions (Johnson 1997).

Phospholipid vesicles (liposomes) were first reported by Bangham et al. in 1965. They studied the chemistry of lipids and their relation to biological membranes (Bangham et al. 1965). There are different types of lipids that form the building blocks of biomembranes (Bergstrand 2003).

This liposomal derivation technology is an important component of bionanotechnology (LeDuc et al. 2007). Novel phospholipid liposomes and their characteristics of entrapping material offer numerous applications, including their use in cosmetics and pharmaceutical industries. When liposomes are inhaled, the non-irritant properties of phospholipids may ensure the delivery of therapeutic molecules with controlled release properties to the target area in the lung (Alsarra et al. 2005, Parthasarathy et al. 1999). The special property of a liposome is its ability to act as an amphiphile, which makes it vital in the field of nanotechnology and drug delivery (Bergstrand 2003). However, one limitation is the instability of liposomes due to oxidation and hydrolysis of the

Published by Woodhead Publishing Limited, 2013

phospholipids (Kensil and Dennis 1981, Riaz 1995, Vemuri and Rhodes 1995).

9.2 Composition and properties of liposomes

Liposomes mainly consist of phospholipids, which can be either derived from natural sources or synthesized in laboratories. Phospholipids play a fundamental role with their unique properties of being amphiphilic and their self-assembly to encapsulate therapeutic agents which can then be targeted to the lung via inhalation.

9.2.1 Phospholipids

Phospholipids play a major role in cell membranes. They generally consist of diglycerides, a phosphate group (a molecule of phosphoric acid) and an organic molecule (choline) (Figure 9.1). A diglyceride is a glyceride composed of two fatty acid chains that are covalently bound to a single glycerol molecule via an ester linkage. Glycerol ($C_3H_8O_3$), containing three hydroxyl groups (–OH), is responsible for the solubility of phospholipid molecules in water. Glycerol acts as a backbone by its attachment to both fatty acids (hydrocarbon) chains and a phosphate group (Vemuri and Rhodes 1995). Fatty acid molecules are either saturated or unsaturated and are insoluble in water. Thus, the phospholipid molecule is composed of a hydrophobic moiety comprising two fatty acid chains, and a hydrophilic head made of glycerol and phosphate. The bilayer structure is formed when the fatty acid moiety of one layer faces the fatty acid moiety of another layer and the head groups face the water.

Published by Woodhead Publishing Limited, 2013

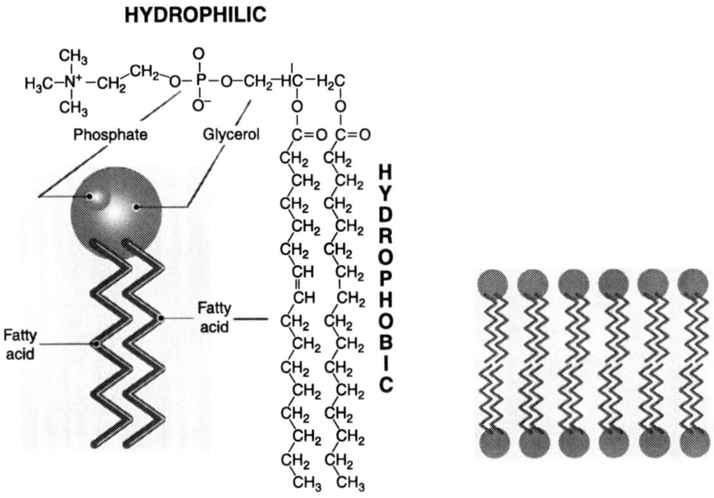

Figure 9.1 Structure of phospholipid and bilayer

Source: http://textbookofbacteriology.net.

Phospholipids are either natural or synthetic. Naturally occurring phospholipids include soya phosphatidylcholine (SPC) and egg phosphatidylcholine (EPC), while synthetic phospholipids include dipalmitoyl phosphatidylcholine (DPPC) and dimyrestoyl phosphatidylcholine (DMPC).

9.2.2 Cholesterol

Cholesterol is used in preparation of liposomes (Figure 9.2) in order to enhance the liposome bilayer properties, i.e. modifying fluidity and reducing molecular (water-soluble) permeability across the bilayer membranes (Kirby et al. 1980) Liposomes consisting of cholesterol and phospholipid can be utilized to improve the penetration of liposome-encapsulated drugsthrough the skin (Coderch et al. 2000). In addition, cholesterol enhances the stability and rigidity of liposomes. (Kirby et al. 1980).

Published by Woodhead Publishing Limited, 2013

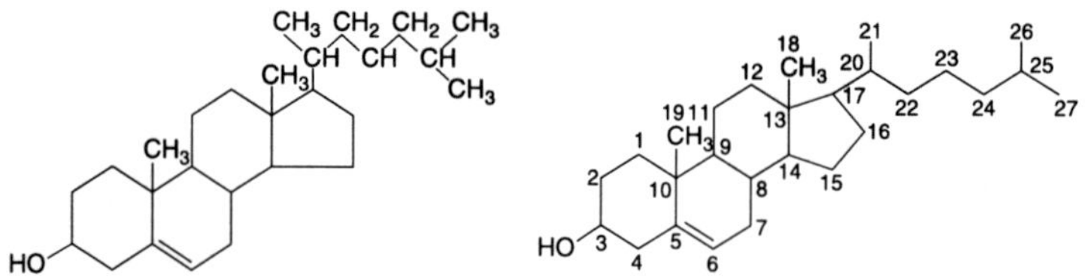

Figure 9.2 Structure of cholesterol

Source: Bagiński et al. (1989).

9.2.3 Amphiphiles

The term 'amphiphile' indicates that a single substance exhibits dual properties, such as having a polar or water-soluble head group (hydrophilic) and non-polar or lipid-soluble tail group (lipophilic). The amphiphilic characteristic of phospholipids makes them applicable in numerous fields (Blazek-Welsh and Rhodes 2001a, Darwis and Kellaway 2001).

9.2.4 Self-assembly

Phospholipids have a unique property which is their spontaneous aggregation in aqueous environments (called self-assembly) (Bergstrand 2003). This property was first observed by Bangham and co-workers (1965). In aqueous solutions, amphiphiles dissolve as monomers. However, as their concentration increases they start to assemble themselves (Figure 9.3) (Jesorka and Orwar 2008). These amphiphiles arrange themselves in a thermodynamically stable manner in the form of sheets (Israelachvili et al. 1977). The formation of sheets in amphiphiles is due to the high entropy of the system. This is due to the forces of interaction caused by water with the hydrophobic hydrocarbon chains (Bergstrand 2003). Therefore, this flat sheet of amphiphile buds off

Published by Woodhead Publishing Limited, 2013

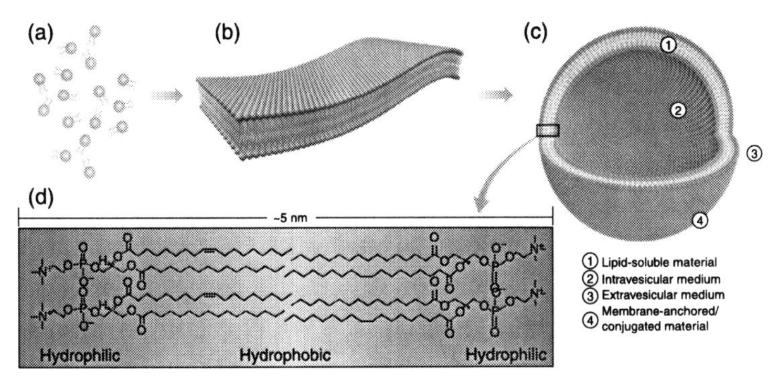

Figure 9.3 Schematic presentation of liposome self-assembly: (a) phospholipids, (b) sheet of phospholipids, (c) liposome and (d) phospholipid chemical form

Source: Jesorka and Orwar (2008).

slowly and converts into geometrical spheres with no edges. The resultant self-assembly is due to the energy produced by heat or agitation (Charles 1972, Jesorka and Orwar 2008). This explains why appropriate formation of liposomes requires hand shaking which is one form of energy input into the dispersed phospholipid system.

9.3 Liposomes

Liposomes have the ability to entrap both hydrophilic and lipophilic molecules (Payne et al., 1986a,b; Sharma and Sharma, 1997; (Blazek-Welsh and Rhodes 2001a, Darwis and Kellaway 2001, Payne et al. 1986b, Payne et al. 1986a, Sharma and Sharma 1997). In general, unilamellar liposomes are preferred for entrapment of hydrophilic drugs while multilamellar liposomes are preferred for entrapment of lipophilic drugs (Blazek-Welsh and Rhodes 2001a, Hu and Rhodes 2000). Drug entrapment in liposomes may enhance

Published by Woodhead Publishing Limited, 2013

the therapeutic outcome when compared to the outcome elicited by conventional dosage forms of the drug (Payne et al. 1986a, Schreier et al. 1994).

As mentioned earlier, liposomes consist of natural and/or synthetic lipids, i.e. phospholipids and sphingolipids in combination with cholesterol and other polymers (Sharma and Sharma 1997). Liposome vesicle size ranges from 20 nm to 20 μm (Taylor and Morris 1995). The composition of liposomes makes them a suitable carrier system due to their biocompatibility and biodegradability. Liposomes have been used as carriers for a variety of active pharmaceutical ingredients, e.g. antimicrobial drugs, vaccines, antineoplastic agents and steroidal drugs (Gregoriadis and Florence 1993). Liposomes are also used to decrease the toxicity, side-effects and degradation of drugs by the systemic metabolism and they can also prolong the drug release time (Kirby et al. 1980, Szoka and Papahadjopoulos 1980).

Formation of liposomes by hydration can be achieved above the phase transition temperature (T_m) of the phospholipid used. At this temperature an ordered/packed gel state (first phase) is converted into a less-ordered/packed liquid crystalline state (second phase), where the phospholipid bilayers become more flexible and leaky (M'Baye et al. 2008, Taylor and Morris 1995).

9.3.1 Classification of liposomes

Liposomes can be classified on the basis of their composition or mechanism of delivery, e.g. small unilamellar, large unilamellar, oligolamellar, multilamellar or pH-sensitive liposomes, long-circulating liposomes, cationic liposomes and conventional liposomes (Sharma and Sharma 1997). These are classified as shown in Figure 9.4 and the basis of their lamellarity (morphology) will be described.)

Published by Woodhead Publishing Limited, 2013

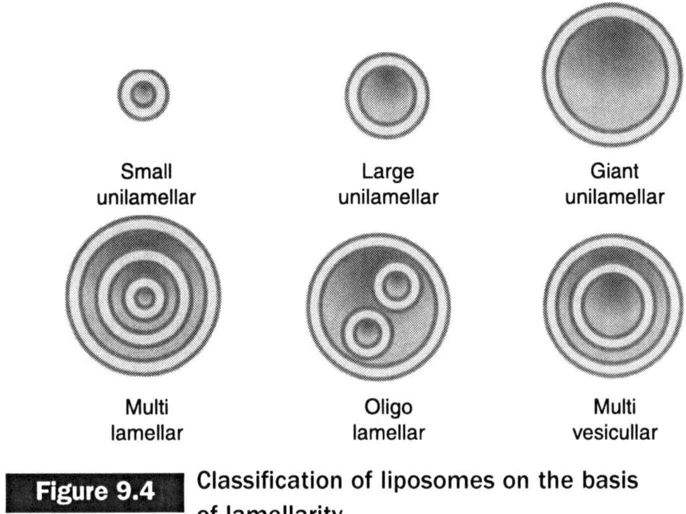

Figure 9.4 Classification of liposomes on the basis of lamellarity

Source: Jesorka and Orwar (2008).

Small unilamellar vesicles (SUVs)

Small unilamellar liposome vesicles (SUVs) have a size range between 20 and 100 nm (Lasic 1988). A solvent injection method can be employed for the preparation of SUVs (Vemuri and Rhodes 1995). In this method, an ethanolic solution is injected into a warm aqueous solution whose temperature is above the phase transition (T_m) to obtain SUVs The liposomes produced are around 25 nm in size (Batzri and Korn 1973, Pons et al. 1993).

Large unilamellar vesicles (LUVs)

LUVs consist of a single phospholipid bilayer and offer high entrapment of hydrophilic materials in the liposome-internal aqueous spaces. LUVs are larger than SUVs, i.e. 0.1–1 μm (Lasic 1988, Szoka and Papahadjopoulos 1980). Reverse-phase evaporation (RPE) (du Plessis et al. 1996, Paternostre et al. 1988) is used for LUV preparation with 60–65% drug

Published by Woodhead Publishing Limited, 2013

entrapment efficiency. In RPE, a buffer in the organic phase causes the formation of a water-in-oil emulsion of the phospholipid. Organic solvent is removed under reduced pressure, and then water and lipid are sonicated to obtain a gel that contains the LUVs (Vemuri and Rhodes 1995).

Multilamellar vesicles (MLVs)

MLVs consist of a number of successive phospholipid bilayers. Their size range is 0.1–20 μm (Lasic 1988). Multilayer liposomes were first described by Bangham and co-workers (1965). They can be prepared by the thin film hydration method (Bangham and Horne 1964, Bangham et al. 1965, du Plessis et al. 1996, Szoka and Papahadjopoulos 1980). Lipids are dissolved in an organic solvent and a thin film (Figure 9.5) is formed in the

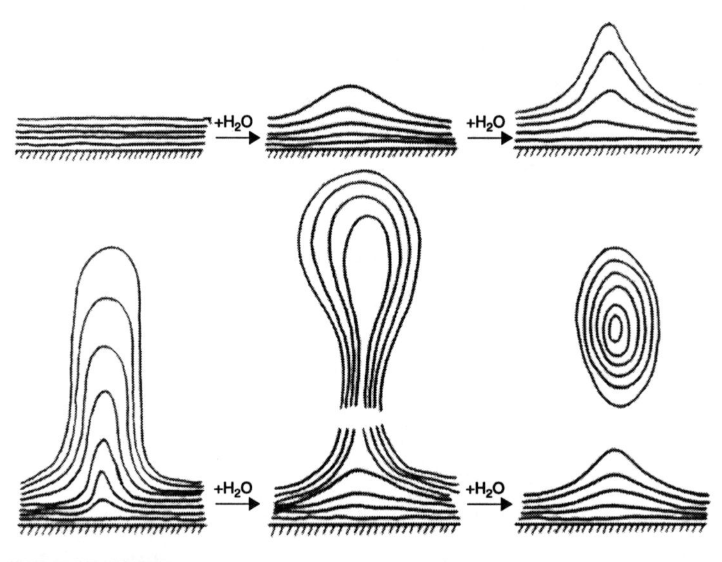

Figure 9.5 **Schematic presentation of MVL formation**

Source: Lasic (1988).

Published by Woodhead Publishing Limited, 2013

round-bottom flask connected to a rotary evaporator under vacuum. After complete evaporation of the organic solvent and formation of a thin film of lipid on the inner walls of the flask, an aqueous phase (buffer) is added with vigorous hand shaking at a temperature above the phase transition (T_m) to produce MLVs. In addition, the hydration time plays a vital role in the formation of liposomes. The entrapment of the drug may increase by slow hydration and moderate mixing of the lipid dispersion (Vemuri and Rhodes 1995).

Multivesicular liposomes (MVLs)

A number of liposomes are mixed together to form MVLs, which comprise a number of liposomes enclosed by a larger liposome vesicles. A dual emulsification technique is used to prepare the MVLs. According to this method, a water-in-oil emulsion is prepared by mixing the phospholipid, cholesterol, triolein, chloroform and diethyl ether with an aqueous solution containing the drug (Kim et al. 1983). A small volume of this emulsion was taken to make a double or second emulsion by placing it in a flask containing the aqueous solution, where the organic solvent (chloroform and diethyl ether) is removed by flushing with nitrogen gas (Zhong et al. 2005).

9.4 Stability of liposomes

Liposomal stability is important to ascertain during storage and before administration. In stability studies, both qualitative and quantitative properties of liposomesshould be checked. Aggregation, sedimentation (Wong and Thompson 1982) and rapid leakage of the active pharmaceutical

Published by Woodhead Publishing Limited, 2013

ingredient (API) from the vesicles are major problems (Payne et al. 1986a). Many formulation factors such as solvent, buffer and pH can affect the stability of liposomes.

9.4.1 Chemical stability (hydrolysis and oxidation)

Phospholipids are the primary constituent that is liable to hydrolysis or oxidation (Hunt and Tsang 1981). Oxidation is caused by the unsaturated fatty acid of phospholipids (Riaz 1995), and if oxidation happens it may change the permeability of liposomes and their shelf life (Vemuri and Rhodes 1995). Liposomes are most unstable when stored in the form of aqueous dispersions. The peroxidation of lipids can be decreased by addition of an antioxidant such as a-tocopherol or butylated hydroxytoluene, and by keeping liposomes away from light (Vemuri and Rhodes 1995). Phospholipid hydrolysis causes the formation of lyso-phosphatidylcholine (lyso-lecithin), which increases the permeability of liposomes (Kensil and Dennis 1981, Riaz 1995, Vemuri and Rhodes 1995).

9.4.2 Physical stability of liposomes

Problems associated with physical properties and stability of liposomes are important to consider when examining the appearance, size and size distribution of liposomes (Payne et al. 1986b, Payne et al. 1986a). Several methods are used to check these parameters (Vemuri and Rhodes 1995). A protocol was adopted to check liposome size of less than 1 μm by using electron microscopy and light scattering techniques (Szoka and Papahadjopoulos 1980). The stability of liposomes can be increased by changing the aqueous phase

Published by Woodhead Publishing Limited, 2013

into solid phase by freeze drying, spray drying or spray-freeze drying.

9.4.3 Freeze drying

Freeze drying, also called lyophilization, is employed to minimize the rate of lipid hydrolysis during storage (Nounou et al. 2005). However, freeze drying itself may cause a damage to the liposome structures because it involves two stressful stages, namely freezing at which ice crystals can pierce the liposomes and drying at which vacuum is applied to sublime the ice. This stressful operation might result in aggregation or fusion of liposomes and subsequent leakage of the originally entrapped material. The damaging effect of freeze drying can be minimized by the addition of cryoprotectants (e.g. carbohydrates) prior to freezing the liposomes (Nounou et al. 2005, Stark et al. 2010). Thus, cryoprotectants like lactose, trehalose, sucrose and other sugars are necessary in freeze drying (lyophilization) to guard the liposomes against aggregation, fusion and leakage of the originally entrapped material. The phase transition alterations that can possibly happen to liposomes following freeze drying are measured by using differential scanning calorimetry (DSC) (Elhissi A. M. et al. 2006b, Vemuri and Rhodes 1995). The freeze-dried product can be reconstituted by rehydration to get liposomes prior to administration. However, it is important to bear in mind that freeze drying is time-consuming and expensive.

Liposome preparations did not show any physical change before or after freeze drying. However, it increased stability and decreased reconstitution time ((Elhissi A. M. A. and Taylor 2005, Lee et al. 2007).

Published by Woodhead Publishing Limited, 2013

9.4.4 Spray drying

Spray drying is a technique where a solution containing therapeutic agents is converted into a dry fine powder, giving more stability than other techniques that take more time and affect the resultant product (Johnson 1997, Skalko-Basnet et al. 2000). Sucrose, mannitol, lactose and trehalose can be used as an excipients as well as carrierin a spray drying for drug formulation (Naini et al. 1998). Proteins and peptides are effectively converted from solutions into fine powders. Thermolabile molecules can be converted into fine powder without degradation as the drying air (of high temperature) and the large surface area help in drying the liposomes in 100 ms to 1 s (Johnson 1997). Spray drying parameters play an important role in the characteristics and spherical-shaped properties of the resultant powder (Johnson 1997).

A more conventional and economic technology than freeze drying and spray drying is the proliposome technology. Proliposomes have been introduced as a formulation approach that can overcome the instability problems of liposomes prepared as aqueous dispersions. Proliposomes are of two types: particulate-based proliposomes (Payne et al. 1986b, Payne et al. 1986a) and alcohol-based proliposomes (Perrett et al. 1991).

9.5 Proliposomes

Proliposomes were first introduced by Payne and co-workers (1986a;b) as dry phospholipid formulations (Hu and Rhodes 2000) and are more stable than liposomeliquid dispersions. The ease of transportation of proliposomes makes them a useful and economic delivery system. Proliposomes comprise water-soluble carrier particles that are coated with phospholipid and cholesterol (Payne et al. 1986b, Payne et al. 1986a). Proliposomes are good for entrapment of both lipophilic and hydrophilic drugs (Payne et al. 1986b, Payne et al. 1986a). Later in 1991, the concept of proliposomes was expanded to include liquid phospholipi formulations that can generate liposomes upon addition of aqueous phase (Perrett et al. 1991). These may be referred to as 'ethanol-based proliposomes' and are concentrated ethanolic solutions of phospholipid (Elhissi A. M. et al. 2006a, Elhissi A. M. et al. 2006b)

9.5.1 Preparation of proliposomes

As concluded from the previous section, proliposomes are two types, which are particulate-based proliposomes and alcohol (solvent)-based proliposomes. Thus, proliposomes can be generally defined as powdered or liquid lipid formulations that can generate liposomes upon addition of aqueous phase and shaking.

Particulate-based proliposomes

Selection of a suitable carrier is an important factor for formulation of particulate-based proliposomes. The carrier should be selected on the basis of its porosity and ability to accommodate phospholipids on its surface. To prepare particulate-based proliposomes, the selected carrier is placed in a round-bottom flask (Elhissi A. M. et al. 2006a) and attached to a rotary evaporator under reduced pressure (Payne et al. 1986b, Payne et al. 1986a). A solution of organic solvent with phospholipid and/or cholesterol is sprayed in portions (0.5–1 ml) on the carrier. Thus, a thin film of phospholipid is coated onto the carrier surface (Jesorka and Orwar 2008) and the organic solvent is

Published by Woodhead Publishing Limited, 2013

evaporated to obtain a dry granular material (i.e. proliposomes). This formulation should be stored after that in the freezer. Proliposomes can be converted into liposomes by the addition of aqueous solution above the phase transition temperature (T_m) of the lipid followed by shaking (Elhissi A. M. et al. 2006a).

The production of proliposomes can be scaled up by fluidized-bed coating (Chen and Alli 1987, Kumar et al. 2001), fluid-energy micronization (jet-milling) (Desai et al. 2003, Desai et al. 2002) or spray drying (Rojanarat et al. 2011). In the fluidized-bed coating method, the carrier selected is first passed through a mesh sieve with the desired size and then placed in the fluidized bed coating pan. The therapeutic agent is then dissolved in an organic solvent and sprayed in time intervals on the carrier particles using an in situ fitted spray gun and the dust formation in the coating pan is removed to make the coat layer on the carrier particles smooth and uniform. This procedure is carried out until the drug solution is completely used. The carrier particles are allowed to dry at room temperature (Kumar et al. 2001). The final product is hydrated to generate liposomes. The other method is the encapsulation of the drug by mixing it with phospholipid and carrier particles, followed by processing in an air-jet mill for micronization. Liposomes are formed by the hydration of the micronized particles with aqueous phase (Desai et al. 2003, Desai et al. 2002).

Solvent-based Proliposomes

Proliposomes are prepared by using an organic solvent that dissolves lipids and at the same time is miscible with water (e.g. ethanol). In this method a high concentration of phospholipid in ethanol is prepared and the resultant liposomes are generated by dispersion into aqueous solution

Published by Woodhead Publishing Limited, 2013

(Perrett et al. 1991). The presence of phospholipid, ethanol and water first makes a precipitated (stacked) bilayer that converts into liposomes by hydration.

The original method can be modified by increasing the cholesterol concentration in the lipid phase. It also increased the ethanol in the ratio of ethanol/phospholipid to facilitate lipid dissolution (Elhissi A. M. et al. 2006b). Phospholipid and cholesterol are dissolved in ethanol by placing them in a glass vial. A clear solution is formed and kept at 70 °C for 1 min. The therapeutic agent is then dissolved in an isotonic/ saline solution and poured into the ethanol solution of the lipid. The solution is shaken vigorously to generate the liposomes (Elhissi A. M. et al. 2006b, Perrett et al. 1991).

9.6 Pulmonary drug delivery

The most common routes of drug delivery are the oral, topical and parenteral.

The field of drug delivery to the lungs by inhalation for treatment of respiratory diseases has been growing over the last few decades. The pulmonary route (Figure 9.6) is most promising for local therapeutic action within the lung for treatment of acute or chronic respiratory diseases. Research in this area has been gaining prominence in the last few decades to make it a vital route of administration (Labiris and Dolovich 2003). This route offers a large surface area (up to 100 m^2) and the extremely thin (0.1–0.2 μm) mucosal membrane of the lung epithelium enhances drug absorption to the systemic circulation, thus also offering a means for treatment of systemic diseases. The absorption of drugs in the lung from the alveolar region directly to the blood circulation means that theGIT can be bypassed and hence hepatic deactivation of the drug can be avoided (Huang and Wang

Published by Woodhead Publishing Limited, 2013

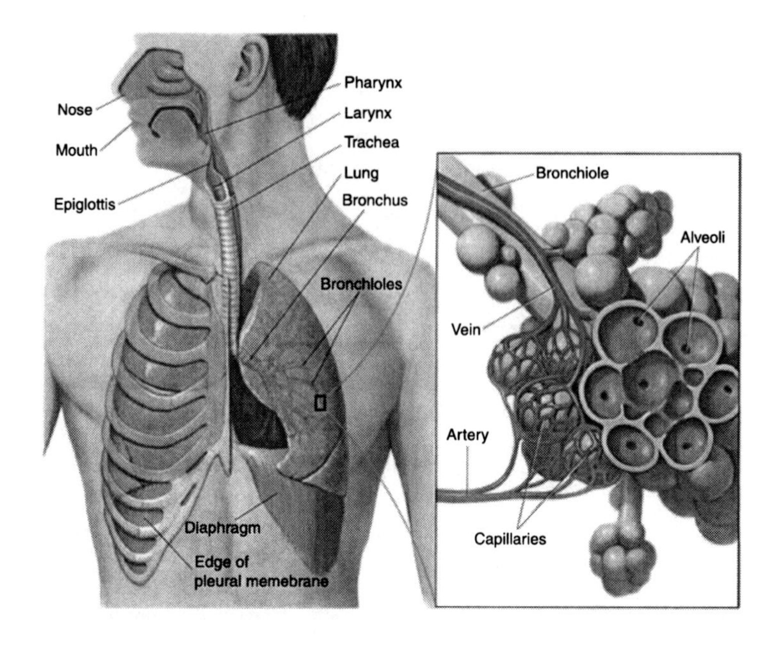

Figure 9.6 **Schematic presentation of the human respiratory system (human respiration, excretion and locomotion)**

Source: http://www.goldiesroom.org/Note%20Packets/13%20Human%20Other/00%20Human%20Other%20Systems-WHOLE.htm.

2006). Injectable drugs are now being formulated as inhalable aerosols. Historically, the lungs have been used for a very long time for inhalation of nicotine in tobacco, and also this route was used centuries ago for the treatment of coughs, e.g. using *Atropa belladonna* (Grossman 1994, Machira et al. 2011). The respiratory system consists of two major parts – the upper and lower respiratory regions (Finlay 2001).

Air enters and leaves the respiratory system and this makes the air moist and warm. Mucus is secreted by the goblet cells, which also entrap foreign particles. Cilia do the rest by moving insoluble particles outwards to be cleared from the respiratory system. The air passes to the mouth and pharynx (a funnel shaped tube). The pharynx consists of three parts, i.e. the nasopharynx, oropharynx and hypopharynx (Bassett 2005, Kent et al. 2009). The next part is the larynx (voice box), and then the epiglottis that opens during respiration and leads the air to the trachea. The trachea is made of flexible cartilage and is the part at which the lung divides into two parts, i.e. the right and left lungs. The right lung is further divided into three lobes whilst the left lung is divided into two lobes (Bassett 2005). The trachea leads to the right and left lungs by the carina into the main or primary bronchi ('first generation'). The main bronchi take the air into the secondary bronchi (lobar bronchi), the second generation, and in turn to the third generation, called the bronchioles (Bassett 2005, Kent et al. 2009). The bronchioles then continue from the small branches into the terminal bronchioles where the air and gas exchange region begins. The final part is the alveolar region where alveolar sacs are present and particles smaller than 2 μm settle there (Stahlhofen et al. 1980).

9.7 Mechanism of particle deposition

The manner in which the particles are deposited at the targeted area depends on particle size in terms of aerodynamic diameter (particle mass density and geometric diameter) (Bennett and Smaldone 1987). Secondary deposition is affected by the physical characteristics of the airway (lung geometry) and the breathing patterns of the patient (Carvalho et al. 2011). The deposition in all these regions (upper, central and alveolar parts) depends upon particle size and flow rate of the particles in the pulmonary system (Labiris and Dolovich 2003, Pilcer and Amighi 2010). The deposition patterms of particles are shown in Figure 9.7.

Published by Woodhead Publishing Limited, 2013

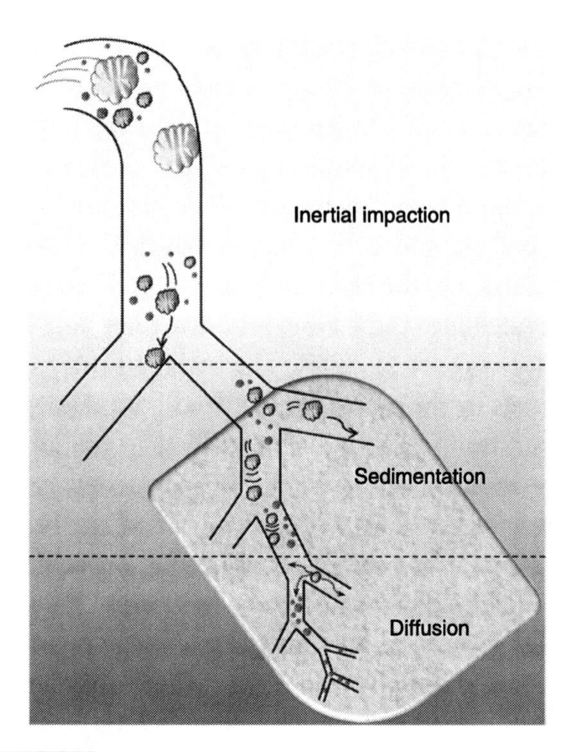

Figure 9.7 **Schematic presentation of particle deposition**

Source: Carvalho et al. (2011).

Five mechanisms cause the deposition of particles in the lungs: inertial impaction, sedimentation, Brownian diffusion, interception and electrostatic precipitation (Carvalho et al. 2011).

9.7.1 Inertial impaction

In this mechanism particles are deposited where the airways bifurcate. The deposition happens due to the large size and high mass (density) of the particles or because of the high velocity of inhaled air in the upper respiratory tract

Published by Woodhead Publishing Limited, 2013

(Pilcer and Amighi 2010). During breathing a particle enters the respiratory tract at a very high speed. This possibly makes the particle unable to change its flow track within the pulmonary airways, and hence it is likely to deposit in the upper respiratory tract. Impaction in the upper respiratory tract is most common for particles that are larger than 5 μm (Darquenne and Prisk 2004, Pilcer and Amighi 2010).

9.7.2 Sedimentation

Sedimentation is the time-dependent deposition of particles due to gravity in both the central and alveolar regions of the lung (Carvalho et al. 2011, Darquenne and Prisk 2004). Sedimentation can be increased by holding the breath (Byron 1986) and the absence of inspiration/expiration causes the particles to move due to gravitational force (Carvalho et al. 2011). Particles in the size range of 0.5–5 μm are likely to deposit by sedimentation (Darquenne and Prisk 2004, O'Callaghan and Barry 1997, Pilcer and Amighi 2010, Stahlhofen et al. 1980).

9.7.3 Brownian diffusion

By this mechanism the deposition of small particles happens when random motion in the alveolar region occurs via the bombardment of particles (Carvalho et al. 2011); this process is called Brownian diffusion. In the alveolar region the velocity of air is almost zero. At this point the movement of individual particles occurs via diffusion and particles that may reach this region are smaller than 2μm (Darquenne and Prisk 2004, Pilcer and Amighi 2010).

Published by Woodhead Publishing Limited, 2013

9.8 Clearance of deposited particles

Particle deposited in the respiratory airways can be cleared completely or translocated to other parts by two mechanisms. One is called the fast phase, which is completed in one day and clears insoluble particles by the mucociliary transport system; the other is the slow phase that represents the clearance of soluble particles from the alveolar system (Asgharian et al. 2001, Lippmann et al. 1980, Stahlhofen et al. 1990). However, it is vital to know that site of particle deposition and physicochemical properties of particles (Lippmann et al. 1980) are very important at determination of particle's fate. Ciliated cells are located on the epithelium terminal bronchioles to the larynx and their function is to move rhythmically. These movements facilitate the removal of particles from the lower part to the upper part of the lung, and coughing may expel the particles from and mucus may take them to the stomach. However, soluble particles might be absorbed into the blood by active or passive transport systems (McClellan and Henderson 1995).

Alveolar macrophages (Farr et al. 1985) are active in clearing particles from the alveolar regions (Kent et al. 2009). In normal humans, only 3–5% of the alveolar cells are alveolar macrophages. The absence of mucociliary cells in the alveolar region may decrease the clearance especially for insoluble particles, resulting in slower clearance of deposited material (Asgharian et al. 2001). (Lippmann et al. 1980)

9.9 Pulmonary diseases

Various types of diseases are associated with the pulmonary system, and liposome preparations are used for prophylaxis or treatment of these conditions depending on the type of the

Published by Woodhead Publishing Limited, 2013

drug included in the liposome formulation. In this chapter the use of liposomes in pulmonary delivery is discussed in only two types of lung disease which are asthma and tuberculosis.

9.9.1 Asthma

Corticosteroid aerosols have been used since the early 1950s for the treatment of asthma (Klein et al. 1977). Asthma is the inflammation of both the small airways (diameter less than 2 mm) and large airways, causing the development of high response in the airways, as manifested by bronchoconstriction and excessive production of mucus (Scichilone et al. 2010).

Inflammation of the lung tissues causes chest tightness, wheezing, irregular breathing and coughing, and signs of obstruction in breathing are usually attributed to asthma (Bjermer 2001). In asthma the peripheral/smaller airways are the primary places for respiratory obstruction when the flow and pressure of bronchioles are measured (Yanai et al. 1992). The uncontrolled inflammation may cause narrowing/closure of the smaller airways (distal airways), resulting in development of asthma that is difficult to control (Burgel et al. 2009). In asthma the airway muscles tighten and become narrow, followed by inflammation that makes them very narrow and consequently the mucus secretion causes complete obstruction of the airways and exacerbates the asthmatic attack.

Jet nebulizer has been used for the delivery of both free and liposome entrapped sodium cromoglicate (SCG) to human volunteers. The entrapped drug achieved a reasonable blood plasma concentration, which was also detected after 24 h, while the free drug achieved seven times higher plasma concentrations, but after 24 h it was no longer detected in

Published by Woodhead Publishing Limited, 2013

the plasma (Taylor et al. 1989). This clearly indicates that the lung could retain the drug for longer when the drug is entrapped in liposomes.

9.9.2 *Mycobacterium tuberculosis*

Tuberculosis is a fatal disease that is caused by *Mycobacterium tuberculosis* which is a slow-growing bacteria (El-Ridy et al. 2007). The disease can affect any site, but the main route is the lung where the bacteria grow and spread. A short 6-months course is recommended for the treatment of tuberculosis: rifampicin, ethambutol, pyrazinamide and isoniazid (El-Ridy et al. 2007), but prolonged drug therapy may cause drug resistance (Adams et al. 1999). Liposomes can be used to encapsulate the drug, and can overcome a number of obstacles by enhancing the efficacy and lowering the toxicity of the liposome encapsulated drug (Swenson et al. 1988). Delivery of antitubercular drugs in liposome formulations via inhalation has shown good results using BALB/c mice (Kurunov Iu et al. 1995). Entrapped drugs in liposomes also increased the retention time in the lung tissues and hence improved the therapeutic efficacy of the drug. Liposomal clofazimine (CLF) is effective by showing bactericidal activity in both liver and spleen, and hence it can be used for the treatment of *Mycobacterium. tuberculosis* (Adams et al. 1999). CLF encapsulated in liposomes has shown 95–100% efficiency of killing cultures collected from American strains of *M. tuberculosis, M. avium* and *M. intracellular* (Mehta et al. 1993). The experimental animal studies showed that liposome formulation of pyrazinamide was much more effective than that of the conventional non-liposomal preparation of the drug (El-Ridy et al. 2007). The study carried by (Suresh et al. 2010) showed that the liposome entrapment efficiency was around 79% and 47%

Published by Woodhead Publishing Limited, 2013

for rifampicin and isoniazid, respectively. The average size of liposome vesicles was 14.66 μm.

9.10 Pulmonary drug delivery devices

The pulmonary route has been used for 4000 years when *A. belladonna* was employed with smoking leaves to cure coughing. (Grossman 1994, Machira et al. 2011).Modern technologies of pulmonary drug delivery have employed new devices for targeting the drug in the form of aerosols to the lung for both prophylaxis and treatment of diseases. Pulmonary drug delivery devices are divided into three types which are pressurized metered dose inhalers (pMDIs), dry powder inhalers (DPIs) and nebulizers (Telko and Hickey 2005).

9.10.1 Pressurized metered dose inhalers (pMDIs)

pMDIs are widely used for treatment of asthma, chronic obstructive pulmonary diseases (COPD) and other respiratory tract disorders. Aerosol delivery by pMDIs started in the 1950s (Brand et al. 2008, Clark 1995). Different types of pMDIs are available nowadays in the market and they consist of three major parts which are a canister, a metering valve and an actuator (Figure 9.8). The canister is a disposable chamber containing the formulation and made of aluminum or stainless steel (Hess et al. 2011). pMDIs should have the capability to resist a pressure of 3–5 atm and can hold 15–30 ml of liquefied formulation (Dunbar 1997). The canister should be solid and light to make it more portable. Most of the pMDI formulation (e.g. 80%) is a propellant such as chlorofluorocarbon (CFC). However, the use of CFCs

Published by Woodhead Publishing Limited, 2013

as propellants has been prohibited by the regulatory authorities of many countries because this type of propellant causes depletion of the ozone layer and hence employing alternative propellant systems is necessary (Vervaet and Byron 1999). Other class of propellants are hydrofluoroalkanes (HFAs), which are non-toxic and chemically stable (Dolovich and Dhand 2011). The actuator is a plastic case composed of a mouth-piece, nozzle and body. The metering valve must have the properties of reproducibility, accuracy and uniform drug dose delivery. The therapeutic agent is dissolved in the liquefied propellant, and upon actuation the metering valve delivers a precise aerosolized dose of the drug through the mouth-piece. The effectiveness of the metering valve is vital to deliver an accurate and reproducible dose of the drug, which is typically 25–100 µl (Hess et al. 2011, Newman 2005).)

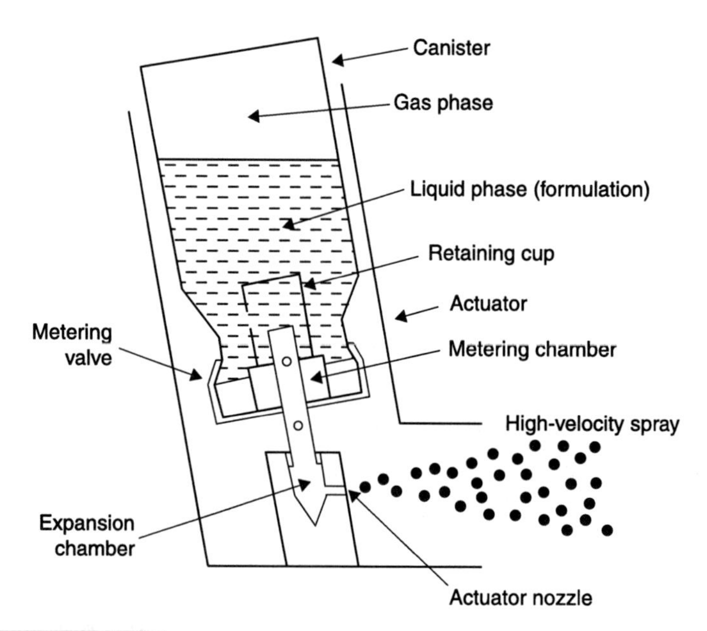

Figure 9.8 Schematic diagram of a pMDI

Source: Oliveira et al. (2010).

Published by Woodhead Publishing Limited, 2013

Proper training of the patient by health care professionals is vital. Nose breathing may also cause partial inhalation of aerosol, so a spacer is required for children and elderly patients to overcome this problem (Ganderton 1999, Rubin and Fink 2005). Holding breath and generation of aerosols having particle size less than 4.5 μm can enhance drug deposition in the peripheral airways especially in the alveolar region.

9.10.2 Dry powder inhaler (DPI) devices

Dry powder inhalers (DPIs) are dry free-flowing powdered formulations of the drug, which can be prepared by either spray-drying or micronization of a blend consisting of the drug and a suitable inert carrier. The resultant drug particles should act locally in the upper respiratory tract or into the deep lung. DPI formulations are delivered as aerosols by using DPI devices. Thus, a DPI device typically consists of a metering system, an actuator and the dry formulation (Figure 9.9). The bulk chamber contains the formulation and is covered by an over-cap, while the mouth-piece is covered by a dust-cap to prevent contamination. The metering valve has a reproducible measuring property, and pulls the powder from the chamber and forwards it to the mouth-piece for inhalation. A negative inhalation is required by the patient in order to deliver the medication as 'respirable' aerosol; however, this technique is not easy for elderly, childrenand patients having shallow breathing patterns (Dolovich and Dhand 2011).

Particles pass through the respiratory tract according to their size and velocity. The specific site of deposition can be controlled by formulating relatively large particles (above 5 μm) for deposition in the upper respiratory tract or smaller particles (e.g. below 4 μm) for deposition in the lower respiratory tract(Telko and Hickey 2005).

Published by Woodhead Publishing Limited, 2013

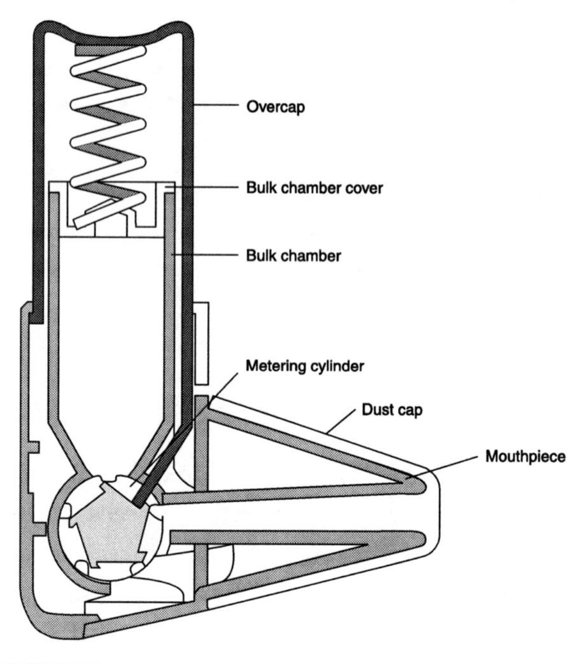

Figure 9.9 Schematic presentation of a DPI

Source: Juntunen-Backman et al. (2002).

Dry powders of liposomes can be prepared first as aqueous dispersions that can then be converted into dry formulations by spray drying. The dry formulation can be stored in a dry place or a desiccators to prevent moisture absorbance, as the micronized powders tend to aggregate (Pedersen 1996). DPIs are free from propellant and are more stable than aqueous formulations. Different types of DPI devices include the Rotahaler, Turbuhaler, Spinhaler and Diskhaler (Clark 1995, Pedersen 1996).

9.10.3 Nebulizers

Nebulizers have been developed for the administration of aerosols that can be delivered to the deep lung. A continuous

Published by Woodhead Publishing Limited, 2013

delivery is effectively used for both prophylaxis and treatment of respiratory diseases (Dhand 2003). Nebulizers can be more desirable than pMDIs and DPIs as they can be used easily by both elderly and children with no skills required to inhale the medication. Also, no propellant or dry procedures are needed for preparation of nebulizer formulations (Hess 2000, Taylor and McCallion 1997). Factors that may affect nebulization of liposomes include particle size of vesicles and surface tension, viscosity and density of the formulation. Medical nebulizers are classified into three main types which are air-jet, ultrasonic and vibrating-mesh nebulizers.

Air-jet nebulizer

Air-jet nebulizer consists of a compressor forcing gas through a plastic bottle (i.e. the nebulizer reservoir) (i.e. nebulizer reservoir) and a T-shaped mouth piece (Waldrep and Dhand 2008). A plastic tube is used to connect both the nebulizer reservoir with the compressor (Figure 9.10). The nebulizer has vital functional parts which are the baffles and the venture nozzle (O'Callaghan and Barry 1997).

Medication solution is placed in the plastic bottle and high-pressure compressed gas is applied with high velocity (making a cone shape) to pass through a narrow hole called the 'venturi' nozzle, to develop a negative pressure on the top of the medical liquid (Bernoulli effect) in order to convert it into inhalable droplets (Figure 9.11) (Hamilton and Guz 1991, Labiris and Dolovich 2003, McCallion et al. 1996). Formation of droplets is caused by the surface tension of the liquid and baffles of the nebulizer (Elhissi A. M. A. and Taylor 2005). The small aerosol droplets move towards the mouth-piece for inhalation by the patient and the large droplets are deflected by the baffles for further atomization into smaller inhalable droplets (Niven and Brain 1994, Smye et al. 1991).

Published by Woodhead Publishing Limited, 2013

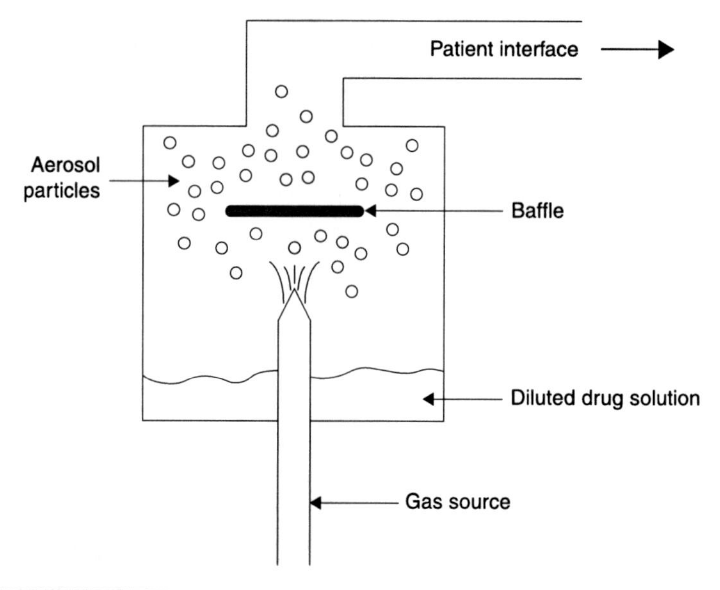

Figure 9.10 Jet nebulizer

Source: Muchão and Silva Filho (2010).

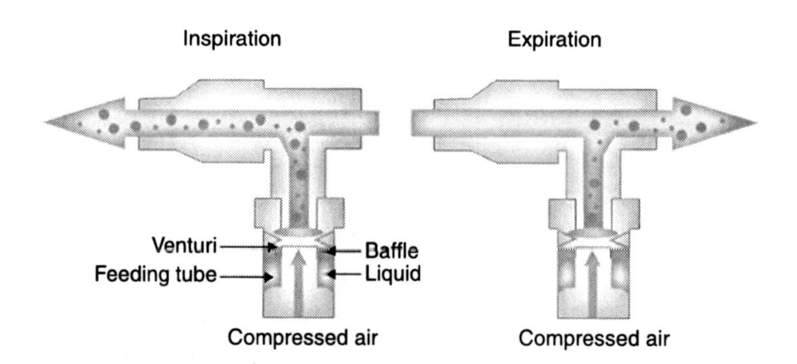

Figure 9.11 Schematic presentation of a conventional nebulizer

Source: Adapted from Medscape (23 January 2012) http://www.google.co.uk/imgres?q=jet+nebuliser&um=1&hl=en&rls=com.microsoft:en-gb&rlz=1I7GGLL_en-GBGB370&biw=1280&bih=786&tbm=isch&tbnid=grXt0poC1-cjgM:&imgrefurl=http://www.medscape.com/viewarticle/579507_4&docid=YHC1MaQRku3ivM&imgurl=http://img.medscape.com/fullsize/migrated/579/507/ers579507.fig1.gif&w=500&h=259&ei=sy5BT_TLC6K-0QWwjeWPDw&zoom=1.

Published by Woodhead Publishing Limited, 2013

Jet nebulizers are very economical and easy to use by patient; however, there is loss of drug during the exhalation caused by the inhalation patterns. High residual or dead volume in the plastic bottle is a possible drawback of jet nebulizers, and can be minimized by minimizing the solute concentration (Hess et al. 2011, Hess et al. 1996). There are a few different types of air-jet nebulizers, which are the open-vent nebulizer, breath-enhanced open-vent nebulizer and breath-actuated nebulizer.)

Open-vent nebulizer

The mechanism of producing aerosols using the open-vent devices is similar to that of conventional nebulizers.

However, in the open-vent design, there is a small vent at the top of the nebulizer reservoir to allow additional air into the device, resulting in delivery of smaller droplets for inhalation (Figure 9.12). A drawback of this technique is that it may not be suitable for children to cope with the extra high flow rate of air in inhalation and ultimately this may result in some loss of the drug. To control this drawback another nebulizer was introduced called the Intermittent Pari LL nebulizer. This nebulizer contains a side button to control the air flow, permitting the aerosol to be inhaled over time intervals (O'Callaghan and Barry 1997).

Breath-enhanced open-vent nebulizer

Breath-enhanced open-vent nebulizers work by the same principle as the open-vent nebulizer with the continuous production of aerosol. However, the high amount of drug loss during patient inspiration and expiration is reduced when using the breath-enhanced design of jet nebulizers as

Published by Woodhead Publishing Limited, 2013

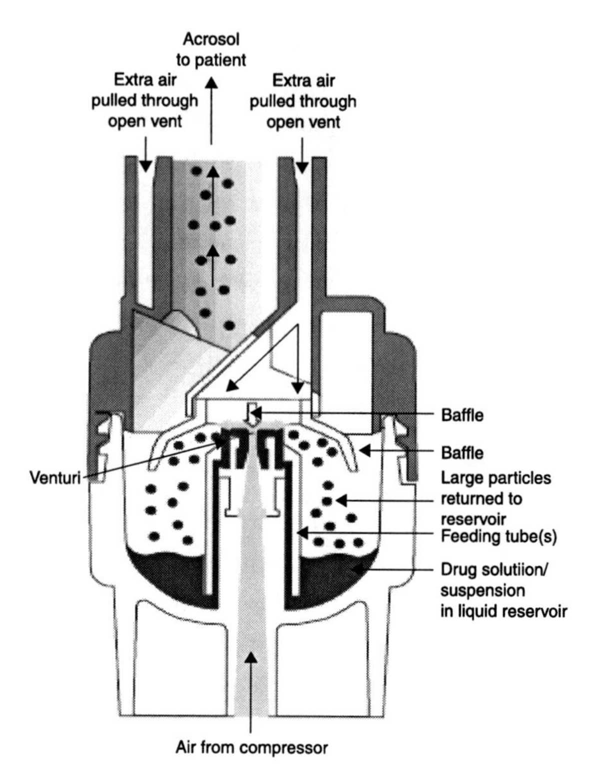

Figure 9.12 **Schematic presentation of an open-vent nebulizer**

Source: O'Callaghan and Barry (1997).

compared to the conventional jet nebulizer design (Figure 9.13).

The design of breath-enhanced jet nebulizers involves a valve near the mouthpiece, the valve remains closed during inspiration and opens during expiration. The open vent at the top opens for the air flow during inspiration and closes itself during expiration. Thus, the open vent and the valve work in opposition to each other to minimize the aerosol losses. This additional air flow enhances the generation of small droplets and hence enhances droplet deposition in the peripheral airways. Thus, a low compressed air

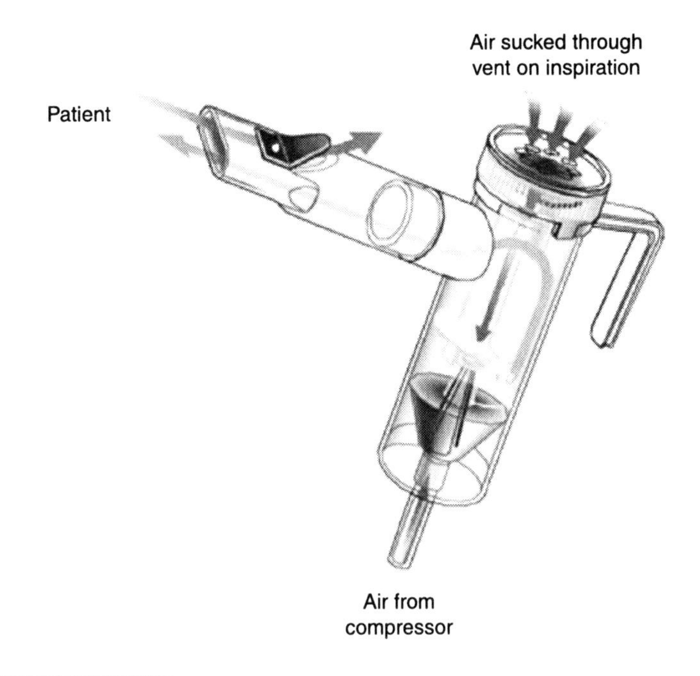

Figure 9.13 Breath-enhanced open-vent nebulizer

Source: Hess (2000).

flow can be used to generate the droplets, allowing the use of economical compressors. However, for high viscous solutions, high-power compressed gas is required to minimize the nebulization time. The breath-enhanced open-vent nebulizer produces higher particle deposition in the pulmonary system and has a shorter nebulization time when compared with the conventional jet nebulizer (Devadason et al. 1997, O'Callaghan and Barry 1997).

Breath-actuated nebulizers

Breath-actuated nebulizers are advanced nebulizers containing a sensor that recognizes the patient's breathing patterns and produces aerosol for inhalation accordingly.

Published by Woodhead Publishing Limited, 2013

This minimizes wastage of medication. The formulation in the reservoir is effectively converted into a small mist (droplets) for inhalation to deposit in the deep lung.

Ultrasonic nebulizers

Ultrasonic nebulizers do not employ compressed gas; instead, a piezoelectric crystal is used to create energy within the stagnant aqueous formulation to convert the solution into small droplets for inhalation (Clark 1995, Khatri et al. 2001, Labiris and Dolovich 2003, Rau 2002). The ultrasonic nebulizer consists of a piezoelectric crystal, a baffle system and a fan that may assist inhalation by patient (Figure 9.14). The medication solution is placed in the nebulizer chamber and the system is connected to a power supply. This electric current causes the piezoelectric crystal to produce vibrations with a high frequency (1–3 MHz), thus allowing the solution to form fountain-like structures (Sollner 1936). Large particles are produced at the apex of the fountain while smaller droplets are generated at the bottom (Elhissi A. M. A. and Taylor 2005). The larger droplets remain in the reservoir because they are deflected by the baffles and are then fragmented into smaller droplets to be ready for nebulization as inhalable aerosols.

There are two mechanisms that produce aerosol droplets: the cavitational bubble method and capillary wave method. In the cavitational method, the piezoelectric crystal produces low-energy vibrations that cause the formation of bubbles inside the solution. Upon reaching the interface these bubbles burst; the internal and external pressure becomes equal, causing the formation of small aerosol droplets. In the capillary wave method, high energy is produced, causing formation of a liquid jet, which breaks to produce small aerosol droplets (Taylor and McCallion 1997).

Published by Woodhead Publishing Limited, 2013

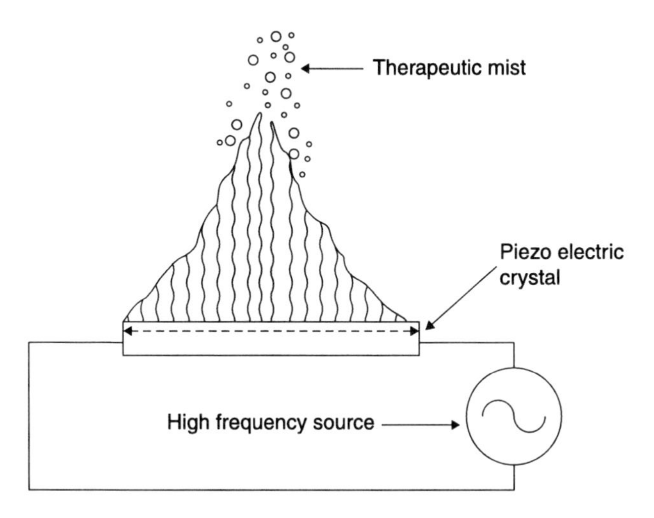

Figure 9.14 Schematic presentation of an ultrasonic nebulizer

Source: Taylor and McCallion (1997).

The ultrasonic nebulizer generates heat where the temperature goes up by 20°C within a few minutes of operation (Phipps and Gonda 1990). This heat is detrimental for thermo-labile materials; however, it may enhance the solubility of poorly soluble drugs.

Vibrating-mesh nebulizer

The vibrating mesh nebulizer consists of a perforated plate (mesh) which vibrates upwards and downwards to extrude the liquid and generate slow moving small aerosol droplets (Newman and Gee-Turner 2005). This technology of nebulization offers very high nebulization output (Dhand 2009). Smooth and consistent nebulization can be achieved easily, and the nebulizer can be operated manually by using batteries as power source, which as a result enhances the portability of the device. There are different types of vibrating-mesh nebulizers and they operate using different

Published by Woodhead Publishing Limited, 2013

mechanisms. Vibrating-mesh nebulizers are either passively vibrating-mesh or actively vibrating-mesh nebulizers.

Passively vibrating-mesh nebulizers

An example of passively vibrating-mesh nebulizers is the Omron Micro Air NEU22 device.

The aperture plate of the Omron NE-U22 (Figure 9.15) consists of 6000 accurately distant tapered holes; each hole

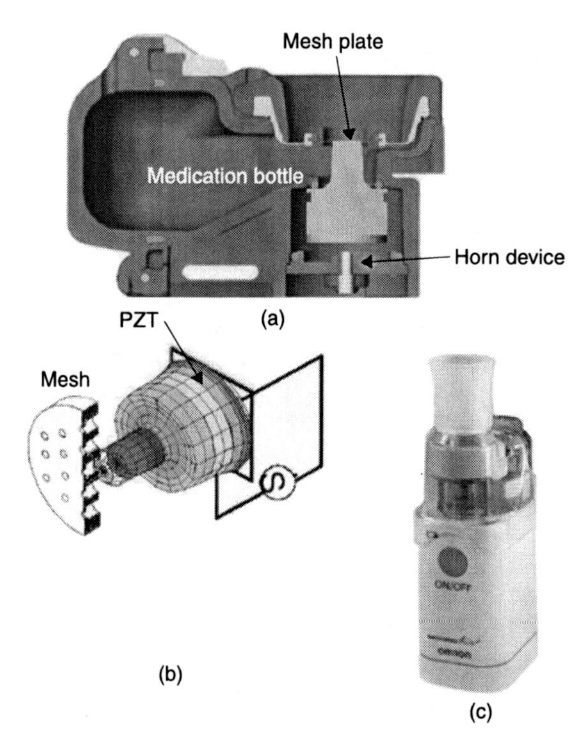

Figure 9.15 Omron NE-U22 nebulizer. (a) Formulation is placed in the medicated bottle covered with mesh, (b) the piezoelectric crystal (PZT) produces vibrational energy and is transferred via transducer horn, which pushes the liquid to pass through mesh (c)

Source: Dhand (2003).

Published by Woodhead Publishing Limited, 2013

is cone-shaped and 3 μm in diameter (Elhissi A. et al. 2007). The vibrations produced by a piezoelectric crystal are transferred via a transducer horn to the mesh that drives the medication through the holes. Passive and silent movement of the mesh produces a smaller droplet size and high aerosol output (Newman and Gee-Turner 2005, Waldrep and Dhand 2008).)

Actively vibrating-mesh nebulizer

In the active vibrating-mesh nebulizer, the vibrating-mesh is a cone-shaped perforated plate having 1000 small holes, surrounded by a piezoceramic vibrational element that causes the mesh to generate aerosols by using a 'micropump' action (Hess et al. 2011). The size of droplets can be controlled by controlling the aperture size of the mesh. There

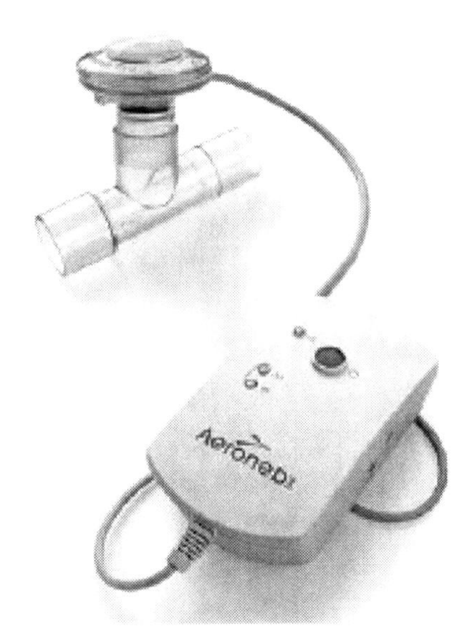

Figure 9.16 Aeroneb Pro

Source: Dhand (2003).

Published by Woodhead Publishing Limited, 2013

are different types of active vibrational mesh nebulizers, and these act differently on the basis of their principle, such as the Aeroneb Pro and Aeroneb Go and Aeroneb Solo. For mechanical ventilation, Aeroneb Pro is very effective and can be linked into the aspiratory limb of the ventilator circuit (Waldrep and Dhand 2008). Aeroneb Pro shows (Figure 9.16) shorter nebulization time than Omron NE-U22 when viscous solutions are used (Ghazanfari et al. 2007).

9.11 References

Adams L B, Sinha I, Franzblau S G, Krahenbuhl J L, Mehta R T (1999), 'Effective treatment of acute and chronic murine tuberculosis with liposome-encapsulated clofazimine', *Antimicrob Agents Chemother* **43**: 1638–1643.

Alsarra I A, Bosela A A, Ahmed S M, Mahrous G M (2005), 'Proniosomes as a drug carrier for transdermal delivery of ketorolac', *Eur J Pharm Biopharm* **59**: 485–490.

Asgharian B, Hofmann W, Miller F J (2001), 'Mucociliary clearance of insoluble particles from the tracheobronchial airways of the human lung', *Journal of Aerosol Science* **32**: 817–832.

Bagiski M, Tempczyk A, Borowski E (1989), 'Comparative conformational analysis of cholesterol and ergosterol by molecular mechanics', *European Biophysics Journal* **17**: 159–166.

Bangham A D, Horne R W (1964), 'Negative staining of phospholipids and their structural modification by surface-active agents as observed in the electron microscope', *Journal of Molecular Biology* **8**: 660–IN610.

Bangham A D, Standish M M, Watkins J C (1965), 'Diffusion of univalent ions across the lamellae of swollen phospholipids', *J Mol Biol* **13**: 238–252.

Published by Woodhead Publishing Limited, 2013

Bashoff E C, Beaser R S (1995), 'Insulin therapy and the reluctant patient. Overcoming obstacles to success', *Postgrad Med* **97**: 86–90, 93–86.

Bassett S (2005), *Anatomy and Physiology*. Hoboken, NJ, USA: Wiley.

Batzri S, Korn E D (1973), 'Single bilayer liposomes prepared without sonication', *Biochim Biophys Acta* **298**: 1015–1019.

Bennett W D, Smaldone G C (1987), 'Human variation in the peripheral air-space deposition of inhaled particles', *J Appl Physiol* **62**: 1603–1610.

Bergstrand N (2003), *Liposomes for Drug Delivery from Physico-chemical Studies to Applications*, Uppsala University, Faculty of Science and Technology, Sweden.

Bjermer L (2001), 'History and future perspectives of treating asthma as a systemic and small airways disease', *Respir Med* **95**: 703–719.

Blazek-Welsh A I, Rhodes D G (2001a), 'Maltodextrin-based proniosomes', *AAPS PharmSci* **3**: E1.

Brand P, Hederer B, Austen G, Dewberry H, Meyer T (2008), 'Higher lung deposition with Respimat Soft Mist inhaler than HFA-MDI in COPD patients with poor technique', *Int J Chron Obstruct Pulmon Dis* **3**: 763–770.

Burgel P R, et al (2009), 'Update on the roles of distal airways in asthma', *Eur Respir Rev* **18**: 80–95.

Byron P R (1986), 'Prediction of drug residence times in regions of the human respiratory tract following aerosol inhalation', *J Pharm Sci* **75**: 433–438.

Carvalho T C, Peters J I, Williams R O, 3rd (2011), 'Influence of particle size on regional lung deposition—what evidence is there?', *Int J Pharm* **406**: 1–10.

Charles T (1972), 'Hydrophobic free energy, micelle formation and the association of proteins with amphiphiles', *Journal of Molecular Biology* **67**: 59–74.

Published by Woodhead Publishing Limited, 2013

Chen C M, Alli D (1987), 'Use of fluidized bed in proliposome manufacturing', *J Pharm Sci* **76**: 419.

Clark A R (1995), 'Medical Aerosol Inhalers: Past, Present, and Future', *Aerosol Science and Technology* **22**: 374–391.

Coderch L, Fonollosa J, De Pera M, Estelrich J, De La Maza A, Parra J L (2000), 'Influence of cholesterol on liposome fluidity by EPR. Relationship with percutaneous absorption', *J Control Release* **68**: 85–95.

Darquenne C, Prisk G K (2004), 'Aerosol deposition in the human respiratory tract breathing air and 80:20 heliox', *J Aerosol Med* **17**: 278–285.

Darwis Y, Kellaway I W (2001), 'Nebulisation of rehydrated freeze-dried beclomethasone dipropionate liposomes', *Int J Pharm* **215**: 113–121.

Desai T R, Hancock R E, Finlay W H (2003), 'Delivery of liposomes in dry powder form: aerodynamic dispersion properties', *Eur J Pharm Sci* **20**: 459–467.

Desai T R, Wong J P, Hancock R E, Finlay W H (2002), 'A novel approach to the pulmonary delivery of liposomes in dry powder form to eliminate the deleterious effects of milling', *J Pharm Sci* **91**: 482–491.

Devadason S G, Everard M L, Linto J M, Le Souef P N (1997), 'Comparison of drug delivery from conventional versus "Venturi" nebulizers', *Eur Respir J* **10**: 2479–2483.

Dhand R (2003), *New Nebuliser Technology – Aerosol Generation by Using a Vibrating Mesh or Plate with Multiple Apertures*, USA: University of Missouri Hospital and Clinics, for Omron Healthcare, Inc. Report no.

Dhand R (2008), 'Aerosol delivery during mechanical ventilation: from basic techniques to new devices', *J Aerosol Med Pulm Drug Deliv* **21**: 45–60.

Dolovich M, Dhand R (2011), 'Aerosol drug delivery: developments in device design and clinical use? Authors' reply', *The Lancet* **378**: 1032–1045.

du Plessis J, Ramachandran C, Weiner N, Müller D G (1996), 'The influence of lipid composition and lamellarity of liposomes on the physical stability of liposomes upon storage', *International Journal of Pharmaceutics* **127**: 273–278.

Dunbar C A (1997), 'Atomization mechanisms of the pressurised metered dose inhaler', *Particulate Science and Technology* **15**: 253–271.

El-Ridy M S, Mostafa D M, Shehab A, Nasr E A, Abd El-Alim S (2007), 'Biological evaluation of pyrazinamide liposomes for treatment of Mycobacterium tuberculosis', *International Journal of Pharmaceutics* **330**: 82–88.

Elhissi A, Faizi M, Naji W F, Gill H S, Taylor K (2007), 'Physical stability and aerosol properties of liposomes delivered using an air-jet nebulizer and a novel micropump device with large mesh apertures', *International Journal of Pharmaceutics* **334**: 62–70.

Elhissi A M, O'Neill M A, Roberts S A, Taylor K M (2006a), 'A calorimetric study of dimyristoylphosphatidylcholine phase transitions and steroid-liposome interactions for liposomes prepared by thin film and proliposome methods', *Int J Pharm* **320**: 124–130.

Elhissi A M, Karnam K K, Danesh-Azari M R, Gill H S, Taylor K M (2006b), 'Formulations generated from ethanol-based proliposomes for delivery via medical nebulizers', *J Pharm Pharmacol* **58**: 887–894.

Elhissi A M A, Taylor K M G (2005), 'Delivery of liposomes generated from proliposomes using air-jet, ultrasonic, and vibrating-mesh nebulisers', *Journal of Drug Delivery Science and Technology* **15**: 261–265.

Farr S J, Kellaway I W, Parry-Jones D R, Woolfrey S G (1985), '99m-Technetium as a marker of liposomal deposition and clearance in the human lung', *International Journal of Pharmaceutics* **26**: 303–316.

Published by Woodhead Publishing Limited, 2013

Finlay W H (2001), *The mechanics of inhaled pharmaceutical aerosols: an introduction*, San Diego: Academic Press.

Ganderton D (1999), 'Targeted delivery of inhaled drugs: current challenges and future goals', *J Aerosol Med* **12** Suppl 1: S3–8.

Ghazanfari T, Elhissi A M, Ding Z, Taylor K M (2007), 'The influence of fluid physicochemical properties on vibrating-mesh nebulization', *Int J Pharm* **339**: 103–111.

Gregoriadis G, Florence A T (1993), 'Liposomes in drug delivery. Clinical, diagnostic and ophthalmic potential', *Drugs* **45**: 15–28.

Grossman J (1994), 'The evolution of inhaler technology', *J Asthma* **31**: 55–64.

Hamilton R D, Guz A (1991), 'Jet and ultrasonic nebuliser output: use of a new method for direct measurement of aerosol output', *Thorax* **46**: 151–152.

Hess D (2000), 'Nebulizers: Principles and Performance', *Respir Care* **45**: 609–622.

Hess D, MacIntyre N, Mishoe S (2011), *Respiratory Care: Principles and Practice*, Jones & Bartlett Learning.

Hess D, Fisher D, Williams P, Pooler S, Kacmarek R M (1996), 'Medication nebulizer performance. Effects of diluent volume, nebulizer flow, and nebulizer brand', *Chest* **110**: 498–505.

Hu C, Rhodes D G (2000), 'Proniosomes: a novel drug carrier preparation', *Int J Pharm* **206**: 110–122.

Huang Y-Y, Wang C-H (2006), 'Pulmonary delivery of insulin by liposomal carriers', *Journal of Controlled Release* **113**: 9–14.

Hunt C A, Tsang S (1981), 'α-Tocopherol retards autoxidation and prolongs the shelf-life of liposomes', *International Journal of Pharmaceutics* **8**: 101–110.

Israelachvili J N, Mitchell D J, Ninham B W (1977), 'Theory of self-assembly of lipid bilayers and vesicles',

Biochimica et Biophysica Acta (BBA) – Biomembranes **470**: 185–201.

Jesorka A, Orwar O (2008), 'Liposomes: technologies and analytical applications', *Annu Rev Anal Chem (Palo Alto Calif)* **1**: 801–832.

Johnson K A (1997), 'Preparation of peptide and protein powders for inhalation', *Adv Drug Deliv Rev* **26**: 3–15.

Juntunen-Backman K, Kajosaari M, Laurikainen K, Malinen A, Kaila M, Mustala L, Kaski U, Linna O, Marenk M, Toivanen P (2002), 'Comparison of Easyhaler Metered-Dose, Dry Powder Inhaler and a Pressurised Metered-Dose Inhaler plus Spacer in the Treatment of Asthma in Children', *Clinical Drug Investigation* **22**: 827–839.

Kensil C R, Dennis E A (1981), 'Alkaline hydrolysis of phospholipids in model membranes and the dependence on their state of aggregation', *Biochemistry* **20**: 6079–6085.

Kent G, Rhees V D, Palmer R W, (2009), *Outline of Human Anatomy and Physiology*, 298–314. New York: McGraw-Hill Professional Publishing.

Khatri L, Taylor K M G, Craig D Q M, Palin K (2001), 'An assessment of jet and ultrasonic nebulisers for the delivery of lactate dehydrogenase solutions', *International Journal of Pharmaceutics* **227**: 121–131.

Kim S, Turker M S, Chi E Y, Sela S, Martin G M (1983), 'Preparation of multivesicular liposomes', *Biochim Biophys Acta* **728**: 339–348.

Kirby C, Clarke J, Gregoriadis G (1980), 'Effect of the cholesterol content of small unilamellar liposomes on their stability in vivo and in vitro', *Biochem J* **186**: 591–598.

Klein R, Waldman D, Kershnar H, Berger W, Coulson A, Katz R M, Rachelefsky G S, Siegel S C (1977), 'Treatment of chronic childhood asthma with beclomethasone dipropionate aerosol: I. A double-blind crossover trial in nonsteroid-dependent patients', *Pediatrics* **60**: 7–13.

Kumar R, Gupta R B, Betageri G V (2001), 'Formulation, characterization, and in vitro release of glyburide from proliposomal beads', *Drug Deliv* **8**: 25–27.

Kurunov I N, Ursov I G, Krasnov V A, Petrenko T I, Iakovchenko N N, Svistelnik A V, Filimonov P A (1995), 'Effectiveness of liposomal antibacterial drugs in the inhalation therapy of experimental tuberculosis', *Probl Tuberk*: 38–40.

Labiris N R, Dolovich M B (2003), 'Pulmonary drug delivery. Part II: the role of inhalant delivery devices and drug formulations in therapeutic effectiveness of aerosolized medications', *Br J Clin Pharmacol* **56**: 600–612.

Lasic D D (1988), 'The mechanism of vesicle formation', *Biochem J* **256**: 1–11.

LeDuc P R, et al (2007), 'Towards an in vivo biologically inspired nanofactory', *Nat Nano* **2**: 3–7.

Lee S, Lee J, Choi Y W (2007), 'Characterization and Evaluation of Freeze-dried Liposomes Loaded with Ascorbyl Palmitate Enabling Anti-aging Therapy of the Skin', *Korean Chem. Soc* **28**: 99–102.

Lippmann M, Yeates D B, Albert R E (1980), 'Deposition, retention, and clearance of inhaled particles', *Br J Ind Med* **37**: 337–362.

M'Baye G, Mely Y, Duportail G, Klymchenko A S (2008), 'Liquid ordered and gel phases of lipid bilayers: fluorescent probes reveal close fluidity but different hydration', *Biophys J* **95**: 1217–1225.

Machira E P M, Obimbo E M, Wamalwa D, Gachare L N (2011), 'Assessment of inhalation technique among asthmatic children and their carers at the Kenyatta National Hospital, Kenya', *African Journal of Respiratory Medicine* **7**: 19–22.

Published by Woodhead Publishing Limited, 2013

McCallion O N M, Taylor K M G, Bridges P A, Thomas M, Taylor A J (1996), 'Jet nebulisers for pulmonary drug delivery', *International Journal of Pharmaceutics* **130**: 1–11.

McClellan R O, Henderson R F, eds (1995), *Concepts in Inhalation Toxicology, 2 ed*, Washington, DC: Taylor & Francis.

Mehta R T, Keyhani A, McQueen T J, Rosenbaum B, Rolston K V, Tarrand J J (1993), 'In vitro activities of free and liposomal drugs against Mycobacterium avium-M. intracellulare complex and M. tuberculosis', *Antimicrob Agents Chemother* **37**: 2584–2587.

Muchão F P, Silva Filho L V R Fd (2010), 'Avanços na inaloterapia em pediatria', *Jornal de Pediatria* **86**: 367–376.

Naini V, Byron P R, Phillips E M (1998), 'Physicochemical stability of crystalline sugars and their spray-dried forms: dependence upon relative humidity and suitability for use in powder inhalers', *Drug Dev Ind Pharm* **24**: 895–909.

Newman S (2005), 'Principles of metered-dose inhaler design', *Respir Care* **50**: 1177–1190.

Newman S, Gee-Turner A (2005), 'The Omron MicroAir vibrating mesh technology nebuliser, a 21st century approach to inhalation therapy', *Journal of Appl. Ther. Res.* **5**: 29–33.

Niven R W, Brain J D (1994), 'Some functional aspects of air-jet nebulizers', *International Journal of Pharmaceutics* **104**: 73–85.

Nounou M M, El-Khordagui L, Khallafallah N, Khalil S (2005), 'Influence of different sugar cryoprotectants on the stability and physico-chemical characteristics of freeze-dried 5-fluoracil plurilamellar vesicles', *Daru* **13**: 133–142.

O'Callaghan C, Barry P W (1997), 'The science of nebulised drug delivery', *Thorax 52 Suppl* 2: S31–44.

Published by Woodhead Publishing Limited, 2013

Oliveira R F, Teixeira S, Silva L F, Teixeira J C, Antunes H (2010), 'Study of a pressurized metered-dose inhaler spray parameters in fluent™', Pages 1083–1087.

Parthasarathy R, Gilbert B, Mehta K (1999), 'Aerosol delivery of liposomal all-trans-retinoic acid to the lungs', *Cancer Chemother Pharmacol* **43**: 277–283.

Paternostre M T, Roux M, Rigaud J L (1988), 'Mechanisms of membrane protein insertion into liposomes during reconstitution procedures involving the use of detergents. 1. Solubilization of large unilamellar liposomes (prepared by reverse-phase evaporation) by Triton X-100, octyl glucoside, and sodium cholate', *Biochemistry* **27**: 2668–2677.

Payne N I, Browning I, Hynes C A (1986b), 'Characterization of proliposomes', *J Pharm Sci* **75**: 330–333.

Payne N I, Timmins P, Ambrose C V, Ward M D, Ridgway F (1986a), 'Proliposomes: a novel solution to an old problem', *J Pharm Sci* **75**: 325–329.

Pedersen S (1996), 'Inhalers and nebulizers: which to choose and why', *Respir Med* **90**: 69–77.

Perrett S, Golding M, Williams W P (1991), 'A simple method for the preparation of liposomes for pharmaceutical applications: characterization of the liposomes', *J Pharm Pharmacol* **43**: 154–161.

Phipps P R, Gonda I (1990), 'Droplets produced by medical nebulizers. Some factors affecting their size and solute concentration', *Chest* **97**: 1327–1332.

Pilcer G, Amighi K (2010), 'Formulation strategy and use of excipients in pulmonary drug delivery', *Int J Pharm* **392**: 1–19.

Pons M, Foradada M, Estelrich J (1993), 'Liposomes obtained by the ethanol injection method', *International Journal of Pharmaceutics* **95**: 51–56.

Rau J L (2002), 'Design principles of liquid nebulization devices currently in use', *Respir Care* **47**: 1257–1275; discussion 1275–1258.

Riaz M (1995), 'Review article: stability and uses of liposomes', *Pak J Pharm Sci* **8**: 69–79.

Rojanarat W, Changsan N, Tawithong E, Pinsuwan S, Chan H K, Srichana T (2011), 'Isoniazid proliposome powders for inhalation-preparation, characterization and cell culture studies', *Int J Mol Sci* **12**: 4414–4434.

Rubin B K, Fink J B (2005), 'Optimizing aerosol delivery by pressurized metered-dose inhalers', *Respir Care* **50**: 1191–1200.

Schreier H, Mobley W C, Concessio N, Hickey A J, Niven R W (1994), 'Formulation and in vitro performance of liposome powder aerosols', *S.T.P. Pharma Sciences* **4**: 38–44.

Scichilone N, Battaglia S, Sorino C, Paglino G, Martino L, Paterno A, Santagata R, Spatafora M, Nicolini G, Bellia V (2010), 'Effects of extra-fine inhaled beclomethasone/ formoterol on both large and small airways in asthma', *Allergy* **65**: 897–902.

Sharma A, Sharma U S (1997), 'Liposomes in drug delivery: Progress and limitations', *International Journal of Pharmaceutics* **154**: 123–140.

Skalko-Basnet N, Pavelic Z, Becirevic-Lacan M (2000), 'Liposomes containing drug and cyclodextrin prepared by the one-step spray-drying method', *Drug Dev Ind Pharm* **26**: 1279–1284.

Smye S W, Jollie M I, Littlewood J M (1991), 'A mathematical model of some aspects of jet nebuliser performance', *Clin Phys Physiol Meas* **12**: 289–300.

Sollner K (1936) 'The mechanism of the formation of fogs by ultrasonic waves', *Transactions of the Faraday Society* **32**: 1532–1536.

Published by Woodhead Publishing Limited, 2013

Stahlhofen W, Gebhart J, Heyder J (1980), 'Experimental determination of the regional deposition of aerosol particles in the human respiratory tract', *Am Ind Hyg Assoc J* **41**: 385–398a.

Stahlhofen W, Koebrich R, Rudolf G, Scheuch G (1990), 'Short-term and long-term clearance of particles from the upper human respiratory tract as function of particle size', *Journal of Aerosol Science* 21, ***Supplement*** 1: S407–S410.

Stark B, Pabst G, Prassl R (2010), 'Long-term stability of sterically stabilized liposomes by freezing and freeze-drying: Effects of cryoprotectants on structure', *Eur J Pharm Sci* **41**: 546–555.

Suresh S, Narendra C, Maheshwari D, Kundawala A J (2010), 'Formulation and evaluation of liposomes containing antitubercular drugs by Taguchi's orthogonal array design', *Acta Pharmaceutica Sciencia* **52**: 79–88.

Swenson C E, Popescu M C, Ginsberg R S (1988), 'Preparation and use of liposomes in the treatment of microbial infections', *Crit Rev Microbiol* **15 Suppl** 1: S1–31.

Szoka F, Jr., Papahadjopoulos D (1980), 'Comparative properties and methods of preparation of lipid vesicles (liposomes)', *Annu Rev Biophys Bioeng* **9**: 467–508.

Taylor K M G, Morris R M (1995), 'Thermal analysis of phase transition behaviour in liposomes', *Thermochimica Acta* **248**: 289–301.

Taylor K M G, McCallion O N M (1997), 'Ultrasonic nebulisers for pulmonary drug delivery', *International Journal of Pharmaceutics* **153**: 93–104.

Taylor K M G, Taylor G, Kellaway I W, Stevens J (1989), 'The Influence of Liposomal Encapsulation on Sodium Cromoglycate Pharmacokinetics in Man', *Pharm Res* **6**: 633–636.

Telko M J, Hickey A J (2005), 'Dry powder inhaler formulation', *Respir Care* **50**: 1209–1227.

Published by Woodhead Publishing Limited, 2013

Todo H, Okamoto H, Iida K, Danjo K (2004), 'Improvement of stability and absorbability of dry insulin powder for inhalation by powder-combination technique', *International Journal of Pharmaceutics* **271**: 41–52.

Vemuri S, Rhodes C T (1995), 'Preparation and characterization of liposomes as therapeutic delivery systems: a review', *Pharmaceutica Acta Helvetiae* **70**: 95–111.

Vervaet C, Byron P R (1999), 'Drug-surfactant-propellant interactions in HFA-formulations', *Int J Pharm* **186**: 13–30.

Waldrep J C, Dhand R (2008), 'Advanced nebulizer designs employing vibrating mesh/aperture plate technologies for aerosol generation', *Curr Drug Deliv* **5**: 114–119.

Wong M, Thompson T E (1982), 'Aggregation of dipalmitoylphosphatidylcholine vesicles', *Biochemistry* **21**: 4133–4139.

Yanai M, Sekizawa K, Ohrui T, Sasaki H, Takishima T (1992), 'Site of airway obstruction in pulmonary disease: direct measurement of intrabronchial pressure', *J Appl Physiol* **72**: 1016–1023.

Zhong H, Deng Y, Wang X, Yang B (2005), 'Multivesicular liposome formulation for the sustained delivery of breviscapine', *International Journal of Pharmaceutics* **301**: 15–24.

Published by Woodhead Publishing Limited, 2013

Index

Published by Woodhead Publishing Limited, 2013

Published by Woodhead Publishing Limited, 2013

Published by Woodhead Publishing Limited, 2013

Published by Woodhead Publishing Limited, 2013

Published by Woodhead Publishing Limited, 2013

Published by Woodhead Publishing Limited, 2013

Published by Woodhead Publishing Limited, 2013

Published by Woodhead Publishing Limited, 2013

Published by Woodhead Publishing Limited, 2013

Published by Woodhead Publishing Limited, 2013

Published by Woodhead Publishing Limited, 2013

Published by Woodhead Publishing Limited, 2013

Published by Woodhead Publishing Limited, 2013

CPSIA information can be obtained at www.ICGtesting.com
Printed in the USA
BVOW02*0359030214

343683BV00006B/174/P

9 780857 090171